$64°°

Wayne Hollingshead, D.V.M.

Emergency
Radiology
in
Small Animal
Practice

Emergency Radiology in Small Animal Practice

Charles S. Farrow, D.V.M.

Professor
Department of Veterinary Anesthesiology
Radiology and Surgery
Western College of Veterinary Medicine
University of Saskatchewan
Saskatoon, Saskatchewan

1988
B.C. Decker • Toronto • Philadelphia

Publisher

B.C. Decker Inc
3228 South Service Road
Burlington, Ontario L7N 3H8

B.C. Decker Inc
320 Walnut Street
Suite 400
Philadelphia, Pennsylvania 19106

Sales and Distribution

United States and Possessions	**The C.V. Mosby Company** 11830 Westline Industrial Drive Saint Louis, Missouri 63146
Canada	**The C.V. Mosby Company, Ltd.** 5240 Finch Avenue East, Unit No. 1 Scarborough, Ontario M1S 5P2
United Kingdom, Europe and the Middle East	**Blackwell Scientific Publications, Ltd.** Osney Mead, Oxford OX2 OEL, England
Australia and New Zealand	**Harcourt Brace Jovanovich Group (Australia) Pty Limited** 30–52 Smidmore Street Marrickville, N.S.W. 2204 Australia
Japan	**Igaku-Shoin Ltd.** Tokyo International P.O. Box 5063 1–28–36 Hongo, Bunkyo-ku, Tokyo 113, Japan
Asia	**Info-Med Ltd.** 802–3 Ruttonjee House 11 Duddell Street Central Hong Kong
South Africa	**Libriger Book Distributors** Warehouse Number 8 ''Die Ou Looiery'' Tannery Road Hamilton, Bloemfontein 9300
South America	**Inter-Book Marketing Services** Rua das Palmeriras, 32 Apto. 701 222–70 Rio de Janeiro RJ, Brazil

Emergency Radiology in Small Animal Practice   ISBN 1–55664–031–5

Library of Congress catalog card number: 87–73452

10   9   8   7   6   5   4   3   2   1

To
Debi, Ami, and Travis
and to the great State
of Texas
where this book was written

ACKNOWLEDGMENTS

I wish to thank the radiologists of the Texas Veterinary Medical Center, Texas A&M University, for their professional support and encouragement, especially Dr. Ron Green. My appreciation also to Walter S. Bailey and the editorial department of B.C. Decker Inc. who have taught me much about the publishing process. Special appreciation is also due to Theo Perry of the Editorial Department and to Pamela Wilkie, production assistant.

It is surprisingly difficult, among physicians and veterinarians alike, to reach a consensus about what constitutes a medical emergency. Proposed definitions are even more diverse when the question is put to pet owners. The one point on which there appears to be general agreement is that a medical emergency is a condition that requires immediate treatment or that should at least be seen by a veterinarian. Who decides, the owner or the veterinarian, when immediate treatment is required, especially if the initial discussion is by phone? Must the animal have been hit by a car, be bleeding, have a heart condition, be vomiting, or have diarrhea? Should the age of the dog, the duration of illness, or the time of night be factors? The issue is unexpectedly complex.

After considering this question carefully, I have reached the conclusion that there is no simple, universally acceptable definition of a medical emergency. Rather, like the appreciation of fine art, emergencies are interpreted individually by professional and nonprofessional alike. With this in mind, I have selected the various disorders for this book from the radiology files at the Universities of Saskatchewan and Texas A&M, attempting to include problems that were considered to be of an emergency nature by the receiving clinician, the pet owner, or both.

I must also bring three other matters to the attention of the reader. First, concerning the radioanatomical descriptions in the text, I have deliberately chosen to mix contemporary terms, such as craniocaudal and dorsopalmar, with more traditional descriptions, such as shoulder and elbow joints. This decision was based on both my personal preference and that exhibited by a majority of my professional colleagues. Second, most of the radiographic figures in this book have been printed with the animal's head, or right side, on the viewer's left, again a matter of personal choice. Arrows appear on many but not all figures to aid in rapid identification of the lesion.

Finally, the views expressed in this book are my own or those of fellow radiologists or other specialists with whom I agree. No attempt has been made to include additional viewpoints, divergent or otherwise, since the principal intent of this book is to present my *individual approach* to the radiologic management of medical emergencies.

CONTENTS

I
The Thorax

THORACIC WALL AND PLEURAL SPACE

1
Chest Wall Trauma 2

2
Spontaneous Pneumothorax 4

3
Tension Pneumothorax 6

4
Pleuropneumonia 8

5
Pleural Abscess 10

THE MEDIASTINUM

6
Cranial Mediastinal Mass:
Lymphoma 12

7
Perihilar Lymphadenopathy:
Middle Mediastinal Mass 14

8
Caudal Mediastinal Mass 16

9
Pneumomediastinum 18

10
Ruptured Subclavian Artery
Producing Hemomediastinum 20

THE TRACHEA

11
Tracheal Perforation 22

12
Tracheal Foreign Body 24

13
Tracheal Stenosis 26

14
Tracheal Collapse 28

15
Carinal Collapse 30

16
Tracheal Hypoplasia 32

17
Peritracheal Tumor 34

THE ESOPHAGUS

18
Esophageal Foreign Body 36

19
Esophageal Perforation 40

20
Congenital Megaesophagus 42

THE DIAPHRAGM

21
Diaphragmatic Hernia 46

22

Pericardioperitoneal Hernia 50

THE LUNG

23

Acute Bacterial Pneumonia 52

24

Acute Inhalation Pneumonia 54

25

Foreign Body Pneumonia 56

26

Lung Lobe Torsion 58

27

Pulmonary Contusion 60

28

Traumatic Bullae 64

29

Pulmonary Metastasis
(Presenting as Acute Dyspnea) 66

30

Feline Asthma 68

31

Pulmonary Infiltrates With
Peripheral Eosinophilia 70

32

Thoracic Gunshot Wound 72

33

Electrocution Producing
Pulmonary Edema 74

34

Strangulation 76

35

Smoke Inhalation 78

36

Near Drowning 80

37

Warfarin Poisoning 82

38

Paraquat Poisoning 84

39

Fluid Overload 86

40

Postural Atelectasis 90

THE HEART

41

Congestive Heart Failure:
Congenital Ventricular Septal Defect
Patent Ductus Arteriosus 94

42

Congestive Heart Failure:
Acquired Mitral Insufficiency 98

43

Cardiomyopathy in the Dog 100

44

Cardiomyopathy in the Cat 104

45

Heartworm in the Dog 108

46

Heartworm in the Cat 112

47

Benign Pericardial Effusion: Tamponade 114

48

Hemangiosarcoma of Right Atrium Producing
Pericardial Effusion 116

49

Heart Base Tumor Producing Heart Failure 118

50

Traumatic Pneumopericardium 120

II

The Abdomen

ABDOMINAL WALL

51

Lateral Abdominal Hernia Producing
Intestinal Herniation 124

52

Inguinal Hernia Producing
Intestinal Herniation 126

53

Bite Wound Producing Peritonitis 128

PERITONEAL CAVITY

54

Ruptured Gallbladder and Bile Duct
Producing Peritonitis 130

55

Abdominal Gunshot Wound 132

56

Spontaneous Pneumoperitoneum 134

57

Peritoneal Foreign Body Secondary to
Gastroesophageal Perforation 136

58

Foreign Body Granuloma Induced by
Surgical Sponge 138

59

Feline Infectious Peritonitis Leading to
Intussusception 140

60

Disseminated Peritoneal Fibrosarcoma 142

THE STOMACH

61

Gastric Foreign Bodies 144

62

Gastrointestinal Foreign Body 148

63

Gastric Dilatation 150

64

Gastric Torsion: Volvulus 152

65

Hemorrhagic Gastroenteritis 154

66

Penetrating Gastric Ulcer 156

67

Incarcerated Hiatal Hernia 158

68

Pyloric Tumor 160

THE INTESTINE

69

Linear Intestinal Foreign Body 162

70

Nonlinear, Intestinal Foreign Body 164

71

Intussusception 166

72

Intestinal Incarceration 168

73

Intestinal Volvulus 170

74

Tumor of the Small Intestine 172

75
Canine Parvoviral Enteritis 174

76
Ruptured Colon 176

77
Post-Traumatic Megacolon 180

URINARY TRACT

78
Ruptured Kidney Producing
Retroperitoneal Hemorrhage 182

79
Renal Abscess 184

80
Ruptured Urinary Bladder
Producing Peritonitis 186

81
Bladder Dislocation: Retroflexion 188

82
Bladder Stones Leading to Obstruction 190

83
Emphysematous Cystitis 192

84
Obstructive Bladder Tumor 194

85
Uremia Secondary to Renal Insufficiency 196

THE PROSTATE

86
Prostatic Abscess 198

87
Ruptured Prostate Producing Peritonitis 200

88
Prostatic Tumor 202

THE UTERUS

89
Dystocia 204

90
Late-Term Fetal Death 206

91
Pyometra 208

92
Necrotic Pyometritis 210

MISCELLANEOUS PROBLEMS

93
Hemorrhaging Liver Tumor 212

94
Hemorrhaging Splenic Tumor 214

95
Pancreatitis Secondary to Penetrating
Foreign Body 216

III
The Skeleton

THE SKULL

96
Dental Fracture 220

97
Dental Infection 224

98
Mandibular Fracture 226

99
Temporomandibular Joint
Fractures and Dislocations 228

100
Maxillary Fracture 232

101
Nasal Cavity Fracture 234

102
Frontal Sinus Fracture 236

103
Zygomatic Arch Fracture 238

104
Orbital Fracture 240

105
Cranial Fracture 242

106
Tympanic Bulla Infection 246

THE SPINE

107
Spinal Fracture 248

108
Disk Herniation 256

109
Subacute and Chronic Spinal Disorders
That May Mimic Acute Conditions 262

PELVIS AND HIP

110
Pelvic Fracture 266

111
Hip Fractures and Dislocations 272

THE HINDLIMB

112
Femoral Fracture 278

113
Patellar Fracture 284

114
Stifle Joint Fractures and Dislocations 286

115
Tibial and Fibular Fractures 290

116
Tarsal Fractures and Dislocations 296

117
Metatarsal Fracture 302

118
Metatarsophalangeal Joint
Fractures and Dislocations 306

119
Digital Fracture 308

THE FORELIMB

120
Scapular Fracture 310

121
Shoulder Joint Fractures and Dislocations 316

122
Humeral Fracture 320

123
Elbow Joint Fractures and Dislocations 326

124
Radial Fracture 334

125
Ulnar Fracture 338

126
Carpal Joint Fractures,
Sprains and Dislocations 348

127
Metacarpal Fracture 354

128
Metacarpophalangeal Joint
Fractures and Dislocations 358

129
Digital Fracture 360

ACCESSORY SKELETON

130
Hyoid Fracture 362

131
Rib Fractures and Dislocations 364

132
Sternal Fracture 366

133
Penis Bone Fracture 368

RELATED SOFT-TISSUE INJURIES

134
Soft-Tissue Injuries 369

INTRODUCTION

This book is designed to be used in the most difficult of clinical situations, the emergency, and specifically involves emergencies in which radiographs are required for diagnosis. Emergency treatment and first aid often assume an intuitive character, prompted by the clinician's experience and the need for rapid clinical response. There is usually little use for reference texts which, because of their length and variable formats, typically require extensive reading time. Accordingly, an emergency reference must be written to be read and understood *rapidly*. An emergency radiology reference text must state which radiographs are required and how they should be made and must illustrate examples of the disorders under discussion.

Thus, to facilitate rapid reference, each chapter of *Emergency Radiology in Small Animal Practice* has an identical format. This standardized format will quickly become familiar to the reader, further accelerating the reference process. Each chapter addresses a specific emergency in which radiographs are likely to be instrumental in diagnosis. The text is concise and brief and is presented under six headings: (1) General Considerations, (2) Major Radiographic Observations, (3) Diagnostic Strategy, (4) Pitfalls, (5) Alternative Diagnoses, and (6) Suggested Reading.

"General Considerations" includes a definition of the disorder described in the chapter heading, its basic pathogenesis, and a brief account of its predicted effect on the animal at the time of presentation. Major complications and prognosis are discussed when appropriate. In the case of appendicular fractures, regional pathology is emphasized.

"Major Radiographic Observations" deals with those radiographic abnormalities that best and most consistently characterize a specific disorder. Secondary or less specific radiographic signs have been omitted. Selected special procedures are included.

"Diagnostic Strategy" describes the optimal radiographic examination for the described condition, including comments on patient positioning, physiological variables, radiographic technique, special radiography, and procedures.

"Pitfalls" deals with potential errors of analysis or interpretation that may be made by the film reader.

"Alternative Diagnoses" includes a short list of conditions sharing one or more of the radiographic features of the considered disorder.

"Suggested Reading" gives readings of a general nature that are not noted in the text. For reader convenience and accessibility, references are taken primarily from major veterinary textbooks. Most are intended as supplementary reading. The few journal articles that are included contain material not found in the recommended texts.

The illustrations I have included are as numerous and varied as space has allowed, which is in keeping with my philosophy that as a predominantly *visual* science, radiology must be taught by example whenever possible. Naturally, not all variations of a given disorder could be included. Illustrative emphasis was deliberately placed on the skeletal section, reflecting the high incidence of fractures encountered in an emergency practice.

Emergency Radiology in Small Animal Practice may be used in a variety of ways, but is mainly intended to function as the basis for radiologic confirmation of a clinically suspected disorder. When diagnosis cannot be refined beyond a specific organ system, *Emergency Radiology* may serve as a reminder of some of the common problems likely to be affecting that system and may suggest the means by which that organ may be further investigated radiologically. *Emergency Radiology* may also function as an atlas of radiologic pathology against which one may compare an abnormal radiograph of questionable interpretation.

I

The
Thorax

THORACIC WALL AND PLEURAL SPACE

1

CHEST WALL TRAUMA

General Considerations

Contusion or bruising of the chest wall may be localized, regional, or diffuse. It may be superficial, involving only the skin and subcutaneous tissues, or it may be deep, involving all the soft-tissue layers up to and including the bony rib cage and the associated intercostal muscles. Emphysema of the chest wall may also be superficial or deep. In the former instance, the gas is usually atmospheric, especially if there are punctures or lacerations of the skin. With deeper accumulations, the air is more likely to have originated from a ruptured lung lobe, pneumothorax, and intercostal tear. Severe chest-wall injuries are often associated with rib fractures and lung contusions. When multiple adjacent rib fractures are present, and there are two or more fractures per rib, the chest wall may be destablized. Breathing may become labored and inefficient. This condition is termed *flail chest* and it may be fatal.

Major Radiographic Observations

Superficial chest-wall injury may show increased soft-tissue density, loss of fascial planes, and localized narrowing of the intercostal spaces. When the skin is disrupted, there is usually subcutaneous emphysema. Deep contusions are associated with the radiographic signs of superficial injury, in addition to some or all of the following: deep cutaneous emphysema, rib fracture, pulmonary contusion, hemothorax, and pneumothorax (Fig. 1–1).

Diagnostic Strategy

Chest wall injuries can be extremely painful. Consequently, patient positioning should be dictated by what is best for the animal. Usually, a lateral view with the affected side up and a minimally extended dorsoventral projection are best. Thoracic wall injuries are often associated with a *position of protection*, i.e., a patient-induced narrowing of the inter-costal spaces on the affected side, an effort to reduce thoracic expansion, which produces pain. Although at times it is necessary, it is diagnostically dangerous to rely solely on a lateral view, since many of the findings described may be seen only in the opposite projection. Be certain not to overpenetrate the thorax, as this may hide subcutaneous gas, fascial detail, and associated pulmonary contusions or pneumothorax. Check the diaphragm carefully for completeness (in both views). Record radiographic techniques in order to produce comparable films in follow-up examinations.

Pitfalls

"Poorly positioned" thoracic radiographs of an animal with chest wall injury are usually the result of injury protection by the patient and are not the fault of the radiographer.

Alternative Diagnoses

Cellulitis or abscessation secondary to bite wounds or other forms of penetrating injury, hematoma, seroma, or migrating (therapeutic) subcutaneous fluids.

Suggested Reading

Jackson DA. Thoracic trauma. In: Binnington AG, Cockshutt JR, eds. Decision making in small animal soft tissue surgery. Toronto: BC Decker, 1988: 76.

Jackson DA. Thoracic wall disease. In: Binnington AG, Cockshutt JR, eds. Decision making in small animal soft tissue surgery. Toronto: BC Decker, 1988: 78.

Root CR, Bahr RJ. The thoracic wall. In: Thrall DE, ed. Textbook of veterinary diagnostic radiology. Philadelphia: WB Saunders, 1986: 236.

Suter PF. Injuries to the thoracic wall and sternum. In: Suter PF, ed. Thoracic radiography. Davis, CA: Stonegate Publishing, 1984: 127.

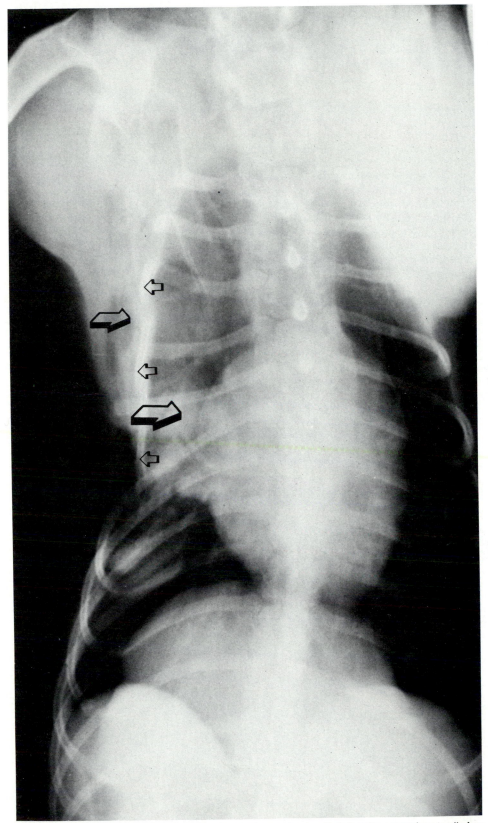

Figure 1–1 Ventrodorsal view of canine thorax shows chest wall deformity secondary to rib fractures and torn intercostal muscles (*small arrows*), deep fascial emphysema (*medium arrow*), and pulmonary contusion (*large arrow*). Diagnosis: chest wall trauma.

SPONTANEOUS PNEUMOTHORAX

General Considerations

Spontaneous pneumothorax is a general term for pneumothorax of unknown origin. It may also be termed *closed pneumothorax,* since there is no associated chest wound. Common causes include ruptured *Paragonimus* lung cysts or pulmonary abscesses, tracheal perforation secondary to *Filarioidea* lesions, visceral pleural tearing following adhesion, and, occasionally, alveolar rupture with retrograde air leakage along the pulmonary vasculature into the mediastinal and pleural spaces. Affected animals may show no clinical signs, or, alternatively, may show overt respiratory distress.

Major Radiographic Observations

Typically, pneumothorax appears as bands or regions of radiolucency located between the inner chest wall and the outer surface of the lung. These areas of reduced density, unlike normal peripheral lung, contain no vasculature. Concomitantly, the collapsing lung increases in density (Fig. 2–1).

Diagnostic Strategy

Medium and large uncomplicated pneumothoraces are easily seen on standard thoracic radiographs. A small pneumothorax, or a complicated pneumothorax that is suspected on survey films, may often be confirmed with postural radiography. Either the animal stands and a horizontal x-ray beam is used, or the animal lies on its side (decubital position) and a horizontal x-ray beam is used.

Pitfalls

Axillary skin folds combined with hypovolemic lungs may mimic pneumothorax in the dorsoventral and ventrodorsal views.

Alternative Diagnoses

Traumatic pneumothorax, tracheal or major bronchial fracture.

Suggested Reading

Cantwell HD. Pneumothorax. In: Farrow CS, ed. Decision making in small animal radiology. Toronto: BC Decker, 1987:144.

Kneller SK. Thoracic radiography. In: Kirk RW, ed. Current veterinary therapy IX. Philadelphia: WB Saunders, 1986:254.

Suter PF. Pleural abnormalities. In: Suter PF, ed. Thoracic radiography. Davis, CA: Stonegate Publishing, 1984:723.

Thrall DE. The pleural space. In: Thrall DE, ed. Textbook of veterinary diagnostic radiology. Philadelphia: WB Saunders, 1986: 275.

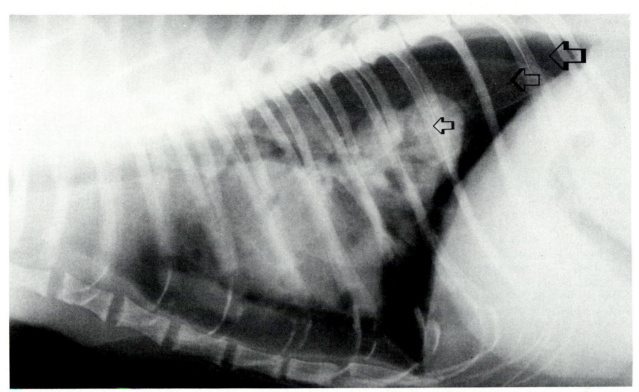

Figure 2–1 Lateral view of feline thorax shows collapsed, consolidated-cavitated lung lobe (*small arrow*), partially collapsed lung lobe (*medium arrow*), and air in the pleural space (*large arrow*). Diagnosis: pneumothorax secondary to a ruptured pulmonary abscess.

3
TENSION PNEUMOTHORAX

General Considerations

Pneumothorax may be classified as open or closed depending on whether or not there is an associated penetrating chest wound. In open chest wounds, air moves through the wound into the pleural space where it compresses the lung to varying degrees. This is termed an *open pneumothorax.* (When the chest wall is intact and there is pneumothorax, the condition is described as *closed pneumothorax.)* A *tension pneumothorax* results when more air enters the pleural space than leaves it, so that the lung is gradually compressed. If unilateral, a tension pneumothorax displaces the heart to the side opposite the lesion. Fully collapsed lung lobes are greatly reduced in size and may appear gray or white radiographically. Both open and closed pneumothoraces may lead to tension pneumothorax. Affected animals usually show severe dyspnea. Tension pneumothorax is usually fatal if not treated shortly after it develops.

Major Radiographic Observations

The lung appears hyperlucent or overexposed, with the heart typically displaced to one side of the chest. The collapsed lung is abnormally dense, resembling consolidation. The thorax is usually widened in the dorsoventral or ventrodorsal view, and the diaphragm is flattened and displaced caudally. Cardiovascular dimensions are often reduced (Fig. 3–1).

Diagnostic Strategy

If severe pneumothorax (possible tension pneumothorax) is suspected clinically, a diagnostic thoracentesis should be performed. If positive, the animal should be treated appropriately until breathing improves and then it should be radiographed. If the chest tap is bloody, negative, or equivocal, thoracic radiographs should be made. Cardiopulmonary-resuscitation equipment and drugs must be close at hand before beginning the radiographic examination. If the patient is severely dyspneic, then whatever view is most comfortable for the animal, usually the dorsoventral projection should

be made. A postural film (standing lateral patient position with a horizontal x-ray beam) is best if the animal prefers to stand. However, this view, like the recumbant lateral projection, does not discriminate between unilateral and bilateral disorders, nor does it identify the abnormal side in the case of a unilateral pneumothorax. A 10 percent reduction in kilovolt peak improves visualization of lung margins, which aids in estimating the size of the pneumothorax.

Pitfalls

A patient in shock often has a hypovolemic (and therefore hyperlucent) lung that closely resembles a severe pneumothorax. Axillary skin folds, especially in deep-chested dogs, also mimic pneumothorax as they pass over the thorax in the dorsoventral or ventrodorsal views.

Alternative Diagnoses

Tension pneumothorax, pulmonary hypovolemia (secondary to blood loss or shock), upper airway obstruction, chronic obstructive lung disease.

Suggested Reading

Cantwell HD. Pneumothorax. In: Farrow CS, ed. Decision making in small animal radiology. Toronto: BC Decker, 1987:144.

Jackson DA. Thoracic trauma. In: Binnington AG, Cockshutt JR, eds. Decision making in small animal soft tissue surgery. Toronto: BC Decker, 1988: 76.

Kneller SK. Thoracic radiography. In: Kirk RW, ed. Current veterinary therapy IX. Philadelphia: WB Saunders, 1986: 254.

Olsson S-E Pneumothorax: In: Olsson S-E, ed. The radiological diagnosis in canine and feline emergencies. Philadelphia: Lea & Febiger, 1973: 36.

Thrall DE. The pleural space. In: Thrall DE, ed. Textbook of veterinary diagnostic radiology. Philadelphia: WB Saunders, 1986: 277.

Suter PF. Trauma to the thorax and the cervical airways. In: Suter PF, ed. Thoracic radiography. Davis, CA: Stonegate Publishing, 1984: 155.

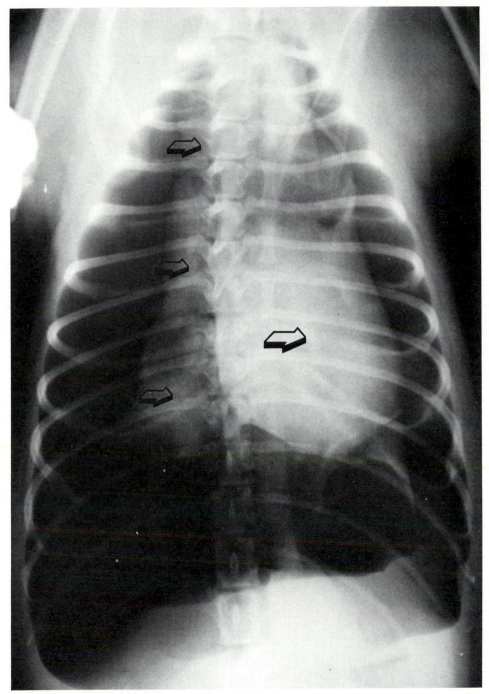

Figure 3–1 Ventrodorsal view of canine thorax shows hyperlucent pleural space, left lateral displacement of the heart—a mediastinal shift (*large arrow*), and collapsed lung lobes (*small arrows*). Diagnosis: tension pneumothorax.

4
PLEUROPNEUMONIA

General Considerations

Pneumonia with extension to the pleural space is termed *pleuropneumonia*. It is most commonly seen in cats. The condition is often fatal because of the severe damage done to the visceral pleural surface. There is a high incidence of recurrence in animals that initially respond to treatment, suggesting that such infections are difficult to eliminate completely. As with most feline respiratory diseases, the clinical signs of pleuropneumonia are variable. However, some degree of dyspnea is usually present.

Major Radiographic Observations

Pulmonary consolidation with associated pleural fluid is most common (Fig. 4–1). A large pleural effusion usually conceals an underlying pneumonia; smaller fluid accumulations often only raise suspicion of pleuropneumonia.

Diagnostic Strategy

Begin with standard thoracic radiographs. If these are inconclusive, make a postural radiograph (erect patient position using a horizontal x-ray beam directed at the sternum) in order to mobilize the pleural fluid away from the obscured lung.

Pitfalls

Pleural effusions often produce abnormal pulmonary inflation patterns, which in turn may mimic pneumonia.

Alternative Diagnoses

Pleural effusion secondary to cardiomyopathy or other forms of heart disease, hemothorax, diaphragmatic hernia, cancer (mediastinal, pulmonary, or pleural), or perforating esophageal foreign body.

Suggested Reading

Suter PF. Pleural abnormalities. In: Suter PF, ed. Thoracic radiography. Davis, CA: Stonegate Publishing, 1984: 703.
Thrall DE. The pleural space. In: Thrall DE, ed. Textbook of veterinary radiology. Philadelphia: WB Saunders, 1986: 268.

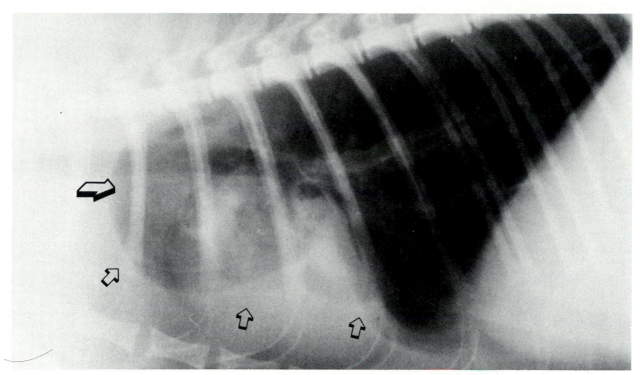

Figure 4-1 Lateral view of feline thorax shows generalized pleural fluid (*small arrows*) and underinflation of the cranial lung lobes (*large arrow*). Diagnosis: pleuropneumonia.

5

PLEURAL ABSCESS

General Considerations

A pleural abscess may result from a penetrating thoracic bite wound, pleuropneumonia, or extension of an infectious lung lesion. They typically form in the caudoventral thorax, probably due to the influence of gravity. Depending on their size, pleural abscesses may interfere with breathing. Some form painful adhesions; others rupture, spreading their contents to the surrounding pleural space. Affected cats may become toxic depending on the size, composition, and duration of the lesion. Clinical signs vary, although many animals are acutely dyspneic at presentation.

Major Radiographic Observations

Large, uncomplicated pleural abscesses usually show clearly as pleural-mass lesions. Some mimic pulmonary lesions because of the way in which they are superimposed on the lung. If pneumonia or pleural fluid is present, the abscess may be obscured (Fig. 5–1).

Diagnostic Strategy

Make standard thoracic radiographs. If a pleural abscess is suspected but cannot be confirmed, make the appropriate postural views, e.g., erect, decubital, and so on.

Pitfalls

Pleural abscesses adjacent to the heart or diaphragm often produce silhouette signs, which may falsely suggest cardiomegaly or diaphragmatic hernia.

Alternative Diagnoses

Extrapleural, pleural, pulmonary, or mediastinal masses. Localized or regional pulmonary consolidation producing a mass effect.

Suggested Reading

Juhl JH. Diseases of the pleura, mediastinum and diaphragm. In: Juhl JH, ed. Paul and Juhl's essentials of roentgen interpretation. 4th ed. Philadelphia: Harper & Row, 1981:1017.

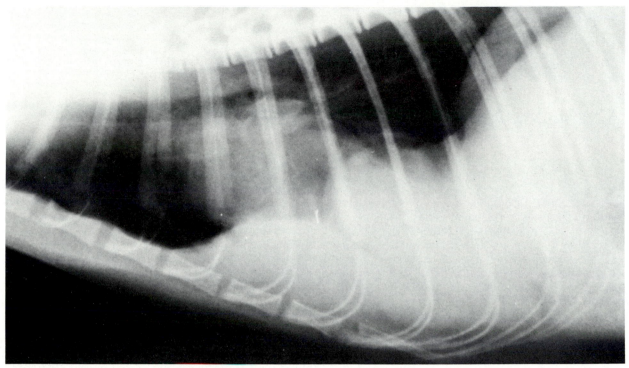

Figure 5–1 Lateral view of feline thorax shows a large, bilobed mass superimposed on the heart and diaphragm (silhouette sign). Diagnosis: pleural abscess.

THE MEDIASTINUM

6

CRANIAL MEDIASTINAL MASS: LYMPHOMA

General Considerations

Mediastinal or thymic lymphoma is a form of malignant lymphoma or lymphoreticular tumor. Other common sites include the alimentary canal, skin, and blood. There is also a multicentric form. Mediastinal lymphoma is more common in the cat than in the dog. In the cat, an associated pleural effusion often develops; in the dog, lymphoma may invade the adjacent lung. Cats with effusions are usually dyspneic or depressed and anorexic. Many are extremely fragile, and some may die, even with gentle handling.

Major Radiographic Observations

Survey radiographs show varying degrees of mediastinal widening, depending on the size of the mass. Most form a positive silhouette sign with the heart cranially. The trachea is usually elevated dorsally and may also be displaced laterally, as seen in the dorsoventral or ventrodorsal view (Fig. 6–1). The cranial and middle lung lobes are often inapparent owing to a combination of compression atelectasis (collapse) and obstruction of view by the radiographically predominant, mediastinal mass density. *Contrast* examinations, employed as marking studies, often show displacement of mediastinal structures such as the esophagus or cranial vena cava; they thereby provide indirect information about the size and location of the mass.

Diagnostic Strategy

The dorsoventral projection provides a more complete image of the cranial mediastinum than the ventrodorsal view does. A *penetrated view* (deliberately overexposed radiograph designed for a better view of cranial mediastinal structures like the trachea, cranial vena cava, and so on—increase kilovolt peak by 20 percent) often reveals displacement of contiguous structures that are obscured with standard exposures. An esophagram or cranial caval venography may also better delineate the limits of the mass. This is especially important if surgery is considered.

Pitfalls

Mediastinal fat, normally quite variable in the dog, may mimic a mediastinal mass. This is especially true of small, round-chested breeds such as Pugs or Boston Bulldogs.

Alternative Diagnoses

Other tumors (e.g., thymoma), mediastinitis (e.g., secondary to esophageal foreign-body perforation), infectious adenopathy associated most commonly with fungal diseases.

Suggested Reading

Cantwell HD. Mediastinal Mass. In: Farrow CS, ed. Decision making in small animal radiology. Toronto: BC Decker, 1987:104.

Suter PF. Mediastinal abnormalities. In: Suter PF, ed. Thoracic radiography. Davis, CA: Stonegate Publishing, 1984: 269.

Thrall DE. The mediastinum. In: Thrall DE, ed. Textbook of veterinary diagnostic radiology. Philadelphia: WB Saunders, 1986: 263.

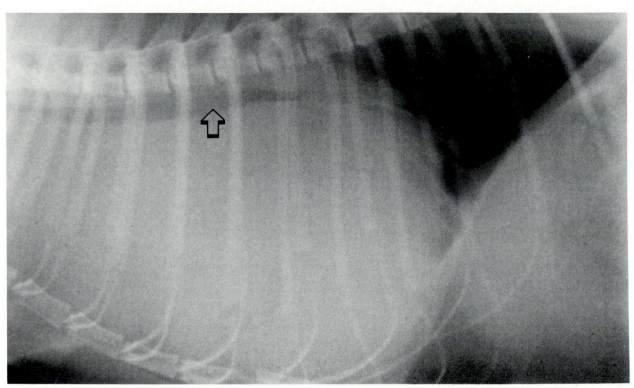

Figure 6-1 Lateral view of feline thorax shows a very large cranial mediastinal mass that blends into the heart, mimicking cardiomegaly. The trachea is displaced dorsally (*arrow*). Diagnosis: cranial mediastinal mass, lymphoma.

7

PERIHILAR LYMPHADENOPATHY: MIDDLE MEDIASTINAL MASS

General Considerations

Hilar adenopathy produces a mass effect centered over the caudal two-thirds of the heart base. Although nodal enlargement of this nature is not etiospecific, it is most frequently encountered with mycotic disorders and lymphoma. Associated lung disease is common. Isolated perihilar adenopathy is unusual. Enlargement of large perihilar vessels (e.g., heartworm disease), the left atrium, and the central esophagus (e.g., foreign-body) lesions may produce a condition termed *pseudoperihilar adenopathy*. Although hilar lymph-node enlargement has been reported to cause coughing by tracheobronchial compression, this does not appear to be common.

Major Radiographic Observations

Lateral *survey* radiographs typically show a large, relatively well-defined mass above the heart (Fig. 7–1). The mass is often poorly defined or invisible in the opposite view unless a high kilovolt-peak technique (penetrated view) is used. *Contrast* examination of the esophagus shows a localized convexity along the dorsal perimeter of the lesion.

Diagnostic Strategy

Standard thoracic views are satisfactory. Check the remaining mediastinum, lung, and skeletal structures for ad-ditional lesions. Esophagography, using barium paste, rules out esophageal disorders, and partially outlines the underlying nodal enlargement.

Pitfalls

Beware pseudoperihilar lesions as described above.

Alternative Diagnoses

In addition to infectious fungal granulomas (coccidioidomycosis, histoplasmosis, blastomycosis in dogs and cryptococcosis in cats) and lymphoma, consider bacterial granulomas (tuberculosis, nocardiosis in dogs, and actinomycosis in dogs and cats), hilar abscesses, cysts, and heart base tumors.

Suggested Reading

Suter PF. Mediastinal abnormalities. In: Suter PF, ed. Thoracic radiography. Davis, CA: Stonegate Publishing, 1984: 277.

Thrall DE. The mediastinum. In: Thrall DE, ed. Textbook of veterinary diagnostic radiology. Philadelphia: WB Saunders, 1986: 263.

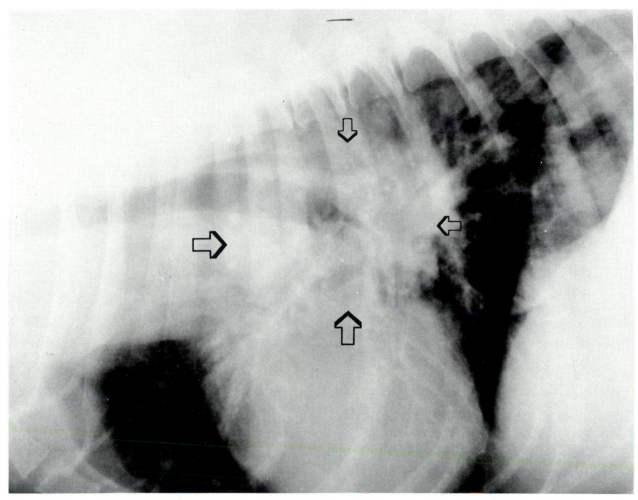

Figure 7–1 Lateral view of canine thorax shows large perihilar mass (*arrows*). Diagnosis: middle mediastinal mass, coccidioidomycosis.

8
CAUDAL MEDIASTINAL MASS

General Considerations

Caudal mediastinal masses often may be further divided into caudodorsal and caudoventral lesions. This subclassification serves to reduce the number of potentially involved structures and, therefore, the number of possible diagnoses. However, many caudal mediastinal lesions defy such classification, because they involve both dorsal and ventral aspects of the caudal mediastinum. Typical of this latter category is disease of the accessory lung lobe, which occupies more than half of the caudal mediastinum. Caudal mediastinal masses may be primary (such as a lung tumor), or secondary (such as a plant-awn abscess that ruptures into the perilobar part of the caudal mediastinal recess. Clinical signs vary from constitutional to organ specific, depending on the nature, size, and location of the mass or mass effect.

Major Radiographic Observations

Survey radiographs typically show increased caudal mediastinal density, accompanied by both cardiac and diaphragmatic silhouette signs (Fig. 8–1). The latter are most evident in the dorsoventral view (Fig. 8–2). Contrast examinations of the esophagus (esophagram), and caudal vena cava (caval venography) may give direct as well as indirect information about the lesion.

Diagnostic Strategy

When pleural fluid obscures the caudal mediastinum, a postural radiograph (made with the dog in a standing position the hindquarters elevated about 25 degrees, and using a horizontal x-ray beam) often provides improved visualization.

Pitfalls

An expiratory radiograph made in the lateral position, with resulting cardiodiaphragmatic overlap, may mimic a caudoventral mediastinal mass.

Alternative Diagnoses

Esophageal disorders (foreign body, granuloma, abscess, tumor, and hiatal or gastroesophageal hernias, diaphragmatic lesions (hernia, abscess, and hematoma) primary caudal mediastinal lesions (infection, abscess, and tumor).

Suggested Reading

Suter PF. Mediastinal abnormalities. In: Suter PF, ed. Thoracic radiography. Davis, CA: Stonegate Publishing, 1984: 277.

Thrall DE. The mediastinum. In: Thrall DE, ed. Textbook of veterinary diagnostic radiology. Philadelphia: WB Saunders, 1986: 263.

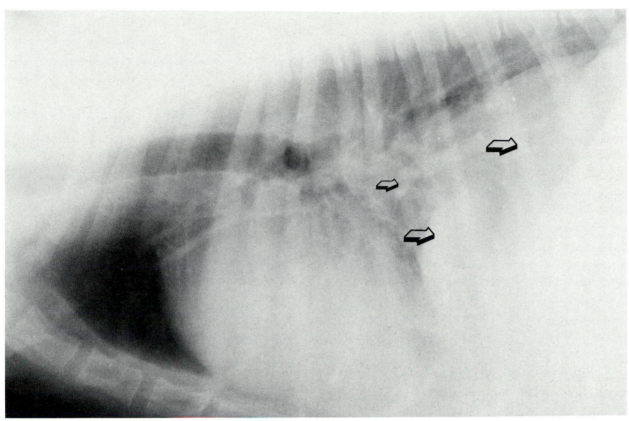

Figure 8–1 Lateral view of canine thorax shows abnormal density caudal to the heart (*arrows*).

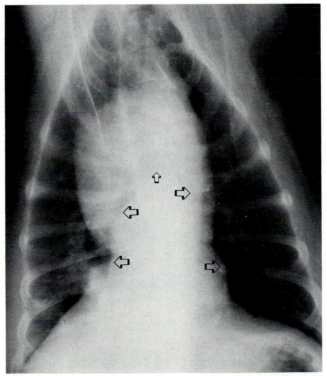

Figure 8–2 Dorsoventral view of Figure 8–1 shows abnormal density to be within the caudal mediastinum (*arrows*). Diagnosis: caudal mediastinal mass, adenocarcinoma of the accessory lung lobe.

9

PNEUMOMEDIASTINUM

General Considerations

The abnormal accumulation of air in the mediastinum, recognized radiographically by the identification of normally invisible mediastinal structures, is termed *pneumomediastinum*. Pneumomediastinum may be classified according to knowledge of its etiology: when the cause is unknown, it is termed *primary*; when the cause is known, it is referred to as *secondary*. Pneumomediastinum is most common in small dogs and cats and is usually caused by the dissection of escaped air along the deep fascial planes of the neck, following perforation of the larynx or cervical trachea. It may also develop after transtracheal wash. Lacerations of the throat and neck can also lead to pneumomediastinum by the same mechanism. Occasionally, a retrograde pneumomediastinum develops following the rupture of alveoli. When there is no associated injury, the condition is termed *spontaneous pneumomediastinum*. Such cases usually resolve spontaneously. Rarely does pneumomediastinum lead to pneumothorax. Radiographic identification of the leakage site is difficult to establish, even with contrast media.

Major Radiographic Observations

The trachea is outlined by air, and normally invisible or barely detectable structures, such as the bracheocephalic and left subclavian arteries, azygos vein, and portions of the esophagus, may become visible. Air is often seen dissecting cranially into the deep fascial planes of the neck and, depending on the volume of escaping air, into the surrounding subcutaneous tissues (Fig. 9–1).

Diagnostic Strategy

Small amounts of mediastinal air are difficult to distinguish from normal thoracic lucencies. Medium volumes are usually seen, provided the film is not overexposed. Large amounts of air are obvious in all but the poorest-quality radiographs. Be certain to include the entire cranial half of the thorax to the level of the thoracic inlet, since this region is typically the most diagnostic.

Pitfalls

Thin or narrow-chested dogs and cats often show outstanding central vascular detail resembling pneumomediastinum. This effect is further enhanced by pulmonary hyperinflation.

Alternative Diagnoses

Perforated esophagus, tracheal rupture secondary to *Filarioidea* infection, and tracheal necrosis secondary to chronic upper-airway infection (primarily in cats).

Suggested Reading

Jackson DA. Thoracic trauma. In: Binnington AG, Cockshutt JR, eds. Decision making in small animal soft tissue surgery. Toronto: BC Decker. 1988: 76.

Suter PF. Mediastinal abnormalities. In: Suter PF, ed. Thoracic radiography. Davis, CA: Stonegate Publishing, 1984: 259.

Thrall DE. The mediastinum. In: Thrall DE, ed. Textbook of veterinary diagnostic radiology. Philadelphia: WB Saunders, 1986: 266.

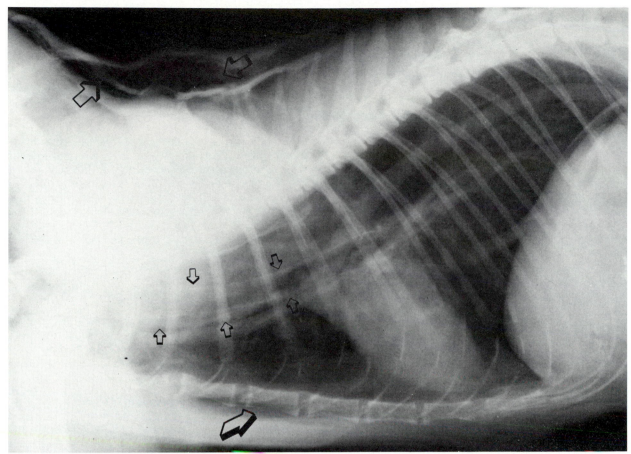

Figure 9-1 Lateral view of feline thorax shows gas within the cranial mediastinum (*small arrows*), beneath the skin (*medium arrows*), and ventral to the sternum (*large arrow*). Diagnosis: pneumomediastinum, deep fascial and subcutaneous emphysema secondary to cervical bite wounds.

10

RUPTURED SUBCLAVIAN ARTERY PRODUCING HEMOMEDIASTINUM

General Considerations

Antemortem data on mediastinal hemorrhage in the dog and cat are minimal. Generally, it is believed that rupture of all but the smaller mediastinal arteries and veins is fatal. It appears that there are exceptions, but it is not possible to say just how many. In my experience, cranial mediastinal hemorrhage is most common, probably owing to the large number of relatively unprotected vessels in this area. Unchecked mediastinal bleeding usually enters the pleural space, producing hemothorax. Varying degrees of hemorrhagic shock dominate the clinical picture.

Major Radiographic Observations

Survey radiographs show increased density of the involved mediastinal compartment (cranial, middle, or caudal) (Fig. 10-1). Dorsoventral or ventrodorsal views typically show widening of the involved mediastinal compartment; lateral projections show increased mediastinal height (Fig. 10-2). Venography or arteriography may reveal leakage of contrast medium at or in the general vicinity of the injury site.

Diagnostic Strategy

Check the cranial mediastinum carefully for widening and increased density, and whether or not there is accompanying pleural hemorrhage. If the mediastinum is suspicious, make an additional pair of thoracic films after 10 minutes, and reevaluate. Selective or semiselective contrast examinations may be diagnostic if performed by an experienced, well-equipped angiographer. Nonselective contrast examinations are better suited to private clinical practice, especially those examinations involving the venous system. For example, if the cranial vena cava is believed to be bleeding, a jugular catheter may be placed and 10 ml of iodinated contrast medium (dose for a medium-sized dog) may be injected. A lateral radiograph centered over the cranial thorax should be made during the injection, just as the last 2 ml are being injected. Keep in mind that iodinated contrast media are anticoagulants as well as diuretics.

Pitfalls

There is considerable normal variation in the width of the canine cranial mediastinum as a result of breed variation and fat deposition. In the context of suspected hemorrhage, such variants could be mistaken for mediastinal bleeding.

Alternative Diagnoses

Cranial mediastinal bleeding caused by neoplastic vascular erosion, anticoagulant poisons such as warfarin, or transthoracic needle biopsies of the cranial mediastinum.

Suggested Reading

Jackson DA. Thoracic trauma. In: Binnington AG, Cockshutt JR, eds. Decision making in small animal soft tissue surgery. Toronto: BC Decker, 1988: 76.

Suter PF, Zinkl JG. Mediastinal, pleural, and extrapleural thoracic diseases. In: Ettinger SJ, ed. Textbook of veterinary medicine. 2nd ed. Philadelphia: WB Saunders, 1983:851.

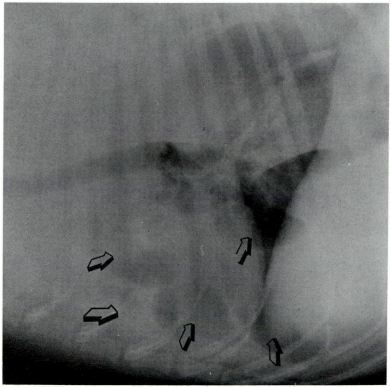

Figure 10–1 Lateral view of canine thorax shows a large volume of pleural fluid (*large arrow*) and partially collapsed lung lobes (*small arrows*).

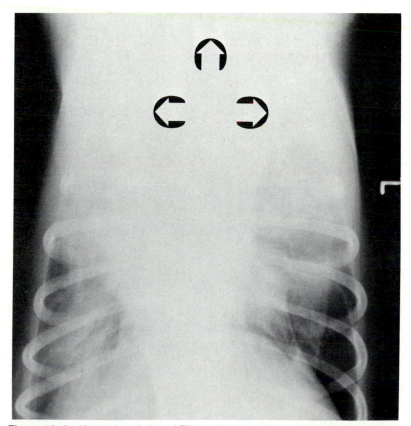

Figure 10–2 Ventrodorsal view of Figure 10–1 shows mass effect in cranial mediastinum (*arrows*). Diagnosis: hemomediastinum, hemothorax secondary to a ruptured left subclavian artery.

THE TRACHEA

11

TRACHEAL PERFORATION

General Considerations

Tracheal perforation is usually caused by bite wounds and is often associated with varying degrees of deep and superficial gas accumulation (emphysema). Tracheal tears, fractures, and avulsions also result in gas accumulation. As with chest wall injuries, deep gas is more likely to be intrinsic than extrinsic. It is often difficult or impossible to locate the injury site because of extensive associated soft-tissue injuries. Radiographic efforts to locate the site(s) of leakage usually fail. Consequently, many perforations are treated conservatively, at least initially. As might be expected, most such cases are seen as emergencies, and many are fatal.

Major Radiographic Observations

Peritracheal gas, regional deep and superficial emphysema, and pneumomediastinum may be seen, depending on the perforation site and the volume of escaped air (Fig. 11–1).

Diagnostic Strategy

Excepting such major injuries as laryngotracheal avulsion and large tracheal tears (most of which prove rapidly fatal), most tracheal perforations escape detection. Accordingly, secondary radiographic signs such as peritracheal gas, pneumomediastinum, and soft-tissue swelling must be sought. Lateral views of the injury site (as indicated by physical findings) are best and are easiest on the animal. These are im-aged optimally using soft-tissue technique. When soft-tissue swelling is great, use of a grid is advisable. When there is a great deal of superficial gas, the radiographic technique should be reduced by 20 percent to avoid overpenetration. Tracheography is rarely useful.

Pitfalls

Large superficial gas accumulations may mask smaller, deep gas deposits, especially with darker films.

Alternative Diagnoses

Retrograde dissection of air from a tear in a primary bronchus or the lung; antegrade movement of air from a perforated larynx or pharynx.

Suggested Reading

Suter PF. Mediastinal abnormalities. In: Suter PF, ed. Thoracic radiography. Davis, CA: Stonegate Publishing, 1984:259.

Suter PF. Trauma to the thorax and the cervical airways. In: Suter PF, ed. Thoracic radiography. Davis, CA: Stonegate Publishing, 1984:133.

Thrall DE. The mediastinum. In: Thrall DE, ed. Textbook of veterinary diagnostic radiology. Philadelphia: WB Saunders, 1986:263.

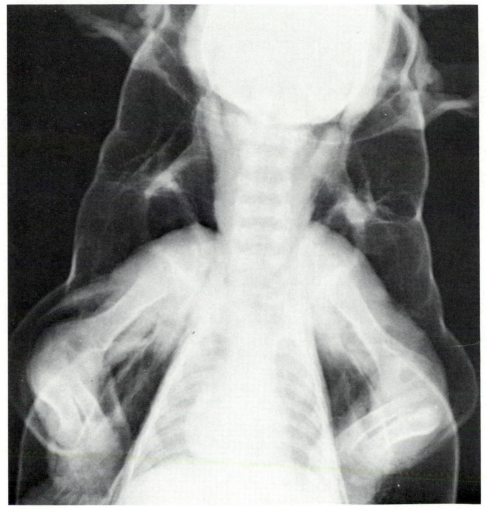

Figure 11–1 Ventrodorsal view of puppy's thorax showing extensive subcutaneous air. Diagnosis: subcutaneous emphysema secondary to cervical tracheal perforation.

12

TRACHEAL FOREIGN BODY

General Considerations

Radiographic detection of tracheal (or bronchial) foreign bodies is dependent on many factors, but primarily upon density. From a functional standpoint, foreign-body location, size, contour, and consistency are the more important concerns. Like esophageal foreign bodies, most tracheal foreign bodies are fixed in position at the time of radiographic identification. As with other occlusive disorders of the trachea, the radiographic appearance of both the trachea and the lung may be variably altered with inspiration and expiration. The later findings may be the only radiographic abnormalities observed in cases of translucent tracheal foreign bodies. Although the majority of animals with tracheal foreign bodies present with acute cough or dyspnea, some do not. Therefore, a chronic course alone is not sufficient evidence upon which to rule out tracheal foreign body.

Major Radiographic Observations

Most radiodense tracheal foreign bodies are easily seen on lateral radiographs (Fig. 12–1). Some may be obscured by overlying or adjacent hard or soft tissues. Large radiolucent foreign bodies are often associated with a regional tracheal dilatation proximal to the point of obstruction on radiographs made during inspiration and with trapped air seen on radiographs made during expiration.

Diagnostic Strategy

Make at least two lateral, inspiratory radiographs: one of the thorax, the other of the cervical trachea including the larynx. Be sure the thoracic inlet and heart base are sufficiently penetrated to allow complete assessment. If these projections are negative and a tracheal foreign body is still suspected, make these views again on expiration and compare the two film series for indirect evidence of obstruction (see above). Contrast examination is potentially dangerous, because it may worsen the obstruction, at least temporarily.

Pitfalls

End-on views of large, central blood vessels may be superimposed over the terminal trachea and carina tracheae mimicking foreign bodies. The caudal edge of the scapula may simulate a bony foreign body when superimposed over the thoracic trachea in the lateral view.

Alternative Diagnoses

Tracheal tumor or parasitic granuloma (*Filarioidea*), diphtheroid membrane (in cats following chronic upper-airway infection), and superimposed esophageal or medially located lung lesions.

Suggested Reading

Cantwell HD. Tracheal foreign body. In: Farrow CS, ed. Decision making in small animal radiology. Toronto: BC Decker, 1987:120.

Suter PF. Diseases of the nasal cavity, larynx, and trachea. In: Suter PF, ed. Thoracic radiography. Davis, CA: Stonegate Publishing, 1984:240.

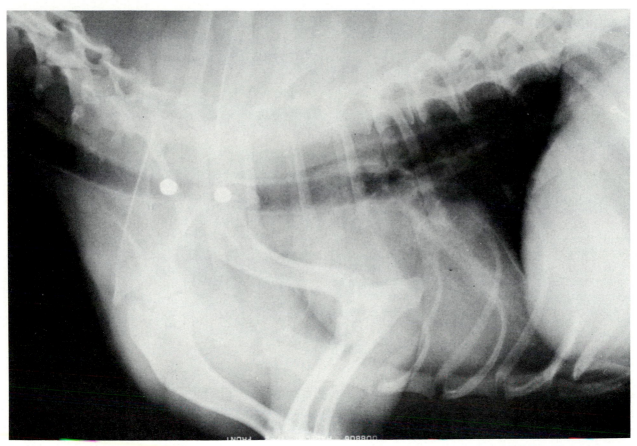

Figure 12–1 Lateral view of canine thorax shows a pair of metallic tracheal foreign bodies. Diagnosis: inhaled fishing line and sinkers.

13

TRACHEAL STENOSIS

General Considerations

Tracheal stenosis may be primary or secondary. Primary lesions usually result from scar formation (cicatrix) secondary to bite wounds, surgery, or intubation injury (pressure-induced ischemic necrosis). Intubation-related injuries are now more common than in the past because of the increased use of inhalation anesthesia. Secondary lesions typically arise from extrinsic, often constrictive masses such as peritracheal tumors. Apparent tracheal narrowing, as judged by decreased vertical diameter, consistently underestimates the actual degree of stenosis, which is a function of cross-sectional area. Affected animals often behave as though they have tracheal collapse, but usually without a comparable degree of sensitivity to tracheal palpation. Syncope may occur in severe cases.

Major Radiographic Observations

Focal and occasionally regional tracheal narrowing are readily identified in survey radiographs (Fig. 13–1). Since tracheal stenosis may be altered by the respiratory phase, both inspiratory and expiratory films are recommended.

Diagnostic Strategy

Survey radiographs (lateral and penetrated ventrodorsal views) show most lesions. Contrast examinations are useful in thoracic-inlet lesions, in which the trachea often is partially obscured by the esophagus.

Pitfalls

The trachea is highly variable at the thoracic inlet, especially in immature and older dogs; this variability often mimics tracheal stenosis. Hyperflexion of the head and neck often result in a regional narrowing of the cervical trachea in a similar location.

Alternative Diagnoses

Congenital localized or regional tracheal stenosis, atypical tracheal collapse.

Suggested Reading

Suter PF. Diseases of the nasal cavity, larynx, and trachea. In: Suter PF, ed. Thoracic radiography. Davis, CA: Stonegate Publishing, 1984:238.

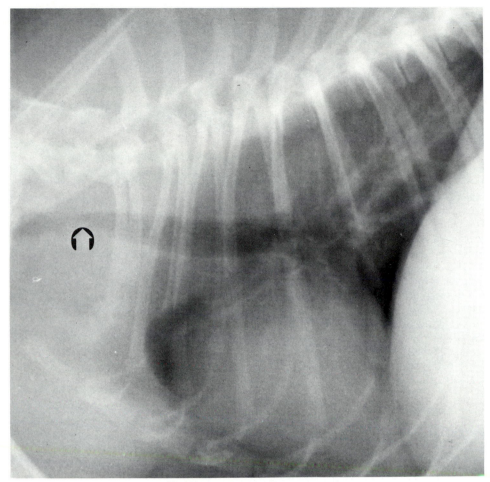

Figure 13–1 Lateral view of canine thorax shows localized tracheal narrowing (*arrow*). Diagnosis: tracheal stenosis secondary to endotracheal-tube injury.

TRACHEAL COLLAPSE

General Considerations

Tracheal collapse may occur as a congenital or an acquired disorder and is most often seen in older, small-breed dogs. Typically, tracheal collapse is a regional phenomenon, involving the cervical, thoracic inlet or thoracic areas (bronchial or carinal collapse is treated elsewhere as a separate discussion). Occasionally, the entire trachea may collapse, but this is exceptional. It is common to see the affected tracheal part change from normal to abnormal, and to see it shift from one region of the trachea to another, depending on whether one makes an inspiratory or expiratory radiograph. When structural weakening is severe, the trachea may become wider than normal; this is termed *ballooning*. Like collapse, ballooning is influenced greatly by respiratory phase. A typical clinical presentation consists of a chronic, dry, often honking cough; exacerbation with excitement or exercise; and provocation with gentle tracheal palpation or massage. Many affected animals have been diagnosed previously as having bronchitis. Collapse occasionally occurs following paroxysmal coughing.

Major Radiographic Observations

Lateral survey radiographs typically show narrowing of the cervical trachea on inspiration, with comparable change in the thoracic segment on expiration (Fig. 14–1). Many variations exist.

Diagnostic Strategy

Comparison of lateral inspiratory-expiratory radiographs is sufficient for diagnosis in most cases. Avoid overexposure of the cervical area when including the neck and thorax on the same film. A natural head position is superior to hyperextension of the head and neck, because it eliminates major positional variations that may mimic collapse. Tangential, cross-sectional views of the hyperextended trachea are difficult to produce consistently, and they normally show varying degrees of apparent deformity, which is often incorrectly interpreted as collapse. For these reasons, I prefer not to use this view. Fluoroscopy is superior to other imaging methods because of its ability to show dynamics; however, it is very difficult to restrain toy breeds beneath an image intensifier without exposing those holding the dog. Esophagography is sometimes useful in separating esophageal overlay of the cervical trachea from true collapse. Tracheography, popular for a brief time in the past, is now rarely used in the diagnosis of tracheal collapse.

Pitfalls

Cervical or thoracic-inlet esophageal overlay often mimics tracheal collapse.

Alternative Diagnoses

Tracheal hypoplasia, bronchoconstrictive disease (immunologic?).

Suggested Reading

Cantwell HD. Tracheobronchial collapse. In: Farrow CS, ed. Decision making in small animal radiology. Toronto: BC Decker, 1987:122.

Suter PF. Diseases of the nasal cavity, larynx, and trachea. In: Suter PF, ed. Thoracic radiography. Davis, CA: Stonegate Publishing, 1984:243.

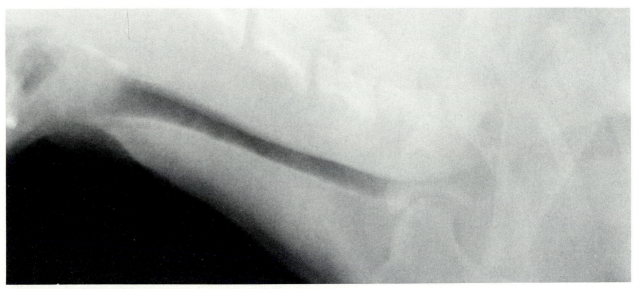

Figure 14–1 Lateral detail view of canine cervical trachea shows regional narrowing; compare with larynx and thoracic part of trachea. Diagnosis: tracheal collapse.

15

CARINAL COLLAPSE

General Considerations

Collapse of the principal bronchi, or carinal collapse, may be an isolated condition, but more usually it is associated with total or subtotal tracheal collapse. This latter relationship suggests that carinal collapse may be an integral part of tracheal collapse or alternatively, may be secondary to abnormal tracheal air flow and associated pressure disturbances. Like tracheal collapse, carinal collapse is typically associated with cough and is usually seen in older toy breeds.

Major Radiographic Observations

Survey radiographs typically show marked narrowing of the terminal thoracic trachea and the principal bronchi, on expiration (Fig. 15–2). An inspiratory film shows a relative widening of the bronchi. (Fig. 15–1). Contrast examinations are unnecessary.

Diagnostic Strategy

As with the demonstration of tracheal collapse, an inspiration-expiration sequence is required. The x-ray beam should be centered over the heart base with the animal in the lateral position. Avoid overpenetration.

Pitfalls

Normal principal bronchi usually appear less distinct on expiratory radiographs, owing to a combination of decreased air content, reduced lumen size, and associated vascular crowding and superimposition. This normal variation must be distinguished from carinal collapse.

Alternative Diagnoses

Hilar adenopathy, abscessation, or neoplasia.

Suggested Reading

Cantwell HD. Tracheobronchial collapse. In: Farrow CS, ed. Decision making in small animal radiology. Toronto: BC Decker, 1987:122.

Suter PF. Diseases of the nasal cavity, larynx, and trachea. In: Suter PF, ed. Thoracic radiography. Davis, CA: Stonegate Publishing, 1984:243.

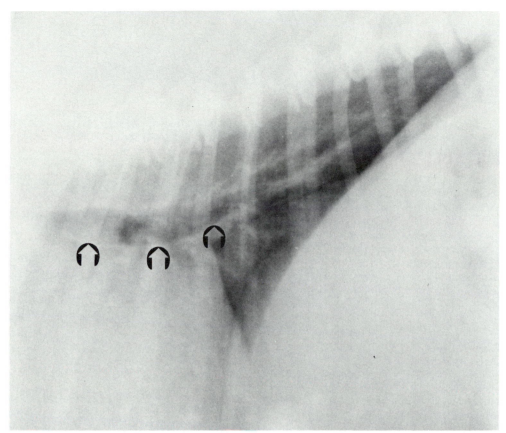

Figure 15–1 Lateral detail view of canine distal trachea and proximal bronchi (carina), made during inspiration, shows relative widening (*arrows*).

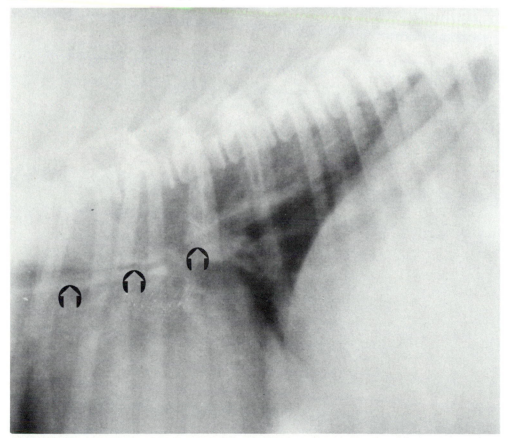

Figure 15–2 Lateral detail view of Figure 15–1, made during expiration, shows severe narrowing (*arrows*). Compare with Figure 15–1. Diagnosis: carinal collapse.

16

TRACHEAL HYPOPLASIA

General Considerations

Tracheal hypoplasia is a congenital condition of English Bulldogs (and occasionally other breeds), in which the vertical diameter of the entire trachea is one-half or less the vertical diameter of the larynx. The tracheal cartilages form closed or nearly closed rings with apposition or overlap of the free ends and essentially no dorsal muscle. Affected animals exhibit exertional dyspnea, decreased exercise tolerance, and recurrent respiratory infections. Palpation may reveal a reduced tracheal caliber. Some normal young animals may temporarily show reduced tracheal dimensions mimicking hypoplasia; consequently caution is required in order to confirm this diagnosis.

Major Radiographic Observations

Survey radiographs show a generalized tracheal narrowing in both standard projections (Fig. 16–1). The principal bronchi may be larger in diameter than the trachea. *Contrast* examinations show comparable changes.

Diagnostic Strategy

Because tracheal hypoplasia is a generalized condition, both the cervical and thoracic portions of the trachea must be affected in order to verify the diagnosis. Laryngeal imaging is also necessary for comparative measurement. Use soft-tissue technique for the cervical radiograph.

Pitfalls

Fat dogs falsely enlarge the apparent thoracic size, in turn falsely decreasing the apparent tracheal dimensions.

Alternative Diagnoses

Species and individual variation (cats have a proportionately smaller trachea than dogs), bronchoconstrictive disease, expiration.

Suggested Reading

Suter PF. Mediastinal abnormalities. In: Suter PF, ed. Thoracic radiography. Davis, CA: Stonegate Publishing, 1984:239.

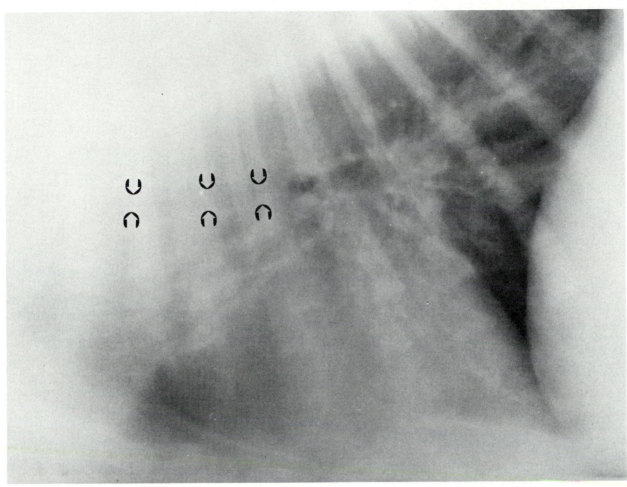

Figure 16–1   Lateral view of thorax of 3-month-old English Bulldog shows uniform narrowing (*arrows*). Diagnosis: tracheal hypoplasia.

17

PERITRACHEAL TUMOR

General Considerations

Peritracheal tumors, like tracheal neoplasms, are rare. Possible origins include the thyroid, esophagus, lung, regional lymph nodes, and regional vascular and aortic chemoreceptors. Clinical signs, such as coughing and gagging, result from luminal narrowing and irritation. Affected animals typically show a gradual onset of signs, although some present with acute illness, associated with cyanosis and collapse. The correct radiograph diagnosis is often missed because of the subtlety of the lesion and a low index of suspicion.

Major Radiographic Observations

Survey radiographs typically show a tapered, localized, or regional reduction in tracheal caliber (Fig. 17–1). Increased luminal density may be present if the lesion is circumferential. The trachea is often displaced, especially with eccentric lesions. Secondarily, there may be pulmonary underinflation if luminal obstruction is great, or if the tracheal wall is weakened. *Tracheography* reveals similar changes.

Diagnostic Strategy

When a peritracheal or tracheal tumor is suspected, lateral views of the thoracic and cervical parts of the trachea should be made, including the larynx and pharynx. Unlike intraluminal tracheal lesions, which are best visualized with lighter radiographic techniques, peritracheal lesions are often better seen with darker exposures. Contrast examinations are most useful when large peritracheal masses obscure the tracheal lumen to the extent that preoperative planning is compromised. Tracheography is best done with a small volume of sterile barium suspension, using a high-contrast technique, and centering on the lesion.

Pitfalls

It is not always possible to separate *peri*tracheal from *para*tracheal lesions. The latter, although not actually invading the trachea, may still produce many of the same radiographic signs. This fact should be kept in mind when making a preoperative prognosis.

Alternative Diagnoses

Superimposition of esophageal, mediastinal, or pulmonary lesions.

Suggested Reading

Suter PF. Diseases of the nasal cavity, larynx, and trachea. In: Suter PF, ed. Thoracic radiography. Davis, CA: Stonegate Publishing, 1984:249.

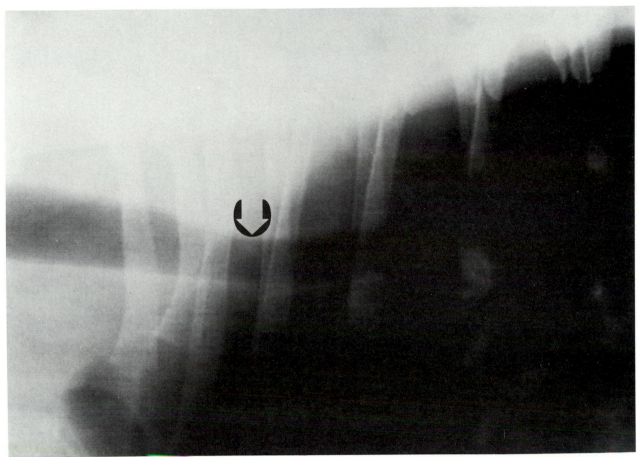

Figure 17–1 Lateral detail view of distal thoracic trachea shows dorsal deformity (*arrow*). Diagnosis: tracheal narrowing secondary to invasive peritracheal tumor.

The Esophagus

18

ESOPHAGEAL FOREIGN BODY

General Considerations

Gristle alone, combinations of bone and gristle, or bone fragments are the most common esophageal foreign bodies in dogs. Typically, they lodge cranial to the diaphragm, between the heart and the diaphragm, or over the heart base. They usually produce varying degrees of esophageal obstruction, irritation, spasm, and inflammation, collectively termed "choking." Retching and regurgitation are common signs of esophageal foreign body; however, these signs may vary depending on the type, location, duration, and obstructive qualities of the lesion. After the immediate concern of obstruction, perforation of the esophagus with resulting mediastinitis is the most important consideration. Esophageal perforation associated with instrument removal of the foreign body must also be considered as a possible complication. Generally, the size and shape of the foreign body, its duration, and the skill and experience of the operator determine the outcome of esophageal extraction procedures.

Major Radiographic Observations

Radiodense esophageal foreign bodies are usually identified without difficulty on *survey* radiographs (Fig. 18–1). The exception is the flat, thin object (such as a cortical-bone fragment), which, when viewed face-on, lacks sufficient density to be recognized. Although of insufficient inherent density to allow for radiographic detection, radiolucent foreign bodies may be inferred from survey radiographs on the basis of localized esophageal fluid or air accumulations (Fig. 18–2). Esophageal perforation may or may not be associated with pneumomediastinum, depending largely on the size of the esophageal opening, its continued patency, and the amount of localized spasm. Mediastinitis, if advanced, is usually associated with diffuse, increased mediastinal density that tends to increase with time. Eventually, pleural fluid forms. *Contrast* studies typically show an esophageal filling defect at the location of the foreign body or occasionally, complete obstruction (Figs. 18–3 and 18–4).

Diagnostic Strategy

Examine the entire esophagus, including the throat. This is especially important in cats, which may have a sewing needle lodged in the pharynx, along with a thread extending into the esophagus, stomach, or intestine. If an esophagram is made, an iodinated contrast medium should be used, anticipating possible mediastinal leakage.

Pitfalls

Air commonly accumulates in the esophagus of anesthetized dogs and cats, mimicking megaesophagus.

Alternative Diagnoses

Esophageal tumor or parasitic granuloma (*Spirocerca sanguinolenta*), hiatal hernia, gastroesophageal intussusception, and acquired megaesophagus.

Suggested Reading

Cantwell HD. Esophageal foreign body. In: Farrow CS, ed. Decision making in small animal radiology. Toronto: BC Decker, 1987:108.

O'Brien TR. Esophagus. In: O'Brien TR, ed. Radiographic diagnosis of abdominal disorders in the dog and the cat. Philadelphia: WB Saunders, 1978:167.

Seim HB III. Cervical esophageal foreign body. In: Binnington AG, Cockshutt JR, eds. Decision making in small animal soft tissue surgery. Toronto: BC Decker, 1988: 14.

Seim HB III. Thoracic esophageal foreign body. In: Binnington AG, Cockshutt JR, eds. Decision making in small animal soft tissue surgery. Toronto: BC Decker, 1988: 16.

Suter PF. Swallowing problems and esophageal abnormalities. In: Suter PF, ed. Thoracic radiography. Davis, CA: Stonegate Publishing, 1984:315.

Watrous BJ. The esophagus. In: Thrall DE, ed. Textbook of veterinary diagnostic radiology. Philadelphia: WB Saunders, 1986:217.

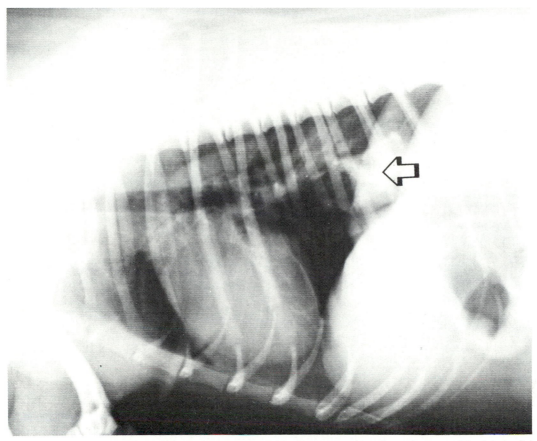

Figure 18–1 Lateral view of canine thorax shows two abnormal densities (bone fragments) in the caudal esophageal field (*arrow*). Diagnosis: esophageal foreign bodies.

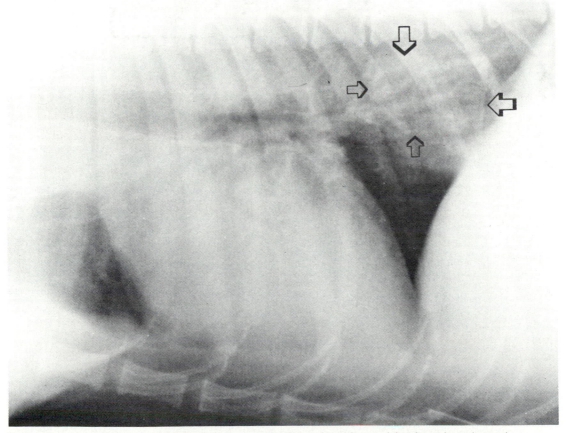

Figure 18–2 Lateral view of canine thorax shows subtle soft-tissue density caudal to heart base (*arrows*).

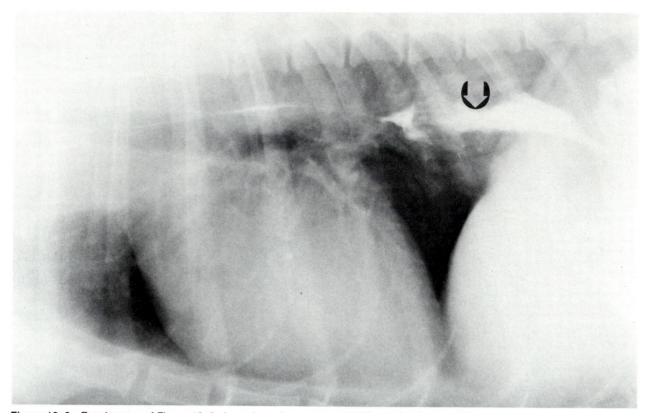

Figure 18-3 Esophagram of Figure 18-2 shows irregular, esophageal filling defect (*arrow*). Diagnosis: esophageal foreign body, thin bone fragment with attached gristle.

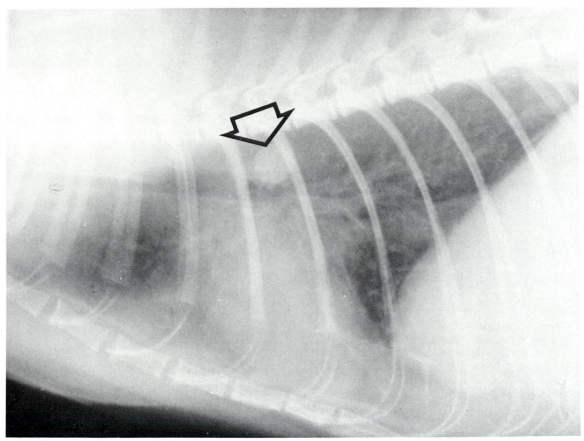

Figure 18–4   Lateral view of feline thorax shows circular, high density shadow dorsal to the heart and within the esophageal field (*arrow*). Diagnosis: esophageal foreign body.

19

ESOPHAGEAL PERFORATION

General Considerations

Esophageal perforation most commonly occurs following operative removal or displacement of an esophageal foreign body, particularly large, irregularly shaped bones or bone fragments. Long-standing esophageal foreign bodies appear to have a greater potential for perforation than acute ones. Possible sequelae to perforation include mediastinitis and pneumomediastinum. The former is usually fatal if not treated successfully; the latter is relatively unimportant (other than for providing visual evidence of possible esophageal perforation). Not all esophageal perforations result in pneumomediastinum or mediastinitis.

Major Radiographic Observations

The perforated esophagus shows no specific radiographic signs. Possibilities range from normal to localized or regional increases in density or lucency. Perforation may be *inferred* from pneumomediastinum or mediastinitis: the former showing increased mediastinal lucency resulting from escaped esophageal air, the latter appearing as an increase in mediastinal density subsequent to esophageal fluid loss (Fig. 19–1). An esophagram (*iodinated contrast media only*) may or may not reveal the leakage site.

Diagnostic Strategy

Make standard thoracic radiographs. Recall that struggling animals and those under sedation or anesthesia may normally show esophageal air. If a foreign body has recently been removed, make an additional lateral spot view over this point, using a 10-percent reduction in kilovolt peak. This may reveal subtle, otherwise obscured esophageal or periesophageal abnormalities. Examine the outer tracheal wall as well as the periesophageal region for small gas accumulations. Check the ventral mediastinum for increased density secondary to inflammation. Esophagrams following esophageal foreign-body removal are often difficult to interpret because there frequently is spasm and some degree of mechanical dysfunction. It is best to wait until the next day to perform the esophagram, unless you strongly suspect perforation, in which case you should proceed without delay. *Be certain to use only organic iodinated contrast media.*

Pitfalls

Early mediastinitis may be undetectable, particularly with small tears or punctures. Consequently, when there is strong suspicion of perforation, and even if the first esophagram is negative, a second esophagram should be performed 24 hours later or sooner, depending on the clinical circumstances.

Alternative Diagnoses

Persistent esophageal density from incomplete foreign-body removal, residual esophageal pathology or transient dysfunction, or fluid retention. Persistent gas from the same causes, as well as from patient discomfort (persistent swallowing) or the influence of drugs.

Suggested Reading

O'Brien TR. Esophagus. In: O'Brien TR, ed. Radiographic diagnosis of abdominal disorders in the dog and the cat. Philadelphia: WB Saunders, 1978:151.

Seim HB III. Cervical esophageal foreign body. In: Binnington AG, Cockshutt JR, eds. Decision making in small animal soft tissue surgery. Toronto: BC Decker, 1988: 14.

Seim HB III. Thoracic esophageal foreign body. In: Binnington AG, Cockshutt JR, eds. Decision making in small animal soft tissue surgery. Toronto: BC Decker, 1988: 16.

Suter PF. Trauma to the thorax and the cervical airways. In: Suter PF, ed. Thoracic radiography. Davis, CA: Stonegate Publishing, 1984:138.

Watrous BJ. The esophagus. In: Thrall DE, ed. Textbook of veterinary diagnostic radiology. Philadelphia: WB Saunders, 1986:218.

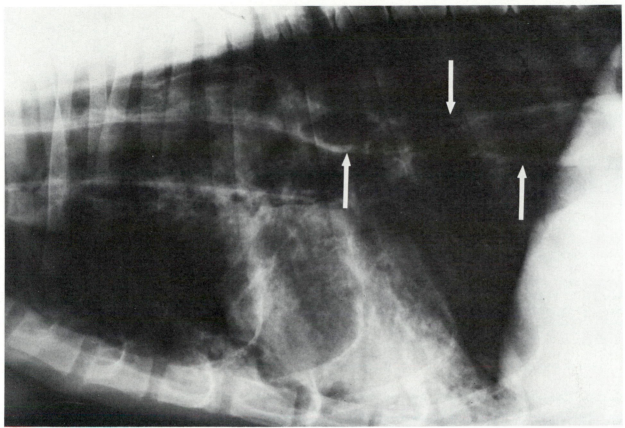

Figure 19–1 Lateral view of canine thorax shows a large-volume pneumomediastinum that allows visualization of both the inner and outer walls of the trachea and esophagus (*arrows*), as well as enhanced detail of the proximal aorta; pulmonary consolidation is present ventrally. Diagnosis: pneumomediastinum, mediastinitis, and inhalation pneumonia secondary to esophageal perforation.

20

CONGENITAL MEGAESOPHAGUS

General Considerations

The term *megaesophagus* is purely descriptive, indicating esophageal enlargement. It may be congenital or acquired, and in either case it is usually associated with ineffective esophageal transport. The latter etiology often results in chronic inhalation pneumonia. With the congenital form of the disease, clinical signs become most evident once solid foods are started.

Major Radiographic Observations

Survey radiographs typically reveal a greatly enlarged esophagus, usually filled with fluid and air. Depending on the extent of esophageal enlargement, the underlying trachea and heart are displaced ventrally (Figs. 20–1 and 20–2). The ventral lung is often pneumonic (Figs. 20–4 and 20–5). Postural radiography (standing lateral position with a horizontal x-ray beam) usually shows an outstanding esophageal fluid level (Fig. 20–3). *Contrast* examination shows the same thing.

Diagnostic Strategy

Little special effort is needed to demonstrate a megaesophagus. When uncertainty exists, postural radiography is as effective as esophagography, and it eliminates the need for a contrast agent. Without fluoroscopy, a motility disorder is inferred on the basis of a distended, fluid-filled esophagus that persists relatively unchanged in sequential films. Contrast examination is largely redundant.

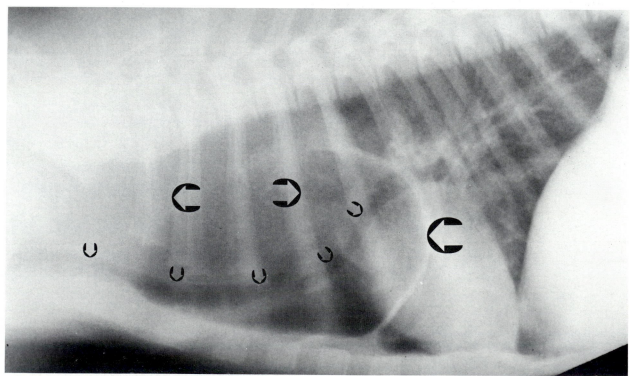

Figure 20–1   Lateral canine thorax of a puppy shows marked ventral displacement of the cervical trachea (*small arrows*), increased cranial mediastinal density (*medium arrows*), caudal heart displacement, and a vertically oriented, curvilinear density superimposed on the heart (*large arrow*).

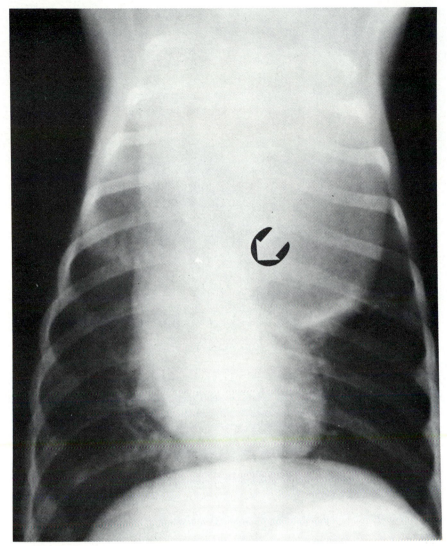

Figure 20–2 Dorsoventral view of Figure 20–1 shows large cranial mediastinal mass-mass effect (*arrow*) displacing the heart laterally. Diagnosis: megaesophagus secondary to persistent right aortic arch.

Pitfalls

Based on existing animal data, there is no factual basis for diagnosing esophageal achalasia (failure of the distal esophageal sphincter to relax) as a result of identifying a megaesophagus.

Alternative Diagnoses

Acquired megaesophagus, congenital vascular ring, fluid retention secondary to distal esophageal obstruction, and gastroesophageal intussusception.

Suggested Reading

Cantwell HD. Esophageal tone deficit. In: Farrow CS, ed. Decision making in small animal radiology. Toronto: BC Decker, 1987:110.

O'Brien TR. Esophagus. In: O'Brien TR, ed. Radiographic diagnosis of abdominal disorders in the dog and the cat. Philadelphia: WB Saunders, 1978:161.

Seim HB III. Megaesophagus. In: Binnington AG, Cockshutt JR, eds. Decision making in small animal soft tissue surgery. Toronto: BC Decker, 1988: 18.

Suter PF. Swallowing problems and esophageal abnormalities. In: Suter PF, ed. Thoracic radiography. Davis, CA: Stonegate Publishing, 1984:321.

Watrous BJ. The esophagus. In: Thrall DE, ed. Textbook of veterinary diagnostic radiology. Philadelpia: WB Saunders, 1986:217.

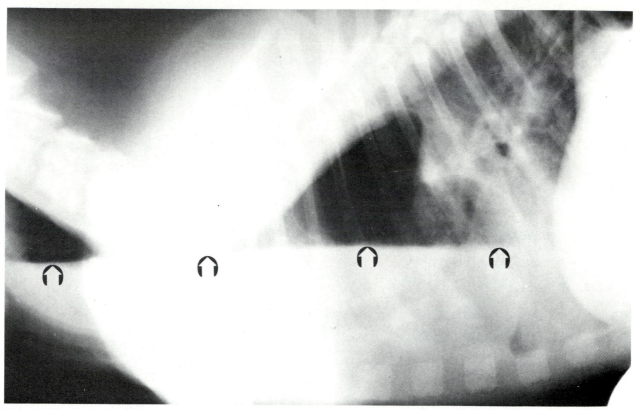

Figure 20–3 Postural radiograph (standing patient position with horizontal x-ray beam) of Figure 20–1 shows air-fluid interface (fluid line) extending from the cervical to the midthoracic esophagus (*arrows*). Note: the enlarged esophagus changes in density according to its content (typically air and fluid), the animal's position (recumbent or standing), and the direction of the x-ray beam (vertical or horizontal).

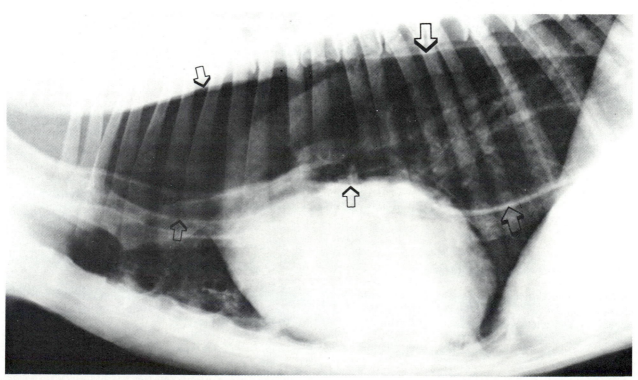

Figure 20–4 Lateral view of canine thorax shows severely dilated esophagus (*small arrows*), ventral displacement of the heart, and mild ventral consolidation. Diagnosis: acquired megaesophagus with mild secondary inhalation pneumonia.

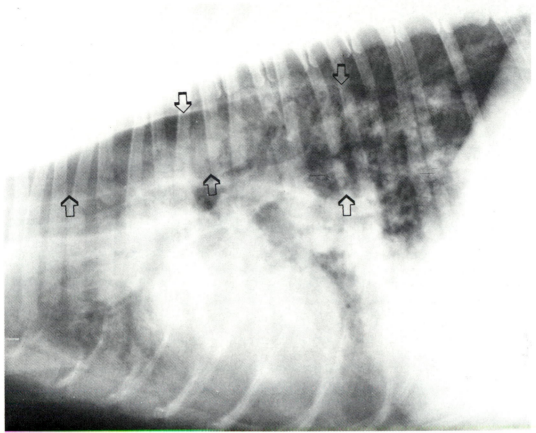

Figure 20–5 Lateral view of canine thorax shows moderately dilated esophagus (*small arrows*) and extensive pulmonary consolidation. Diagnosis: acquired megaesophagus with severe secondary inhalation pneumonia.

THE DIAPHRAGM

21

DIAPHRAGMATIC HERNIA

General Considerations

A diaphragmatic hernia ia a protrusion of abdominal viscera through the diaphragm into the thorax. Diaphragmatic hernias that can be recognized radiographically include traumatic (the most common form), peritoneal-pericardial, hiatal, mediastinal, and congenital diaphragmatic defects. Abdominal trauma, which produces a brief but large increase in intra-abdominal pressure, is responsible for most traumatic diaphragmatic hernias. The size and site of the diaphragmatic tear, as well as the extent of visceral herniation, varies with individual injuries. Associated clinical signs include dyspnea, muffled heart sounds, and decreased abdominal content on palpation. Circulatory or gastrointestinal signs may also develop, depending on the involvement of these organ systems. Some hernias are unassociated with clinical signs and are detected incidentally on thoracic radiography; others are recognized later, when they produce clinical signs. These two types are termed *occult hernias*.

Major Radiographic Observations

Survey films may show one or more of the following: an incomplete diaphragm, a positive or negative cardiac silhouette sign, abnormal thoracic densities or lucencies (representing displaced abdominal viscera), a mediastinal shift (typically to the side opposite the hernia), lung compression (usually on the affected side), pleural fluid, and a partial absence of abdominal content (Figs. 21–1, 21–2, 21–4, 21–5 and 21–6). Sometimes intestine or stomach may be seen extending from the abdomen to the thorax. *Contrast* examination show intrathoracically located elements of the gastrointestinal tract or indirect evidence of hernia in the form of cranial displacement of the stomach or bowel (Fig. 21–3).

Diagnostic Strategy

Make lateral and dorsoventral views of the thorax being certain to include the entire diaphragm. If these films are equivocal, make a lateral abdominal radiograph centered over the caudal part of the thorax and evaluate the cranial abdominal viscera for visibility and location.

Postural radiographs (standing lateral position with a horizontal x-ray beam) often demonstrate intestinal fluid levels within the chest that are not apparent in standard projections. When doubt exists, a barium marking study (approximately one-third the normal upper-gastrointestinal dose) should be done. Lateral views are usually adequate and should be made immediately upon introduction of the barium and every 15 minutes thereafter until the diagnostic question is resolved.

Pitfalls

A positive cardiac silhouette sign may result from contusions in an adjacent lung lobe, instead of from herniated viscera.

Alternative Diagnoses

When medium to large volumes of thoracic fluid are present, diagnosis is often difficult. With history of trauma: hemothorax and lung lobe torsion. Lacking a history of recent injury: heart failure (especially cardiomyopathy in the cat), pleuropneumonia, pulmonary or pleural metastasis, and atrial or mediastinal tumor.

Suggested Reading

Cantwell HD. Diaphragmatic hernia. In: Farrow CS, ed. Decision making in small animal radiology. Toronto: BC Decker, 1987:114.

Jackson DA. Thoracic trauma. In: Binnington AG, Cockshutt JR, eds. Decision making in small animal soft tissue surgery. Toronto: BC Decker, 1988: 76.

Park RD. The diaphragm. In: Thrall DE, ed. Textbook of veterinary diagnostic radiology. Philadelphia: WB Saunders, 1986:251.

Suter PF. Abnormalities of the diaphragm. In: Suter PF, ed. Thoracic radiography. Davis, CA: Stonegate Publishing, 1984:185.

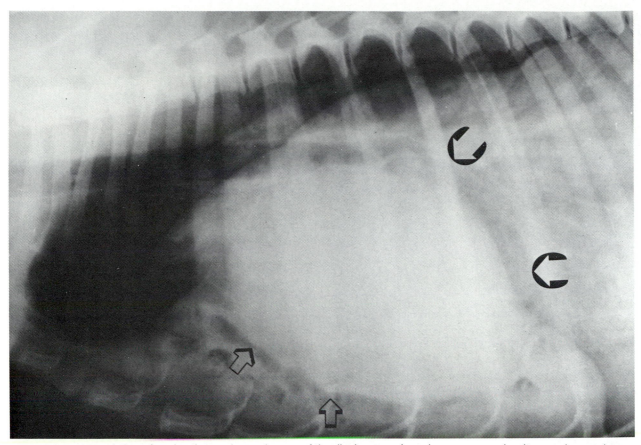

Figure 21–1 Lateral view of canine thorax shows absence of the diaphragm, a large homogeneous density superimposed over the caudal and middle aspects of the thorax (*large arrows*), and cylindrical lucencies ventral to the heart (*small arrows*).

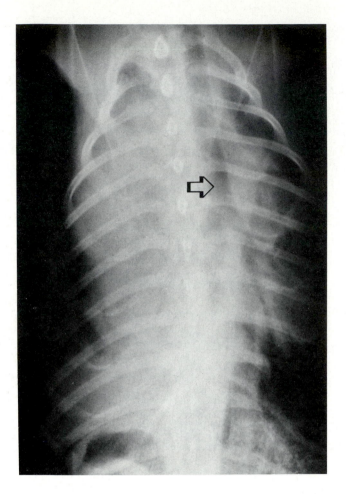

Figure 21-2 Dorsoventral view of Figure 21-1 shows absence of diaphragm, a poorly defined heart shadow, and left lateral tracheal displacement (*arrow*).

Figure 21-3 Dorsoventral gastric marking study of Figure 21-1 shows intrathoracic gastric and intestinal displacement. Diagnosis: large diaphragmatic hernia.

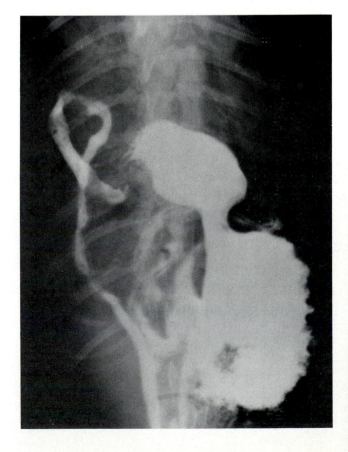

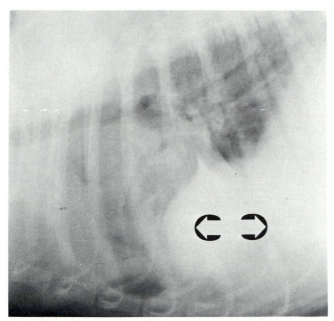

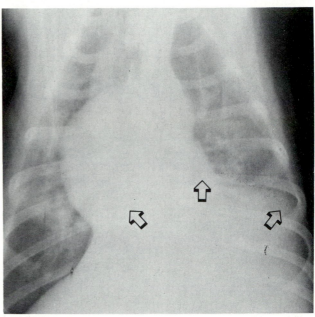

Figure 21-4 Lateral view of canine thorax shows a large abnormal density superimposed over the caudoventral aspect of the heart and diaphragm (*arrows*).

Figure 21-5 Dorsoventral view of Figure 21-4 shows large mass superimposed on the left caudal heart margin and associated hemidiaphragm (*arrows*). Diagnosis: diaphragmatic hernia (left liver lobes).

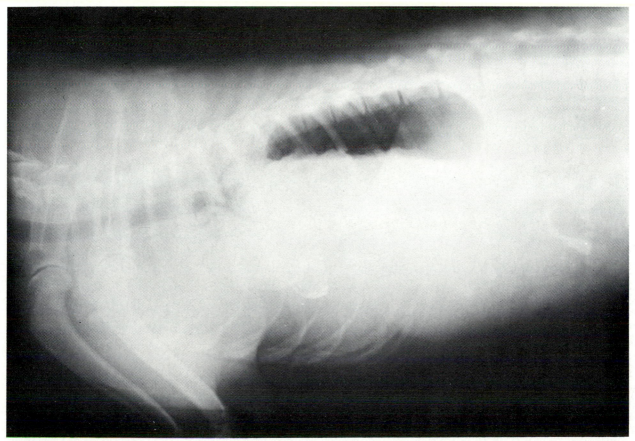

Figure 21-6 Standing lateral view (postural radiograph) of feline thorax and cranial abdomen shows contained gas-capped fluid level centered on the dorsal aspect of the diaphragmatic field. Diagnosis: left-sided diaphragmatic hernia with stomach displaced into thorax.

22

PERICARDIOPERITONEAL HERNIA

General Considerations

Pericardioperitoneal hernias are relatively common congenital disorders in both the dog and cat, in which various abdominal viscera pass through a common opening between the central diaphragm and the caudal aspect of the pericardium. Many are discovered incidentally on physical examination or when viewing thoracic radiographs for other problems. In my experience most affected animals have been without clinical signs, although a wide variety of abnormalities have been reported. It is important not to misdiagnose pericardioperitoneal hernias as cardiac enlargement, and perhaps treat for heart failure. It is for this reason that pericardioperitoneal hernias are discussed.

Major Radiographic Observations

Most but not all survey radiographs show globular cardiomegaly. In the lateral view the heart is often pumpkin shaped, forming a positive silhouette sign with the diaphragm (Fig. 22–1). Occasionally, localized gas shadows representing herniated bowel are seen superimposed over the heart in the same projection. The dorsoventral or ventrodorsal views often show a heart shadow that spans the width of the thorax (Fig. 22–2).

Diagnostic Strategy

Survey radiographs are made in a conventional manner. A barium marking study, using one-third the normal dose, may be used to confirm a hernia directly by identifying bowel within the pericardial sac. Alternatively, this examination may be used indirectly by showing bowel adjacent to the diaphragm, inferring herniation of the liver, which normally occupies this abdominal location.

Pitfalls

A barium marking study is only negative when a sufficient number of films have been made to evaluate the location of the entire small intestine.

Alternative Diagnoses

Central diaphragmatic hernia, cardiomegaly secondary to heart or pericardial disease, caudal mediastinal tumor or abscess, and accessory lung-lobe disease.

Suggested Reading

Cantwell HD. Peritoneopericardial hernia. In: Farrow CS, ed. Decision making in small animal radiology. Toronto: BC Decker, 1987:112.

Park RD. The diaphragm. In: Thrall DE, ed. Textbook of veterinary diagnostic radiology. Philadelphia: WB Saunders, 1986:254.

Suter PF. Abnormalities of the diaphragm. In: Suter PF, ed. Thoracic radiography. Davis, CA: Stonegate Publishing, 1984:194.

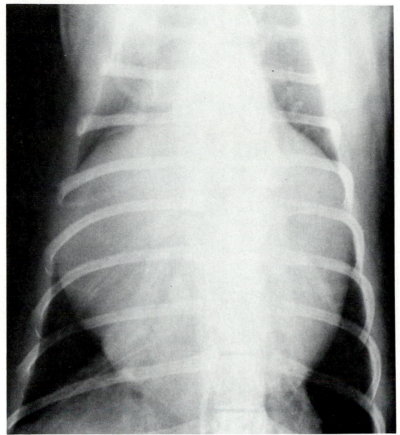

Figure 22-1 Ventrodorsal view of feline thorax shows apparent generalized cardio-megaly.

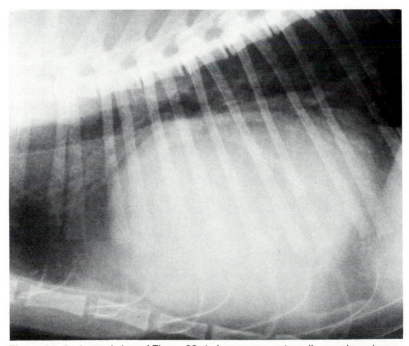

Figure 22-2 Lateral view of Figure 22–1 shows apparent cardiomegaly and merg-ing of the apparent cardiac and diaphragmatic shadows (silhouette sign). Diagnosis: pericardioperitoneal hernia (ultrasound showed the *actual* heart size to be about one-third the apparent radiographic size).

THE LUNG

23

ACUTE BACTERIAL PNEUMONIA

General Considerations

The term *pneumonia* generally refers to inflammation of the lung; pneumonitis is a less desirable synonym. Pneumonia may be further divided according to location (cranial, ventral), area of anatomic involvement (interstitial, alveolar), pathologic distribution (bronchial, lobar), general cause (bacterial, fungal), or specific etiology (streptococcal, blastomycotic). Although most pneumonias are infectious, some are not. The latter include verminous, allergic, and immunologic disorders. Pneumonias may develop suddenly, often with subtle clinical signs. Hemograms can be near normal, and temperatures may be only slightly elevated. Coughing is frequently absent. Pneumonic lungs may initially appear normal, only to develop extensive consolidation 24 hours later. Acute pneumonias resolve rapidly when detected early and treated effectively. Feline pneumonia tends to recur, often becoming chronic.

Major Radiographic Observations

Unilateral, cranial, or middle-lobe consolidation is most common in bacterial pneumonia. Distribution is typically ventral. Cardiac silhouetting is common. If treatment is unsuccessful, the opposite side usually becomes involved in a similar manner (Fig. 23–1). Diffuse pneumonias are often composed of multiple, patchy consolidations that sometimes resemble pulmonary edema or metastasis. Feline pneumonias are often of this type, especially in older cats.

Diagnostic Strategy

Standard thoracic projections are needed initially, with frequent follow-up films until the animal is well.

Pitfalls

Follow-up radiographs must be of *comparable technique* to avoid inaccurate comparisons and resulting errors in diagnosis.

Alternative Diagnoses

Lung abscess or primary tumor.

Suggested Reading

Cantwell HD. Lobar pneumonia. In: Farrow CS, ed. Decision making in small animal radiology. Toronto: BC Decker, 1987:130.

Suter PF. Lower airway and pulmonary parenchymal disease. In: Suter PF, ed. Thoracic radiography. Davis, CA: Stonegate Publishing, 1984:569.

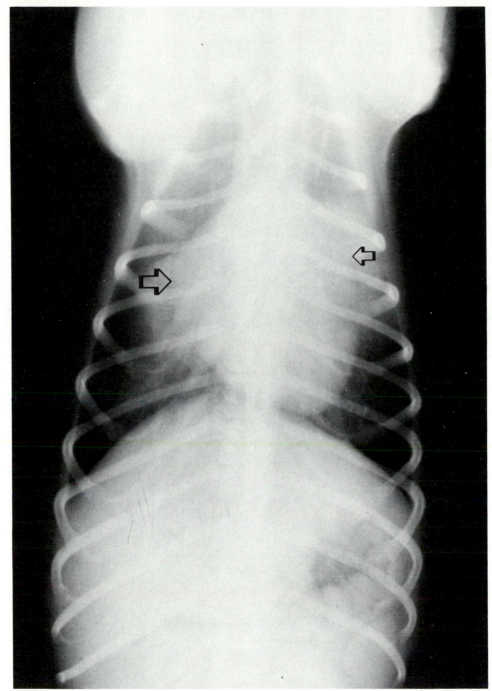

Figure 23–1 Dorsoventral view of canine thorax shows subtotal consolidation of the right middle lung lobe (*large arrow*) and the left cranial lobe (*small arrow*). Diagnosis: acute, bilateral, bacterial lobar pneumonia.

24
ACUTE INHALATION PNEUMONIA

General Considerations

The inhalation of liquid or particulate matter into the tracheobronchial tree is termed *aspiration pneumonia*. There are two forms, acute and chronic. The *acute* form results from the inhalation of foreign material over a short span, causing an acute onset of clinical signs. The aspirate may be either solid or liquid. Solid matter, such as chunks of meat, typically produces bronchial obstruction. Conversely, liquid aspirates often reach the distal airspace, where they commonly produce dyspnea, cyanosis, and, occasionally, shock. Chronic aspiration pneumonia results from repeated episodes of aspiration (as with megaesophagus), which ultimately produce chronic pneumonia. Some aspirates produce a characteristic pathology and are then considered as specific entities, e.g., lipid pneumonia.

Major Radiographic Observations

Findings vary according to the nature and volume of the aspirate. Typically, early radiographs show increased peribronchial densities, often combined with patchy regional consolidation, the latter usually developing in accordance with the animal's position at the time of inhalation (Figs. 24–1 and 24–2). (Fluids move to the most dependent part of the lung.) Later appearances are dictated by the effectiveness of treatment.

Diagnostic Strategy

Make standard thoracic radiographs initially. Repeat within 8 hours if the original films are normal, and again at 24 hours to check for late-developing pathology.

Pitfalls

Postural atelectasis results in a unilateral increase in lung density that mimics pulmonary consolidation.

Alternative Diagnoses

Noninhalation pneumonia (e.g., bacterial, viral), pulmonary abscess, primary lung tumor.

Suggested Reading

Suter PF. Lower airway and pulmonary parenchymal disease. In: Suter PF, ed. Thoracic radiography. Davis, CA: Stonegate Publishing, 1984:632.

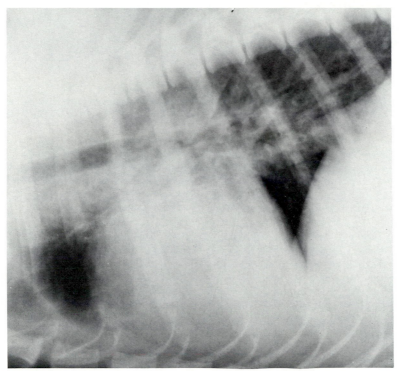

Figure 24–1 Lateral view of canine thorax shows increased lung density dorsally.

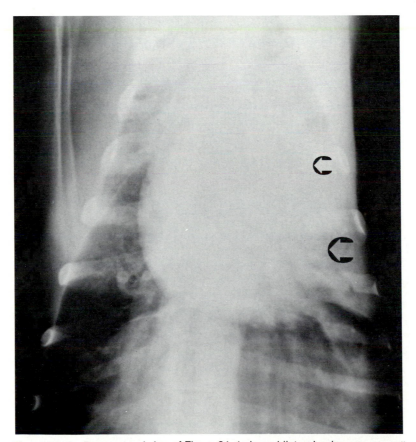

Figure 24–2 Dorsoventral view of Figure 24–1 shows bilateral pulmonary consolidation that is relatively more severe on the left, where it merges with the heart forming a positive silhouette sign (*arrows*). Diagnosis: subacute inhalation pneumonia.

25

FOREIGN BODY PNEUMONIA

General Considerations

Plant awns are the leading cause of foreign-body pneumonia. The caudal lung lobes are reported to be at greatest risk, although I have found the right middle and accessory lobes affected with comparable frequency. Coughing is present in the majority of acute cases. The hemogram and temperature are usually normal. With time, constitutional signs, such as weight loss, begin to develop. The foreign body may penetrate the lung and produce a pleuropneumonia, or remain in place and cause abscessation. Some foreign bodies are isolated within the terminal airspace by natural pulmonary defense mechanisms, thereby eliminating the majority of clinical signs. Weeks or even months later, the foreign body may migrate, producing relapse. This series of events is especially prevalent in hunting dogs, by virtue of their potentially greater exposure.

Major Radiographic Observations

Plant foreign bodies are radiographically invisible. However, acute or subacute foreign-body pneumonias may be inferred from localized pulmonary consolidation (Figs. 25–1 and 25–2). Foreign-body abscess is suggested by recurrent pneumonia, especially if the radiographic appearance is repetitive. Pleural fluid often results when a foreign body penetrates the lung and enters the pleural space, although this is a nonspecific radiographic finding.

Diagnostic Strategy

Standard thoracic views are adequate. Suspect lesions should be viewed from the opposite direction, e.g., left versus right lateral. Make follow-up radiographs as needed, especially if the initial films are normal and the animal's signs persist.

Pitfalls

Early foreign-body pneumonia involving the caudomedial aspect of the right middle lung lobe (dorsoventral or ventrodorsal projections) is often masked by the numerous vascular structures criss-crossing this field.

Alternative Diagnoses

Pneumonia or primary lung tumor.

Suggested Reading

Suter PF. Lower airway and pulmonary parenchymal disease. In: Suter PF, ed. Thoracic radiography. Davis, CA: Stonegate Publishing, 1984:548.

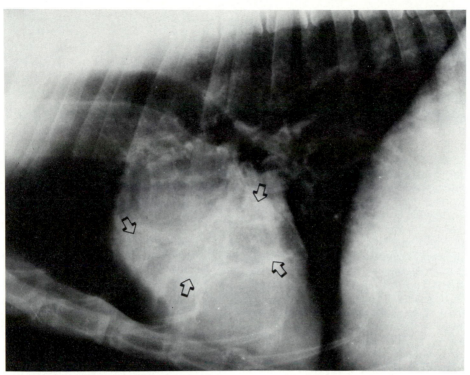

Figure 25-1 Lateral view of canine thorax shows cavitated pulmonary consolidation superimposed on the heart (*arrows*).

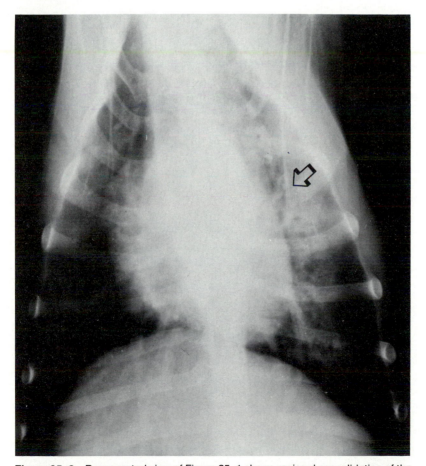

Figure 25-2 Dorsoventral view of Figure 25-1 shows regional consolidation of the left cranial lung lobes (*arrow*). Diagnosis: cavitated pulmonary abscess (secondary to inhalation of a plant awn).

26

LUNG LOBE TORSION

General Considerations

Lung lobe torsion is an axial rotation or twisting of a lung lobe at its point of origin. This results in varying degrees of obstruction of both the incoming and the outgoing blood and air supplies. The affected lobe initially swells as venous blood content increases owing to partial arterial inflow and complete blockage of associated venous return. A substantial pleural transudate (usually hemorrhagic) often develops subsequently. With time, and assuming the animal survives, the torsed lobe gradually shrinks, the pleural effusion is reabsorbed, and the surrounding lung lobes compensatorily hyperinflate. Most affected animals typically show extreme initial distress followed by shock, and they are unlikely to survive without effective surgical treatment. Torsion may occur as a primary disorder or secondary to a pleural effusion. The mechanism is uncertain. The right middle lobe is most commonly involved, followed by the left cranial lobe. Although breed disposition has been reported, I have encountered none. Both cats and dogs may be affected.

Major Radiographic Observations

The data are highly variable. Medium to large pleural effusions are present in most cases (Figs. 26–1 and 26–2). If the affected lobe can be seen, it is typically consolidated; this may often be seen without bronchograms.

Diagnostic Strategy

Make standard thoracic radiographs (lateral and dorsoventral views). If a small pleural effusion is present, make a ven-trodorsal view; this usually provides improved visualization of the heart and lung. Visualization of the cranial half of the thorax can be improved further with postural radiography (erect or standing patient position using a horizontal x-ray beam centered on the heart).

Pitfalls

Abnormal inflation patterns, possibly indicative of lung lobe torsion, are unreliable in the context of pleural fluid, since the latter causes varying degrees of pulmonary atelectasis and flotation.

Alternative Diagnoses

Conditions associated with large pleural effusions: heart failure, pleuropneumonia, pulmonary metastases, diaphragmatic hernia, hemothorax.

Suggested Reading

Suter PF. Lower airway and pulmonary parenchymal diseases. In: Suter PF, ed. Thoracic radiography. Davis, CA: Stonegate Publishing, 1984:635.

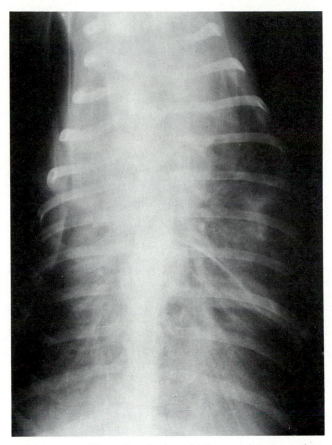

Figure 26–1 Ventrodorsal view (oblique owing to patient resistance) of canine thorax shows a large volume of pleural fluid that "greys" the lung and hides the heart.

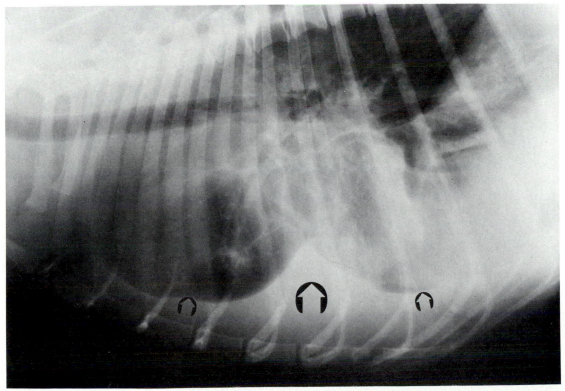

Figure 26–2 Lateral view of Figure 26–1 shows pleural fluid (*large arrow*) and partial lung collapse (*small arrows*); the heart remains obscured. Diagnosis: torsion of the cranial part of the left cranial lung lobe with resulting hemorrhagic pleural effusion.

27

PULMONARY CONTUSION

General Considerations

Pulmonary contusion (intrapulmonary capillary hemorrhage) results in the temporary consolidation of various parts of the lung with blood, which in turn prevents normal ventilation and leads to hypoxemia. Contusions commonly occur following car accidents. They may be localized or diffuse, mild or severe, and are often (but not always) associated with other thoracic injuries such as chest wall bruising, intercostal tearing, rib fracture, hemothorax, pneumothorax, traumatic pulmonary bullae, and diaphragmatic hernia. Depending on their severity, pulmonary contusions may produce no clinical signs; conversely they may lead to marked respiratory distress and even death. Most contusions are radiographically improved in 24 hours and resolve within a week.

Major Radiographic Observations

Contusive injuries show a wide range of increased lung densities, depending on their severity. If they are located in the interstitial part of the lung, contusions often appear as a diffuse, unilateral, veil-like shadow (Figs. 27–1 and 27–2). Air-space hemorrhage, on the other hand, appears as typical pulmonary consolidation (Figs. 27–3 to 27–6). Many contusions are of a mixed nature, having combined interstitial and alveolar components.

Diagnostic Strategy

Make standard thoracic radiographs (lateral and dorsoventral views). Avoid overpenetration, as it often conceals interstitial contusions. Record the radiographic technique in order to make comparable progress films later.

Pitfalls

Axillary skin folds passing across the thorax add to the underlying lung density and resemble interstitial contusions.

Alternative Diagnoses

Pulmonary edema (cardiogenic or noncardiogenic), DIC, warfarin poisoning, pneumonia.

Suggested Reading

Suter PF. Trauma to the thorax and cervical airways. In: Suter PF, ed. Thoracic radiography. Davis, CA: Stonegate Publishing, 1984: 140.

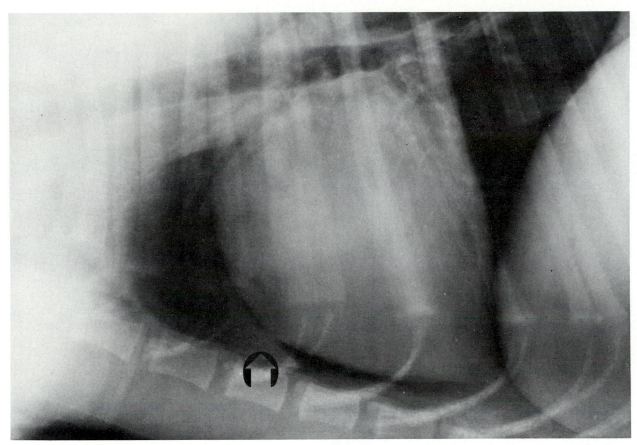

Figure 27-1 Lateral view of canine thorax shows partial consolidation of the ventral aspect of the right cranial lobe (*arrow*). Diagnosis: localized, peripheral pulmonary contusion.

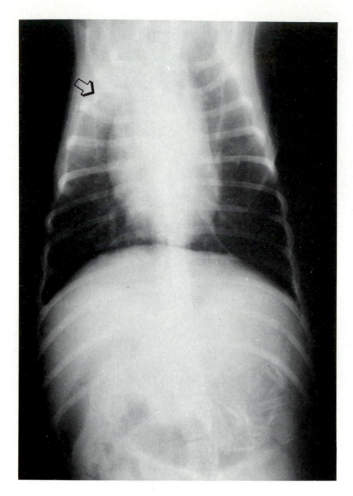

Figure 27–2 Ventrodorasl view of canine thorax shows increased density and volume loss in the right cranial lung lobe with associated pleural fluid (*arrow*). Diagnsois: localized pulmonary contusion and hemothorax.

Figure 27–3 Ventrodorasl view of canine thorax shows complete consolidation of the right cranial lobe (*arrow*). Diagnosis: localized intrapulmonary hemorrhage.

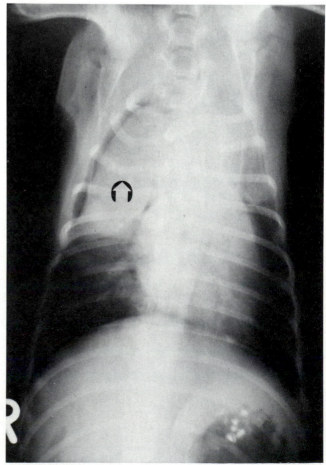

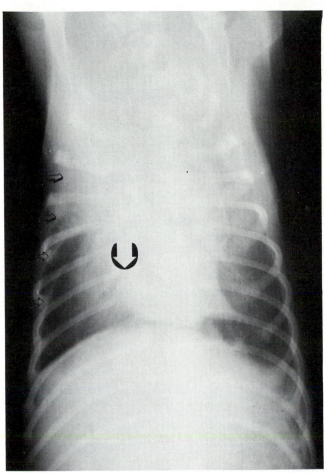

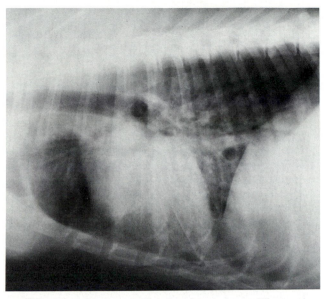

Figure 27–5 Lateral view of canine thorax shows diffuse pulmonary consolidation. Diagnosis: diffuse pulmonary contusions.

Figure 27–4 Ventrodorsal view of canine thorax shows partial consolidation of the right lung lobes resulting in a cardiac silhouette sign (*large arrow*), and pleural fluid causing lobar separation (*small arrows*). Diagnosis: regional pulmonary contusions with associated hemothorax.

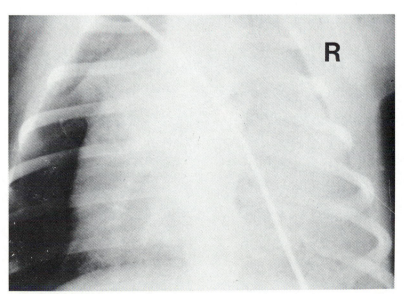

Figure 27–6 Dorsoventral view of canine thorax shows total consolidation of the right side of the lung (*R*) following trauma. An ECG lead passes diagonally across the chest. Diagnosis: severe unilateral pulmonary contusion.

28

TRAUMATIC BULLAE

General Considerations

Traumatic bullae are cavitary lung lesions resulting from blunt thoracic injury. They typically contain air, blood, or a combination of the two. Although bullae may rupture, leading to pneumothorax, this rarely occurs. Most bullae resolve rapidly, usually within a few days of their being identified. There are no specific clinical signs associated with bullae, nor is any treatment required. Because of their potential for rupture, it appears advisable to follow them radiographically until they are no longer apparent.

Major Radiographic Observations

Traumatic bullae typically appear as large, oval, or ring-like shadows within the lung (Fig. 28–1). An intracavitary fluid line may be present in postural films. Other bullae appear as homogeneous, egg-shaped lung densities.

Diagnostic Strategy

Standard thoracic radiographs are required initially, followed by an alternate side lateral view if a bulla is suspect-
ed. If doubt persists, make a postural radiograph using a horizontal x-ray beam, with the animal in the standing or sternal position. The latter view allows detection of a fluid line that would otherwise be inapparent.

Pitfalls

Curved, intersecting blood vessels, especially caudodorsal to the heart in lateral projection, may mimic traumatic bullae.

Alternative Diagnoses

Cavitated lung abscess or tumor.

Suggested Reading

Suter PF. Lower airway and pulmonary parenchymal disease. In: Suter PF, ed. Thoracic radiography. Davis, CA: Stonegate Publishing, 1984:548.

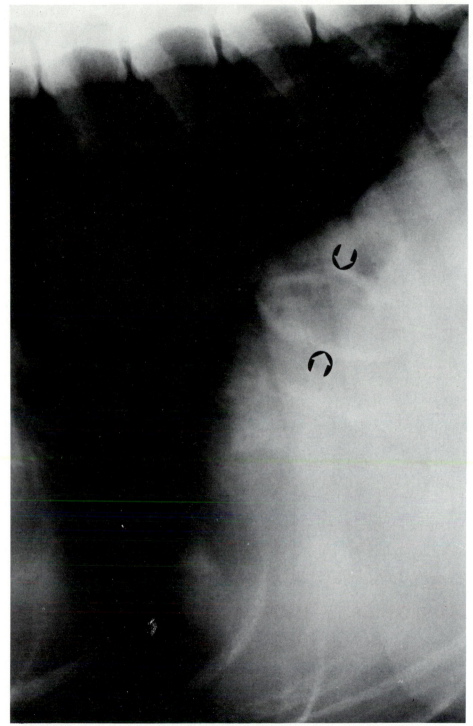

Figure 28–1 Detail lateral view of canine thorax at the level of the diaphragm shows hollow, oval-shaped density (*arrows*). Diagnosis: traumatic bulla.

29

PULMONARY METASTASIS (PRESENTING AS ACUTE DYSPNEA)

General Considerations

Pulmonary metastasis frequently presents as a nonspecific illness associated with an increased respiratory rate or, occasionally with a cough. Rarely is the onset acute. However, when an associated pleural effusion forms, dyspnea is common, and the onset of related clinical signs may be acute. This is especially true in the cat.

Major Radiographic Observations

There is variable presentation, but typically diffuse, structured, spherical lung densities exist, occasionally associated with pleural fluid (Fig. 29–1). If large, the effusion may obscure the metastasis, or at least make metastatic lesions difficult to distinguish from normal vascular shadows.

Diagnostic Strategy

Begin with standard thoracic radiographs. If a large volume of pleural fluid is present, remove it and repeat the films. A diagnosis of pulmonary metastasis should not be made until the suspected lesions can be visualized clearly. The ventrodorsal view of the thorax provides the best opportunity to see the lung when pleural fluid is present. Postural radiography, particularly the standing patient position using a horizontal x-ray beam, not only often provides an unobscured view of the dorsal lung field but also is less stressful to the patient.

Pitfalls

Some pneumonias (especially in the cat) resemble pulmonary metastasis, although most pneumonias are not associated with pleural fluid. Some forms of pulmonary metastasis are difficult to distinguish from nonneoplastic types of interstitial disease.

Alternative Diagnoses

Focus on other potential sources of pleural-fluid formation such as diaphragmatic hernia, pleuropneumonia, mediastinal tumors, heart failure (especially cardiomyopathy in the cat), and ruptured thoracic duct.

Suggested Reading

Cantwell HD. Pulmonary neoplasia. In: Farrow CS, ed. Decision making in small animal radiology. Toronto: BC Decker, 1987:140.

Suter PF. Lower airway and pulmonary parenchymal diseases. In: Suter PF, ed. Thoracic radiography. Davis, CA: Stonegate Publishing, 1984:659.

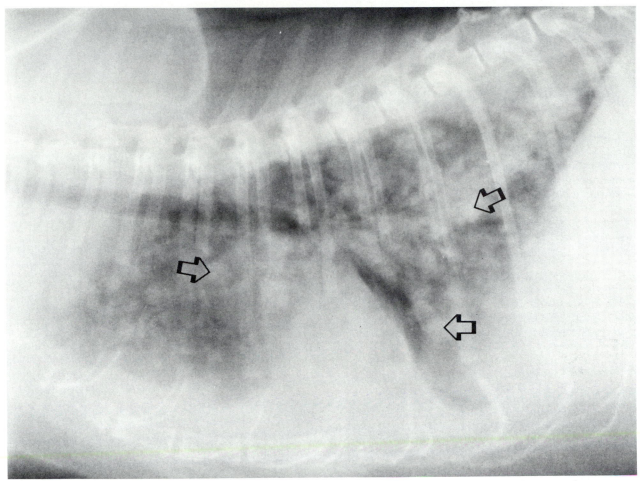

Figure 29–1   Lateral view of feline thorax shows diffuse, small to medium-sized lung densities (*arrows*) with associated pleural fluid. Diagnosis: pulmonary metastasis (breast cancer) with secondary pleural effusion.

30

FELINE ASTHMA

General Considerations

Much controversy exists about the true nature of "feline asthma". Some doubt that it exists at all, at least as a counterpart to asthma in human beings. Much of what appears in contemporary textbooks appears to be based on scant original veterinary observations or, more usually, human literature. The name "feline asthma" is retained here to avoid further confusion. Acutely affected cats show varying degrees of dyspnea.

Major Radiographic Observations

Pulmonary hyperinflation, hyperlucency, and oligemia are the classic signs of human asthma (Fig. 30–1). I believe similar signs should be used in the cat as long as the term asthma is retained.

Diagnostic Strategy

Make standard thoracic radiographs, being careful to avoid overexposure and patient movement.

Pitfalls

An overexposed thoracic radiograph appears abnormally lucent, and therefore mimics feline asthma. Hypovolemic disorders (including shock) are often associated with the same radiographic signs as asthma.

Alternative Diagnoses

Emphysema and other forms of chronic obstructive lung disease (COLD), and obstructive pharyngeal-laryngeal disorders.

Suggested Reading

Suter PF. Lower airway and pulmonary parenchymal disease. In: Suter PF, ed. Thoracic radiography. Davis, CA: Stonegate Publishing, 1984:533.

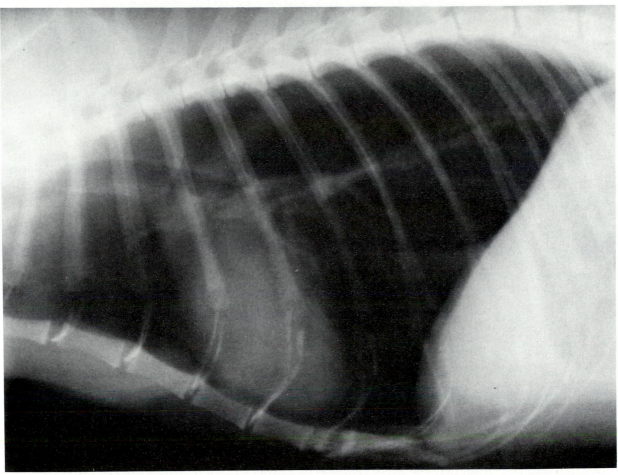

Figure 30–1 Lateral view of feline thorax shows pulmonary hyperinflation, hyperlucency, and pulmonary oligemia. Diagnosis: feline asthma.

31

PULMONARY INFILTRATES WITH PERIPHERAL EOSINOPHILIA

General Considerations

Pulmonary infiltrates with eosinophilia is a broad term to describe numerous human lung disorders that share the common features of diffuse pulmonary infiltrates (consolidation) and eosinophilia. These similar diseases are believed to be immune mediated or, as I prefer to term them, immunopneumonias. Although there is little original veterinary research on the subject, many anecdotal descriptions exist. These describe affected animals as having acute respiratory distress, which is frequently responsive to steroids. Relapse is common, usually at decreasing intervals. Medication often must be increased to control these subsequent attacks. Some animals eventually become refractory to treatment and eventually succumb to their illness. German shepherds are more frequently affected than other breeds in our practice.

Major Radiographic Observations

Typically, there are diffuse interstitial and alveolar lung densities (Fig. 31–1). Associated pulmonary hyperemia often creates the false impression of increased dorsal involvement. With effective treatment the mixed lung pattern becomes interstitial; with ineffective therapy the lung pattern becomes predominantly alveolar.

Diagnostic Strategy

Standard thoracic examination is required. Owing to the highly labile nature of the disorder, frequent follow-up films are advisable.

Pitfalls

The sometimes patchy nature of the consolidations seen in this disease may mimic pulmonary metastasis.

Alternative Diagnoses

Diffuse lung disease including pneumonia (bacterial, fungal, and parasitic), disseminated intravascular coagulation, nonstructured pulmonary metastasis, and intrapulmonary hemorrhage.

Suggested Reading

Cantwell HD. Allergic pneumonitis: pulmonary infiltrate with eosinsophilia. In: Farrow CS, ed. Decision making in small animal radiology. Toronto: BC Decker, 1987:136.

Suter PF. Lower airway and pulmonary parenchymal diseases. In: Suter PF, ed. Thoracic radiography. Davis, CA: Stonegate Publishing, 1984:571.

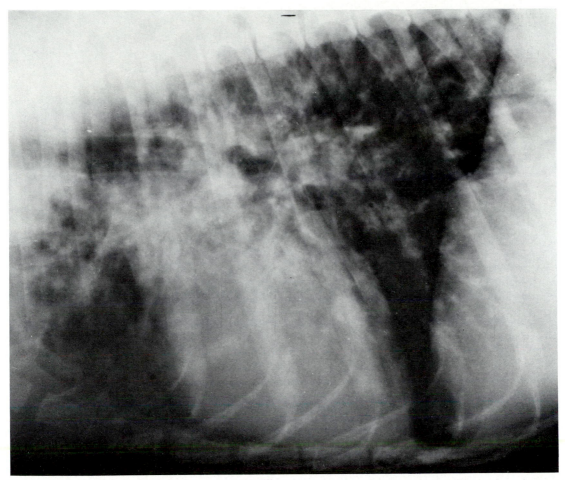

Figure 31–1 Lateral view of canine thorax shows diffuse interstitial and alveolar densities. Diagnosis: pulmonary infiltrates with eosinophilia (PIE).

32

THORACIC GUNSHOT WOUND

General Considerations

The amount of injury caused by a gunshot wound is dependent on a number of factors. These include the speed of the bullet (muzzle velocity); the size of the bullet (caliber); its weight, composition, and configuration; and the distance from the target (range). The wounding capacity of a bullet is fundamentally a function of its kinetic energy, determined by multiplying its mass by its speed. Tissues of relatively high density, such as bones and teeth, often break or shatter following gunshot injury; less dense organs like lung remain intact. The greater density of bone slows or stops the projectile, allowing the bullet to dissipate its stored energy rapidly to its immediate surroundings. Conversely, lung, a tissue of minimal density, does not appreciably slow a missile; however there may be extensive injury caused by the shock wave accompanying the bullet, which momentarily expands and tears the lung adjacent to the wound tract. Most other organs are of an intermediate density and sustain injury accordingly.

Clinically, chest wounds are often complex, involving the chest wall, pleural space, mediastinum, and lung. Abdominal involvement, not always apparent externally, may also occur. Sequelae may include pleural, mediastinal, or pulmonary hemorrhage; tracheobronchial perforation with resulting pneumomediastinum; and lung collapse with associated pneumothorax. Signs of internal thoracic injury are variable, but are most often expressed as dyspnea of one form or another. When wounds occur at close range or with high-velocity weapons, bullets or bullet fragments may not be present, forcing the consideration of other causes. Bullet wounds of the skin are often distinctly circular, resembling punch biopsy sites, and may be very difficult to find in long-haired dogs. Much controversy exists as to whether such wounds should be routinely surgically explored.

Major Radiographic Observations

There is no single, typical radiographic appearance. Possibilities include pleural fluid (hemothorax), increased lung density (pulmonary hemorrhage and/or lung collapse), pneu-

momediastinum, and pneumothorax (Fig. 32–1). This last may produce a mediastinal shift depending on the degree of associated volume loss.

Diagnostic Strategy

Make lateral and dorsoventral thoracic radiographs centered over the heart. Employ the ventrodorsal position if hemothorax is present or suspected, because this allows much of the blood to move to the caudal thorax, improving the central thoracic image. If the animal resists standard recumbent positioning, make a postural radiograph (standing lateral or sternal recumbency, using a horizontal x-ray beam). This improves visualization of the dorsal half of the thorax and makes it easier for the animal to breathe. If active bleeding is suspected, follow-up films must be made regularly until hemorrhaging is confirmed or denied; a similar approach is required for suspected tension pneumothorax.

Pitfalls

Pleural fluid may not only obscure thoracic detail but also mimic thoracic disease. Therefore, it is best to reserve final judgment until the fluid is removed or reabsorbed, and a follow-up radiograph has been evaluated.

Alternative Diagnoses

Diaphragmatic hernia, warfarin poisoning, and penetrating chest wound other than that caused by gunshot.

Suggested Reading

Fraser RG, Pare JAP. Diseases of the thorax caused by external physical agents. In: Fraser RG, Pare JAP, eds. Diagnosis of diseases of the chest. 2nd ed. Philadelphia: WB Saunders, 1979:1609.

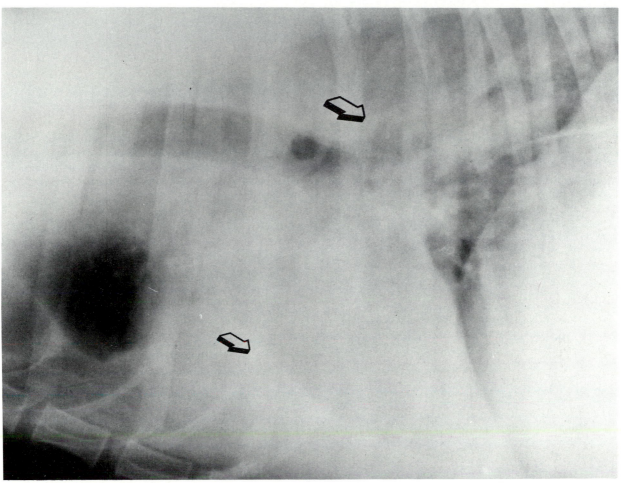

Figure 32–1 Lateral view of canine thorax (expiratory) shows increased lung density dorsocaudally (*large arrow*) and pleural fluid ventrally (*small arrow*). Diagnosis: pulmonary and pleural hemorrhage resulting from a bullet wound.

33

ELECTROCUTION PRODUCING PULMONARY EDEMA

General Considerations

Injuries caused by biting low- and medium-voltage electrical cords may or may not produce pulmonary edema. High-voltage injuries, including lightning strike, are usually fatal. The mechanism of edema formation is largely theoretical, focusing on an increase in systemic blood pressure secondary to hypothalamic injury (anoxia?), an overload of the pulmonary capillary bed, and, ultimately, flooding of the terminal air spaces. When electrocution is suspected but is not witnessed, oral-cavity burns may provide additional circumstantial evidence. However, the absence of visible burns (in the mouth or elsewhere) does not rule out the possibility of electrical injury. Other injuries that may produce pulmonary edema include strangulation and head trauma. Organophosphate poisoning and hypoglycemia may also produce lung edema, possibly by the same mechanism. Dyspnea is the major clinical abnormality. Most deaths occur within the first few minutes following injury; beyond this time, recovery is likely.

Major Radiographic Observations

Typically, there is bilateral pulmonary consolidation of the dorsal aspects of the caudal lung lobes (Fig. 33–1). The heart is normal or mildly enlarged, thereby ruling out cardiogenic edema.

Diagnostic Strategy

Lateral radiographs of the thorax, centered over the heart and normally penetrated, reveal most advanced neurogenic edemas. If the examination is negative and the injury is recent, the edema may not yet be of sufficient magnitude to be detected. Accordingly, an additional lateral thoracic film should be made in the next few hours to be sure the lung remains normal.

Pitfalls

Pulmonary contusions may resemble neurogenic pulmonary edema radiographically and clinically. Neurogenic edema usually resolves more rapidly than contusive injury and is often associated with a rapidly deteriorating clinical course.

Alternative Diagnoses

Pulmonary contusion; noncardiac, nonneurogenic edema; warfarin poisoning.

Suggested Reading

Suter PF. Lower airway and pulmonary parenchymal diseases. In: Suter PF, ed. Thoracic radiography. Davis, CA: Stonegate Publishing, 1984:560.

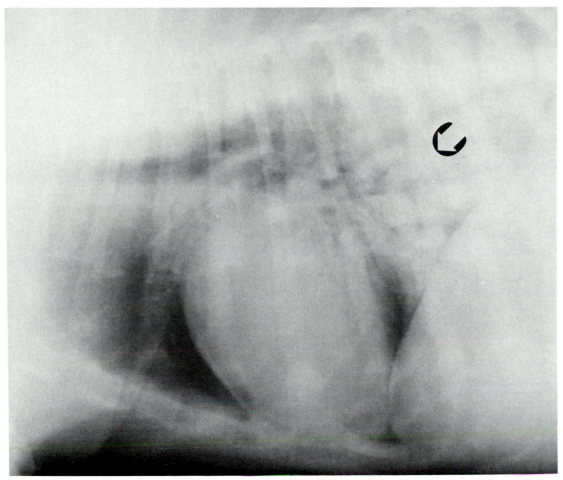

Figure 33–1 Lateral view of canine thorax shows consolidation of the middle and dorsal aspects of the caudal lung lobes (*arrow*). Diagnosis: neurogenic pulmonary edema secondary to electric shock (dog bit satellite-dish cable).

34

STRANGULATION

General Considerations

Strangulation is produced by pressure on the neck and can take different forms. Dogs (especially puppies) may become entangled in restraining devices such as leashes, chains, and ropes. Cats may become ensnared by their collars, particularly when climbing trees. Both may be caught in fences. The pathophysiology of strangulation is imperfectly understood, but it is generally believed to be caused by the following sequence of events: neck pressure to venous obstruction to cerebral anoxia to unconsciousness to decreased muscular tone(neck) to airway and arterial obstruction to death. Animals that survive varying periods of asphyxia associated with strangulation often develop pulmonary edema, which I attribute to central neurogenic causes (see Electrocution). Strangulation may also be complicated by inhalation pneumonia secondary to vomiting.

Major Radiographic Observations

There is no typical appearance. When pulmonary edema is present, it may be found in the interstitium and/or alveoli. It is usually bilateral and located predominantly in the dorsal half of the lung (Fig. 34–1).

Diagnostic Strategy

Make paired thoracic radiographs and assess for neurogenic edema. Handle the animal's head and neck with extreme care, as there may be associated injury to the cervical spine. The latter should be radiographed. If the initial radiographic examination is negative, a second study within 24 hours is advisable to rule out complications such as pneumonia.

Pitfalls

Failure to splint or otherwise support the neck of suspected strangulation patients may lead to aggravation of associated cervical injuries.

Alternative Diagnoses

Pulmonary contusion, inhalation pneumonia, and other causes of neurogenic edema such as electrocution.

Suggested Reading

Iverson KV. Strangulation: a review of ligature, manual, and postural neck compression injuries. Ann Emerg Med 1984; 13:179–185.

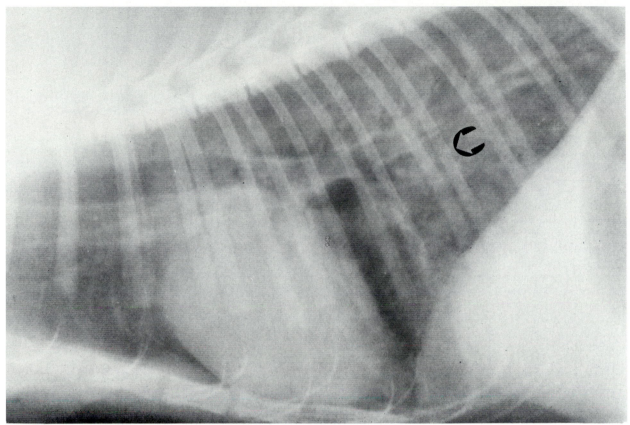

Figure 34-1 Lateral view of feline thorax shows diffuse mixed interstitial-alveolar density throughout the lung, particularly in the caudal lung field (*arrow*). Diagnosis: pulmonary edema secondary to strangulation (cat was caught by neck in garage door-opener for 10 minutes).

35
SMOKE INHALATION

General Considerations

Smoke-inhalation injury results from a combination of factors, including, oxygen deprivation, carbon-monoxide poisoning, heat, and mechanical-chemical irritation. Additionally, toxic gases other than smoke are produced by the combustion process and are also inhaled, producing additional injury. Pneumonia and adult respiratory distress syndrome (ARDS) often develop subsequently. Fatalities may occur as a direct result of the inhalation injury or secondary to its complications. Associated burns worsen the prognosis. Patient presentation may vary from unconsciousness to near normal. Facial burns and the strong smell of smoke on the hair coat are suggestive of severe heat and smoke damage. Cherry-colored mucus membranes support hypoxemia secondary to carbon-monoxide binding of hemoglobin. Fluid lung sounds indicate excessive airway secretions and/or pulmonary edema. Survival is dependent on immediate and correct supportive care. Prognosis should remain guarded until the full extent of the inhalation injury can be assessed, often not before 72 hours. A persistent cough is common in surviving dogs; chronic rhinitis often affects cats.

Major Radiographic Observations

Great variability exists, ranging from normal to interstitial or alveolar lung patterns. Diffuse peribronchial densities are most common, followed by mixed (alveolar-interstitial) patterns (Figs. 35–1 and 35–2).

Diagnostic Strategy

Make standard thoracic radiographs. Initial appearances are often normal; however, they may become abnormal shortly thereafter. For this reason, frequent follow-up films are recommended. They should be made at least daily for the first 3 days following inhalation, and twice weekly thereafter until the animal is discharged.

Pitfalls

Prolonged lateral recumbency, e.g., in an unconscious animal, leads to postural atelectasis, which in turn can mimic pulmonary consolidation. Excessive cardiopulmonary resuscitation may cause lung bruising, which resembles pulmonary edema.

Alternative Diagnoses

ARDS and/or pneumonia, especially if the initial thoracic radiographs are normal, and subsequent examinations become abnormal.

Suggested Reading

Farrow CS. Smoke inhalation. In: Kirk RW, ed. Current veterinary therapy VIII. Philadelphia: WB Saunders, 1985:173

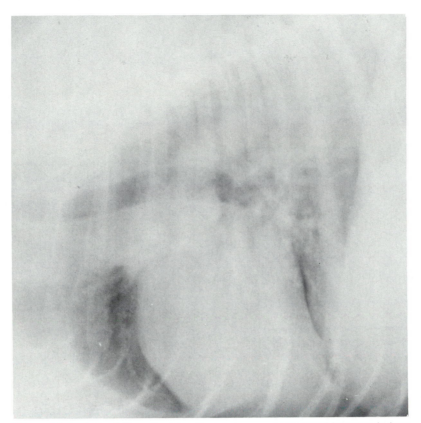

Figure 35–1 Lateral view of canine thorax shows a generalized increase in lung density, especially dorsocaudally.

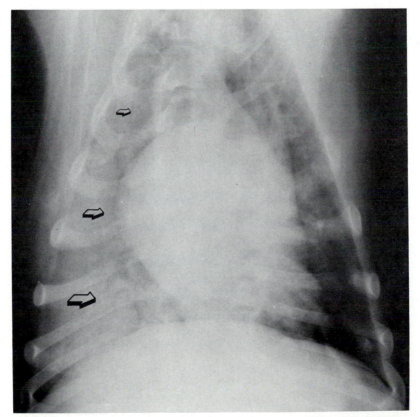

Figure 35–2 Dorsoventral view of Figure 35–1 shows most of the pulmonary consolidation on the right (*arrows*). Diagnosis: pulmonary edema secondary to smoke inhalation.

36

NEAR DROWNING

General Considerations

Near drowning is defined as survival, at least temporarily, following submersion in a fluid medium. Resulting pathophysiologic alterations may arise as a consequence of asphyxia due to reflex laryngospasm or, more commonly, as a result of aspiration of the drowning fluid. Pneumonia or adult respiratory distress syndrome (ARDS) may develop subsequently.

Major Radiographic Observations

Initial radiographs often show pulmonary consolidation centered in the dorsocaudal lung lobes; alternatively, there may be diffuse interstitial lung density (Fig. 36–1). Later films may show resolution of earlier lung densities signifying effective treatment and likely recovery. Spreading of existing lung densities, or a transition from an interstitial to an alveolar pattern, suggests treatment ineffectiveness, complicating pneumonia, or ARDS.

Diagnostic Strategy

In conscious animals, make standard thoracic radiographs. In unconscious animals, or in animals that have re-mained lying on one side for 30 minutes or more, postural atelectasis may mimic pulmonary consolidation or make existing lung density appear relatively worse. If the animal remains unconscious, make follow-up films at least twice daily. If the animal is conscious and improving gradually, make follow-up films daily for the first 3 days, with additional studies as dictated by the animal's clinical progress.

Pitfalls

The radiologic appearance of the lungs does not necessarily reflect the severity of the patient's condition, and there may be a delay of 48 hours before radiographic evidence of pulmonary edema can be seen.

Alternative Diagnoses

Inhalation pneumonia, ARDS.

Suggested Reading

Farrow CS. Near drowning. In: Kirk RW, ed. Current veterinary therapy VIII. Philadelphia: WB Saunders, 1985:167.

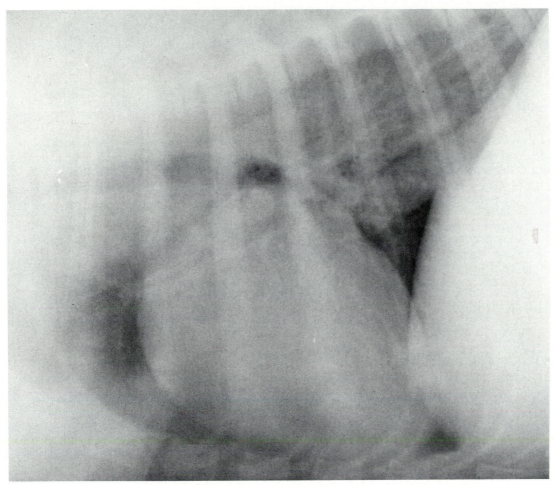

Figure 36–1 Lateral view of canine thorax shows increased interstitial density in the dorsal aspect of the caudal lung field. Diagnosis: pulmonary edema and fresh-water aspiration secondary to near drowning (dog spent an hour in a well before being rescued).

37

WARFARIN POISONING

General Considerations

Warfarin, a common rat poison, depletes the body's store of vitamin K, resulting in internal bleeding. Although hemorrhage may occur anywhere, the pleural space, mediastinum, and lung are the most common sites. The weakness and pallor in affected animals reflect the degree of blood loss, as do organ-specific signs such as dyspnea, epistaxis, hematuria, and melena. Diagnosis may be confirmed historically or by a positive coagulation screen. Warfarin is strongly suspected when thoracentesis produces a hemorrhagic transudate. Vitamin K_1 is the antidote of choice.

Major Radiographic Observations

Mediastinal widening, pulmonary consolidation, and pleural fluid may be present singularly or in any combination (Fig. 37–1). Often these findings are predominantly unilateral.

Diagnostic Strategy

Standard thoracic radiographs are satisfactory. If the animal is markedly dyspneic and will stand, a postural radio-graph (standing lateral using a horizontal x-ray beam) is usually least stressful. Alternatively, a dorsoventral view with minimal restraint is relatively safe.

Pitfalls

Avoid unnecessary stress when possible! The combination of pleural-pulmonary compromise and anemia may prove fatal for the struggling warfarin patient.

Alternative Diagnoses

Disseminated intravascular coagulation, adult respiratory distress syndrome, iatrogenic estrogen overdose, and primary or secondary thrombocytopenia.

Suggested Reading

Suter PF. Lower airway and pulmonary parenchymal diseases. In: Suter PF, ed. Thoracic radiography. Davis, CA: Stonegate Publishing, 1984:567.

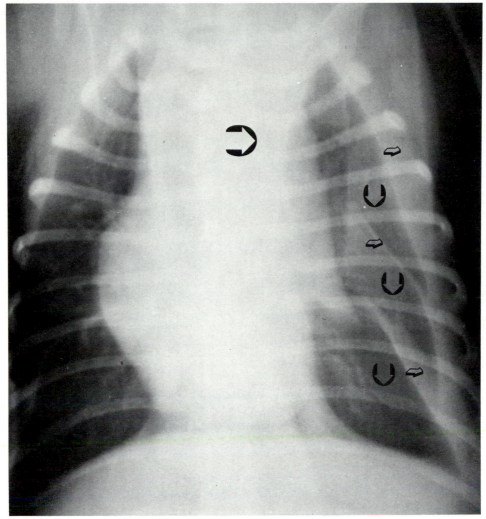

Figure 37–1 Dorsoventral view of canine thorax shows dense, widened cranial mediastinum (*large arrow*); partially collapsed left lung lobes (*medium arrows*); and associated pleural fluid (*small arrows*). Diagnosis: hemothorax-hemomediastinum secondary to warfarin poisoning.

38
PARAQUAT POISONING

General Considerations

The weedkiller paraquat is toxic to plants and animals. It causes acute respiratory distress in animals secondary to alveolar inflammation. Hyaline-membrane formation follows, producing respiratory distress syndrome (RDS). Intrapulmonary fibrosis usually develops within a week. The condition is often fatal, especially if RDS or renal failure develops.

Major Radiographic Observations

Diffuse peribronchial and interstitial lung densities are present initially. Very early cases (a few hours) may appear normal. An interstitial disease pattern usually replaces the previous mixed densities within 24 to 48 hours. The interstitial densities are, in turn, replaced by an alveolar pattern 3 to 5 days following paraquat ingestion (Fig. 38–1). The timing of these findings is largely determined by the extent of intoxication and the effectiveness of treatment.

Diagnostic Strategy

Early pathology is subtle and requires a high-quality radiograph for detection. Avoid respiratory motion by using short exposure times, and avoid overpenetration by referring to a technique guide. Later changes are more obvious. When paraquat poisoning is suspected but unconfirmed, a follow-up film may detect delayed pulmonary fibrosis.

Pitfalls

An initially normal radiograph does not rule out paraquat poisoning.

Alternative Diagnoses

Interstitial pneumonia, disseminated intravascular coagulation, adult respiratory distress syndrome, neurogenic pulmonary edema, permeability pulmonary edema, and coagulation disorders.

Suggested Reading

Gee BR, Farrow CS, White RJ, et al. Paraquat toxicity resulting in respiratory distress syndrome in a dog. JAAHA 1978; 14:256-263.

Suter PF. Lower airway and pulmonary parenchymal diseases. In: Suter PF, ed. Thoracic radiography. Davis, CA: Stonegate Publishing, 1984:564.

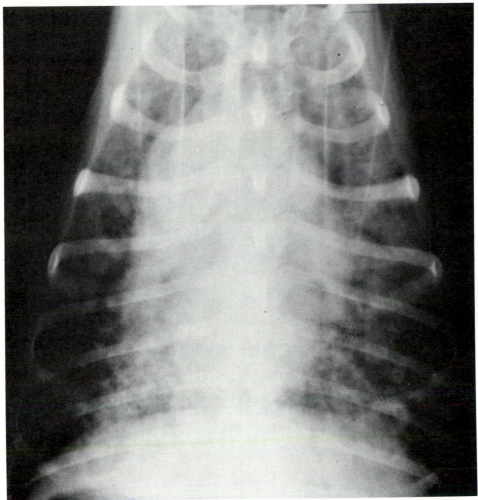

Figure 38–1 Dorsoventral view of canine thorax shows diffuse, patchy pulmonary consolidation. Diagnosis: adult respiratory distress syndrome (ARDS) secondary to paraquat poisoning.

39

FLUID OVERLOAD

General Considerations

Excessive intravenous fluid therapy resulting in pulmonary edema is termed *fluid overload* or *overhydration*. The mechanism of edema formation is not entirely clear, but it centers on the reduced osmotic pressure secondary to volume expansion and the associated increase in capillary pressure. Fluid overload is accelerated by circulatory and renal disorders. In severely affected animals it may closely resemble congestive heart failure; less severely overhydrated animals may only show a mild increase in respiratory rate. Most have moist lung sounds. The hemogram usually shows a reduction in cellular elements as a result of dilution.

Major Radiographic Observations

Mild cases show only increased vascular dimensions; mildly to moderately affected animals also show cardiomegaly, and often vascular indistinctness secondary to interstitial edema (Figs. 39–1 to 39–4). Overhydration in severely affected patients resembles overt heart failure, with cardiomegaly, pulmonary hyperemia, and alveolar edema.

Diagnostic Strategy

Avoid unnecessary patient stress. Make standard thoracic radiographs, paying careful attention to positioning and technique in order to get the examination correct the first time. The dorsoventral position with minimal restraint is easier on the animal than a ventrodorsal view.

Pitfalls

A rapidly breathing dog or cat whose thorax is exposed on expiration may resemble fluid overload owing to vascular crowding and motion-induced vascular blurring.

Alternative Diagnoses

Pulmonary edema of various causes, including congestive heart failure.

Suggested Reading

Suter PF. Lower airway and pulmonary parenchymal diseases. In: Suter PF, ed. Thoracic radiography. Davis, CA: Stonegate Publishing, 1984: 559.

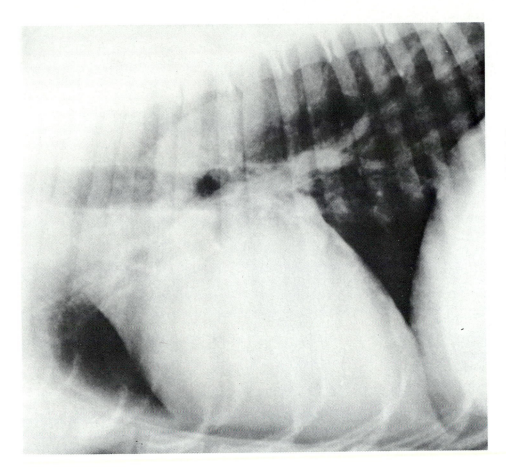

Figure 39–1 Lateral view of canine thorax shows increased cardiovascular dimensions. The dog had recently been struck by a car and was being treated for shock with intravenous fluids.

Figure 39–2 Dorsoventral view of dog shown in Figure 39–1 shows cardiac enlargement and vascular congestion. Diagnosis: cardiomegaly and pulmonary hypervolemia secondary to fluid overload.

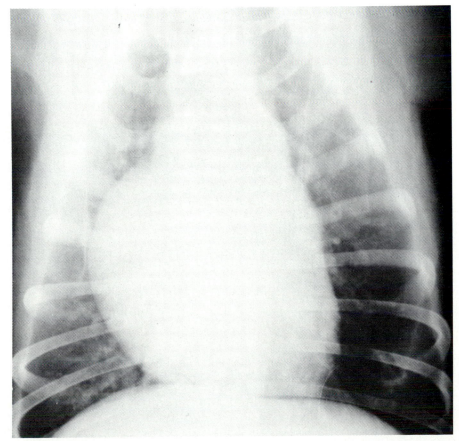

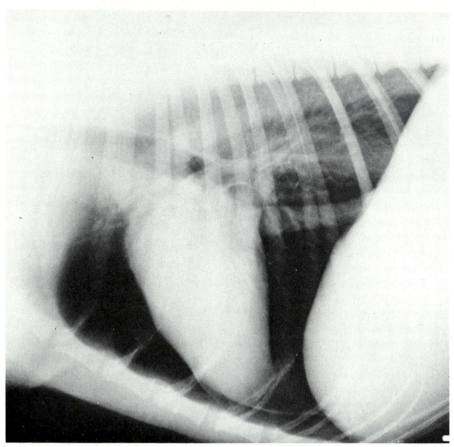

Figure 39–3 Lateral view of canine thorax shortly following automobile accident with related abdominal hemorrhage shows decreased cardiovascular dimensions. Compare this appearance with Figure 39–1.

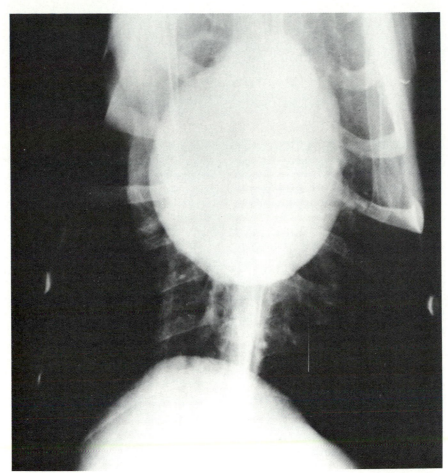

Figure 39–4 Dorsoventral view of dog shown in Figure 39–3 shows hypovascular (and therefore hyperlucent) lung fields and a small round heart. Diagnosis: microcardia and pulmonary hypovolemia secondary to blood loss and shock.

40
POSTURAL ATELECTASIS

General Considerations

Postural atelectasis is the partial loss of air from the dependent lung of an animal that has been lying on one side for a period of time. The specific length of time required to produce this form of atelectasis is variable, ranging from as little as 10 to 15 minutes to an hour or more. This normal pulmonary volume loss is more rapid in onset and greater in degree when an animal is unconscious, such as under anesthesia during surgery, or when there is heart or lung disease. Concomitant venous congestion further reduces ventilatory efficiency, adding to both the amount of atelectasis and the radiographic density. It is important to recognize postural atelectasis as a physiologic phenomenon and to distinguish it from pathologic types of atelectasis, as well as from pulmonary edema and other lung disorders.

Major Radiographic Observations

Typically, postural atelectasis is seen as a uniform, unilateral increase in lung density, with a corresponding mediastinal shift to the affected side of the thorax. The opposite lung is usually more lucent than normal as a result of compensatory overinflation (Figs. 40–1 to 40–4).

Diagnostic Strategy

A well-positioned dorsoventral or ventrodorsal radiograph is required to compare the right and left sides of the lung for density differences, and the mediastinum, for position.

Pitfalls

A dorsoventral or ventrodorsal oblique radiograph may closely mimic postural atelectasis, with one-half of the lung appearing dense and the other side, relatively lucent. However, in the case of obliquity, the heart appears to have shifted to the relatively clear side of the thorax, whereas in postural atelectasis the heart moves toward the denser side of the chest.

Alternative Diagnoses

Pneumonia, including inhalation pneumonia.

Suggested Reading

Suter PF. Lower airway and pulmonary parenchymal diseases. In: Suter PF, ed. Thoracic radiography. Davis, CA: Stonegate Publishing, 1984: 640.

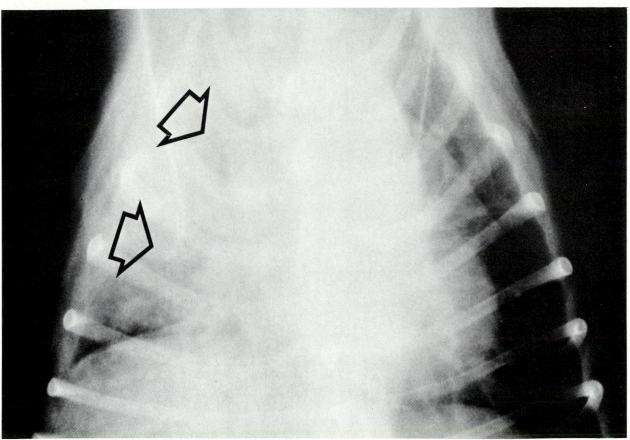

Figure 40–1 Dorsoventral view of canine thorax (made during anesthesia) following head injury, coma, and prolonged right lateral recumbency shows apparent consolidation of the right lung lobes (*arrows*) and an elevated right hemidiaphragm. Secondary pneumonia based on abnormal lung sounds was suspected.

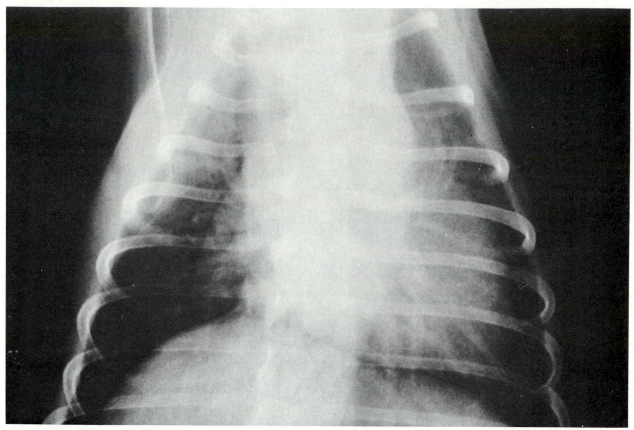

Figure 40-2 Dorsoventral view of dog shown in Figure 40-1 following endotracheal ventilation (bagging) shows marked improvement in inflation of the right lung lobes. Diagnosis: postural atelectasis following prolonged recumbency.

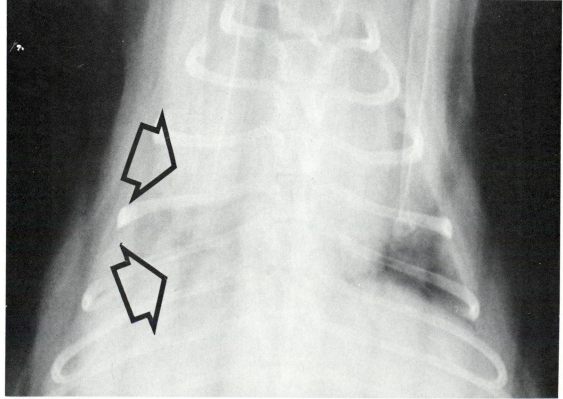

Figure 40-3 Dorsoventral view of canine thorax made following 25 minutes of anesthesia shows apparent consolidation of right middle lung lobes (*arrows*). Overhydration was suspected based on abnormal lung sounds heard during surgery. The parallel dark lines are caused by the heating pad on which the dog was radiographed.

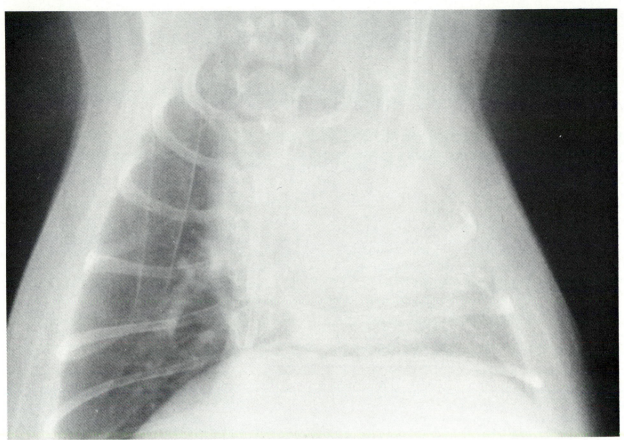

Figure 40–4 Dorsoventral view of dog shown in Figure 40–3 shows greatly improved inflation of the right lung lobes. Diagnosis: postural atelectasis following a brief period of general anesthesia.

THE HEART

41

CONGESTIVE HEART FAILURE: CONGENITAL VENTRICULAR SEPTAL DEFECT PATENT DUCTUS ARTERIOSUS

General Considerations

Congenital heart disease may go undetected until it produces heart failure. Since owners rarely consider heart disease in puppies and kittens, early signs are often missed, ignored, or attributed to other (often nonmedical) causes. Consequently, many such cases are presented as emergencies in the advanced stages of failure. Typical presenting signs may include exercise intolerance, coughing, tachypnea, and respiratory difficulty at rest or following exercise. Physical findings vary according to the nature and extent of the cardiac defect, but they often include a loud heart murmur and abnormal lung sounds. Although insufficient tissue oxygenation is the fundamental problem in congestive heart failure, pulmonary edema (when present) is the most immediate concern. Once this has been alleviated and the heart has been stabilized, the specific source of failure may be sought.

Major Radiographic Observations

Left-sided heart failure typically shows cardiomegaly, and enlarged pulmonary vasculature, and pulmonary edema. *Right-sided* failure is characterized by cardiomegaly, hepatomegaly, and, often, pleural and peritoneal fluid (Figs. 41–1 and 41–2). Combined left- and right-sided congestive heart failure usually produces a combination of changes, dominated by those affecting the left side (Fig. 41–3). Angiocardiography reveals more specific alterations, depending on the nature and location of the lesion. Echocardiography may also be of use. Both procedures require considerable technical skill and experience.

Diagnostic Strategy

Make lateral and dorsoventral radiographs (the latter is easier on most dogs), centered over the heart. Avoid respiratory motion or patient movement, which blurs the radiographic image, often producing an image that resembles interstitial edema. Overpenetration may disguise interstitial fluid. Attempt standard patient positioning, but not at the cost of unnecessary patient stress; a perfectly positioned radiograph is not required to diagnose congestive heart failure. Full inspiration is desirable but difficult to obtain when the animal is breathing rapidly.

Pitfalls

Be aware that the heart is absolutely (and relatively) larger on expiration, resulting in an increased cardiothoracic ratio. This normal physiologic finding may be misinterpreted as cardiomegaly. Puppies have a greater cardiothoracic ratio than adult dogs, which may lead to an incorrect diagnosis of heart disease. Breeds with vertically compressed, rounded chests (Bulldogs); with long bodies and short legs (Basset Hounds); and some toy and minature dogs (Chihuahuas) have rounded hearts compared to other breeds. This normal variation may falsely suggest cardiac abnormality.

Alternative Diagnoses

Congestive heart failure of an acquired nature (e.g., mitral insufficiency), noncardiogenic pulmonary edema with coincidental cardiomegaly, fluid overload. Also see "Pitfalls" above.

Suggested Reading

Cantwell HD. Congenital cardiac disease. In: Farrow CS, ed. Decision making in small animal radiology. Toronto: BC Decker, 1987:148.

Holmberg DL. Patent ductus arteriosus In: Binnington AG, Cockshutt JR, eds. Decision making in small animal soft tissue surgery. Toronto: BC Decker, 1988: 82.

Holmberg DL. Ventricular septal defect. In: Binnington AG, Cockshutt JR, eds. Decision making in small animal soft tissue surgery. Toronto: BC Decker, 1988: 88.

Suter PF. Cardiac diseases. In: Suter PF, ed. Thoracic radiography. Davis, CA: Stonegate Publishing, 1984:371, 474.

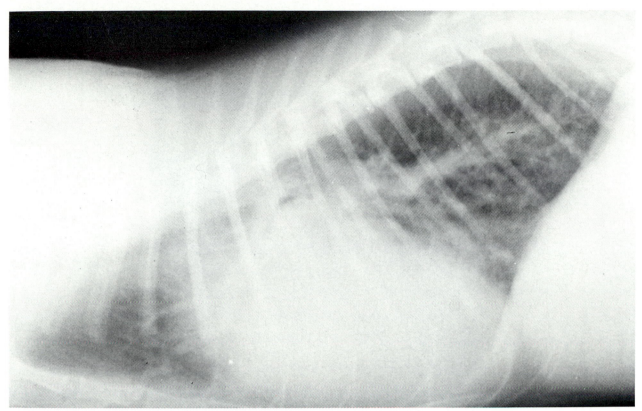

Figure 41–1   Lateral view of feline thorax (6 months old) shows cardiomegaly, increased size and number of pulmonary vessels, and increased interstitial lung density.

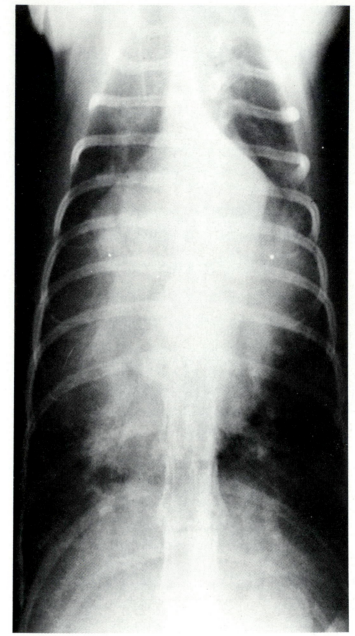

Figure 41–2 Dorsoventral view of Figure 41–1 shows severe cardio-megaly with right-sided emphasis (the cardiac apex is shifted to the right side). Diagnosis: congenital heart disease (ventricular septal defect) resulting in congestive heart failure.

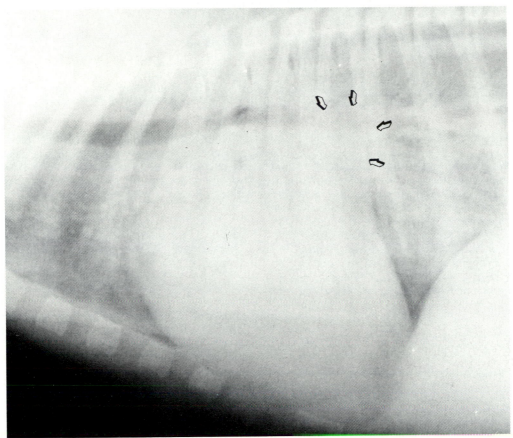

Figure 41–3 Lateral view of canine thorax (4 months old) shows generalized cardiomegaly with left atrial emphasis (*arrows*), increased size and number of pulmonary vessels, and increased alveolar lung density. Diagnosis: congenital heart disease (patent ductus arteriosus, PDA) resulting in congestive heart failure.

42

CONGESTIVE HEART FAILURE: ACQUIRED MITRAL INSUFFICIENCY

General Considerations

Mitral insufficiency secondary to endocardiosis of the mitral valves is the most common cause of congestive heart failure in older dogs. Mitral insufficiency may be divided into various phases according to the severity of clinical and radiographic signs. Although of proven value in human heart patients, such classification appears to be of questionable practical benefit in dogs. Congestive heart failure produced by mitral insufficiency differs little from failure resulting from most congenital heart diseases, insofar as both may present as emergencies associated with exercise intolerance, cough, and dyspnea. Congenital and acquired heart failure may also share such characteristic physical findings as a loud murmur and moist lung sounds.

Major Radiographic Observations

Typically, congestive heart failure secondary to mitral insufficiency shows cardiomegaly (left-sided emphasis), an increased pulmonary vasculature, and lung edema (Figs. 42–1 and 42–2). Pleural effusion, caudal vena cava enlargement, and hepatomegaly may be present in some cases.

Diagnostic Strategy

Make a lateral and a dorsoventral radiograph centered over the heart, being careful to avoid unnecessary patient stress. Avoid respiratory motion, which may mimic pulmonary edema, and avoid overpenetration, which may obscure edema. Repeat films of inferior quality, but not in the extremely ill animal.

Pitfalls

A moderately rotated lateral radiograph makes the heart appear enlarged vertically but does not compromise the detection of pulmonary edema.

Alternative Diagnoses

Congestive heart failure of a congenital nature (e.g., ventricular septal defect), cardiomyopathy, noncardiogenic pulmonary edema with coincidental cardiomegaly, fluid overload. Also see "Pitfalls" above.

Suggested Reading

Cantwell HD. Acquired cardiac disease. In: Farrow CS, ed. Decision making in small animal radiology. Toronto: BC Decker, 1987:150.

Suter PF. Cardiac Diseases. In: Suter PF, ed. Thoracic radiography. Davis, CA: Stonegate Publishing, 1984:371, 483.

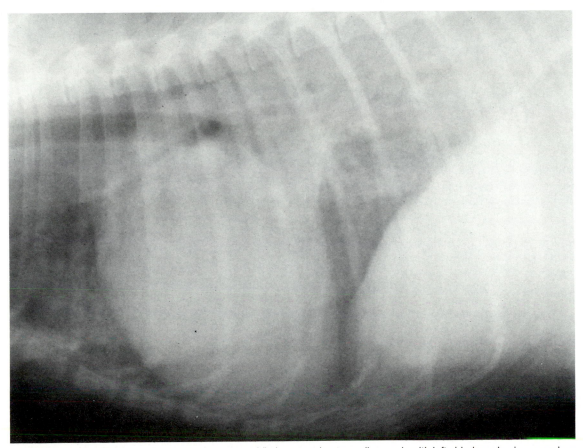

Figure 42-1 Lateral view of canine thorax (9 years old) shows moderate cardiomegaly with left-sided emphasis, secondary dorsal tracheal displacement, and diffuse alveolar lung density.

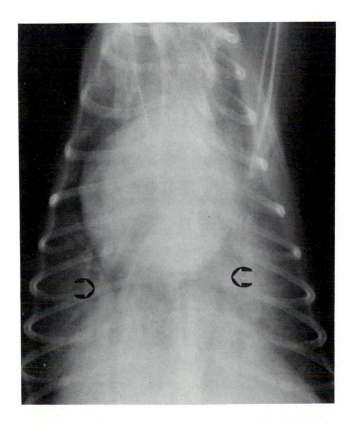

Figure 42-2 Dorsoventral view of Figure 42-1 shows the bilateral density pattern typical of cardiogenic edema (*arrows*). Diagnosis: acquired heart disease (mitral insufficiency) resulting in congestive heart failure.

43

CARDIOMYOPATHY IN THE DOG

General Considerations

Cardiomyopathies in the dog may be most simply divided into congestive and hypertrophic types on the basis of altered myocardial anatomy and/or function. Congestive (now frequently termed *dilated*) cardiomyopathy is common in the dog, where as the hypertrophic form of the disease is rare. Unlike in the cat, thromboembolism in the dog is exceptional. Clinical signs may reflect right, left, or generalized heart failure. Onset may be acute or chronic: the acute form is associated with dyspnea, weakness, or collapse; the chronic variety produces decreased exercise tolerance, lethargy, and, if ascites is present, a pendulous abdomen. Some amount of dyspnea is common; coughing is not. Tachycardia and a gallop rhythm are often detected with auscultation. Murmurs are uncommon and, when present, are mild. Ultimately, most cardiomyopathies prove fatal.

Major Radiographic Observations

Although signs are variable depending on which heart chambers are involved, there is usually obvious cardiomegaly, often with left-sided emphasis. Pulmonary hyperemia is usually present, frequently with pulmonary edema and pleural effusion (Figs. 43–1 to 43–3). Fluoroscopy often shows poor contractility. Angiocardiography typically reveals chamber enlargement, valvular incompetence, and sluggish blood flow. Sonography shows enlargement of the left heart chambers and reduced left ventricular contractility.

Diagnostic Strategy

Avoid unnecessary patient stress! Make dorsoventral and right lateral thoracic radiographs centered on the heart. Use the shortest possible exposure time, since both the heart and respiration rates are usually markedly elevated. A brief period in an oxygen cage prior to radiographic examination is highly desirable. Resuscitation materials should be immediately available in the event of cardiopulmonary arrest. Ultrasound (if available) produces minimal distress and is often diagnostic. Nonselective angiocardiography, although very useful in differentiating the principal forms of cardiomyopathy, should not be performed until the animal's condition has stabilized.

Pitfalls

Pleural fluid (a frequent component of congestive cardiomyopathy) makes assessment of the heart difficult or impossible in a majority of cases. Remove thoracic fluid before making a definite diagnosis.

Alternative Diagnoses

Mitral insufficiency in older dogs, congenital heart disease (patent ductus arteriosus [PDA], aortic stenosis, ventricular septal defect in younger animals).

Suggested Reading

Bonagura JD, Herring DS. Echocardiography: Acquired heart disease. Vet Clin North Am (Small Anim Pract) 1985; 15:1209–1224.

Cantwell HD. Acquired cardiac disease. In: Farrow CS, ed. Decision making in small animal radiology. Toronto: BC Decker, 1987:150.

Suter PF. Cardiac diseases. In: Suter PF, ed. Thoracic radiography. Davis, CA: Stonegate Publishing, 1984:388.

Ware WA, Bonagura JD. Canine myocardial diseases. In: Kirk RW, ed. Current veterinary therapy IX. Philadelphia: WB Saunders, 1986:370.

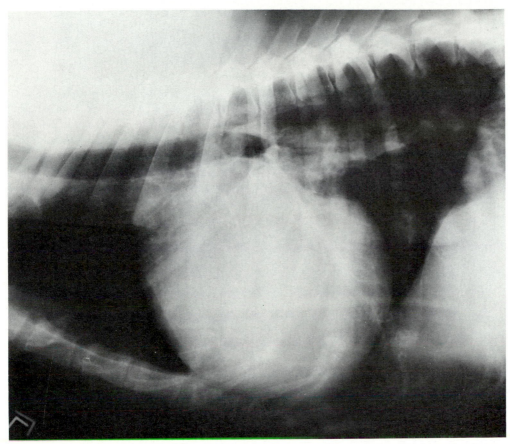

Figure 43–1 Lateral view of canine thorax shows generalized cardiomegaly, increased vascular dimensions, and a clear lung. Diagnosis: cardiovascular enlargement compatible with cardiomyopathy but without congestive heart failure. Sonography confirmed congestive (dilated) cardiomyopathy.

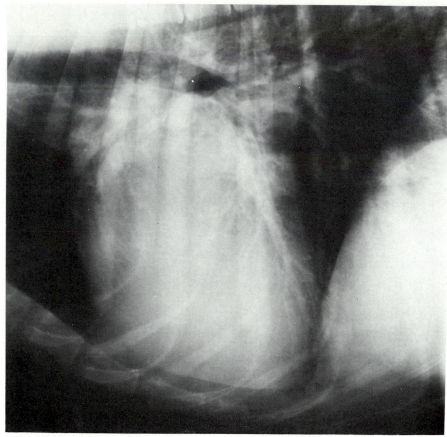

Figure 43–2 Lateral view of canine thorax shows cardiomegaly with left-sided emphasis, increased vascular dimensions, and perihilar edema. Diagnosis: congestive heart failure. Sonography confirmed congestive (dilated) cardiomyopathy.

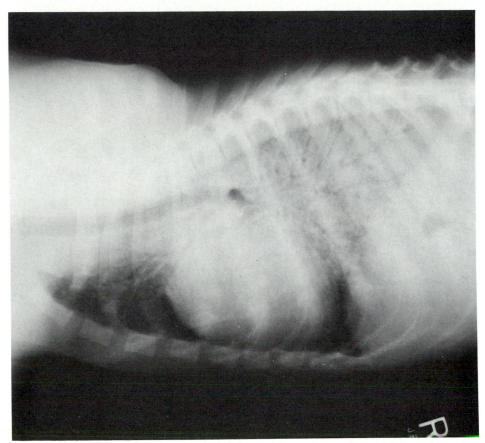

Figure 43–3 Lateral view of canine thorax shows generalized cardiomegaly and diffuse lung edema. Diagnosis: congestive heart failure. Sonography confirmed congestive (dilated) cardiomyopathy.

44

CARDIOMYOPATHY IN THE CAT

General Considerations

Cats may suffer from three distinct forms of cardiomyopathy: *congestive* (dilated, dilatative), *hypertrophic*, and restrictive. In most regions of North America, the congestive form is most common, and *restrictive* cardiomyopathy is rare. Both congestive and hypertrophic cardiomyopathy typically affect male cats of more than 2 years of age. Anorexia, lethargy, and dyspnea are common. Hindquarter weakness or paralysis may be present as a result of thromboembolism. Cardiac abnormalities usually include tachycardia, atrial or ventricular arrhythmia, a gallop rhythm, and a mild murmur best heard over the cardiac apex. Because of these many similarities, it is often difficult to distinguish one type of myopathy from another without the aid of radiography, angiocardiography, or diagnostic ultrasound. Ultimately, the disease is fatal.

Major Radiographic Observations

Congestive cardiomyopathy is typically associated with moderate to severe cardiomegaly, a rounded cardiac apex, and a bulging left atrium (Figs. 44–1 to 44–4). Pleural effusion is common; pulmonary edema is not. Angiocardiography shows chamber enlargement, thin heart walls, poor contractility, and valvular incompetence. Sonography reveals similar findings. *Hypertrophic* cardiomyopathy shows varying degrees of cardiomegaly with left atrial or biatrial emphasis. Because of the disproportionate atrial enlargement,

the heart has a distinctive triangular shape in the dorsoventral or ventrodorsal views. Pulmonary edema frequently is present, often with pleural effusion. Angiographically, the left ventricle is small with a thickened free wall and septum, and it contains hypertrophied papillary muscles. Contractility is normal. The left atrium is typically enlarged with incompetent valves. Sonography confirms these findings.

Diagnostic Strategy

Avoid unnecessary patient stress! Make dorsoventral and right lateral thoracic radiographs centered over the heart (ribs 4 to 7) using the fastest possible exposure times to avoid blurriness resulting from tachycardia and dyspnea. Avoid overexposure of the lungs, which may conceal pulmonary edema and underestimate the amount of pleural effusion. If a large effusion is present, remove it cautiously before attempting to evaluate the heart. If the heart must be assessed immediately, a postural radiograph (erect patient position with a horizontal beam directed at the sternum) should be made. This maneuver allows the pleural fluid to gravitate toward the diaphragm, thus revealing the majority of the heart. Record the radiographic technique, because follow-up films are usually required to evaluate the success of treatment.

Pitfalls

The heart cannot be evaluated in the context of a medium or large pleural effusion. Oblique dorsoventral or ventrodorsal views of the heart often mimic cardiac abnormalities, particularly unilateral atrioventricular enlargement. Avoid overdiagnosis in this regard! Motion blur closely resembles pulmonary edema; it also creates an erroneous impression of cardiac enlargement. Overexposed radiographs of the heart make the heart appear relatively small when compared to normally exposed or underexposed films.

Alternative Diagnoses

Hyperthyroid heart disease, ventricular septal defect, and aortic stenosis (AS) in young cats.

Suggested Reading

Bonagura JD, Herring DS. Echocardiography: Acquired heart disease. Vet Clin North Am (Small Anim Pract) 1985; 15:1209–1224.

Harpster NK. Feline myocardial diseases. In: Kirk RW, ed. Current veterinary therapy IX. Philadelphia: WB Saunders, 1986:380.

Suter PF. Cardiac diseases. In: Suter PF, ed. Thoracic radiography. Davis, CA: Stonegate Publishing, 1984:388.

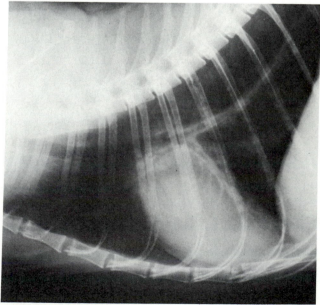

Figure 44–1 Lateral view of feline thorax shows mild cardiomegaly with left-sided emphasis, normal vasculature, and a clear lung.

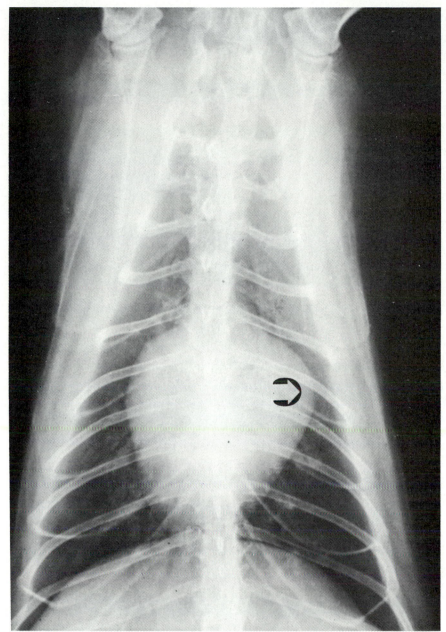

Figure 44–2 Ventrodorsal view of Figure 44–1 shows left atrial enlargement (*arrow*). Diagnosis: cardiac alterations compatible with cardiomyopathy. Sonography confirmed hypertrophic cardiomyopathy.

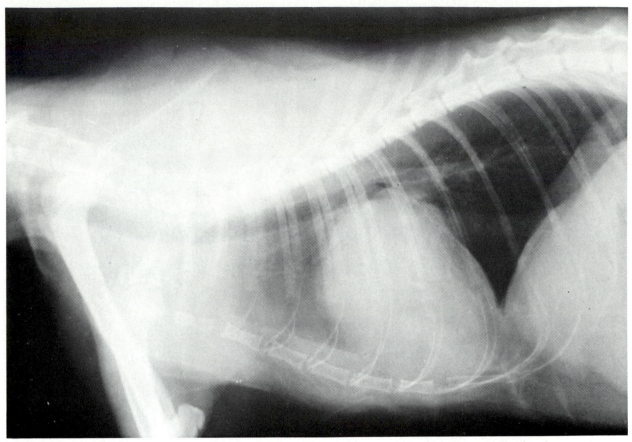

Figure 44–3 Lateral view of feline thorax shows marked generalized cardiomegaly, normal vasculature, and a clear lung.

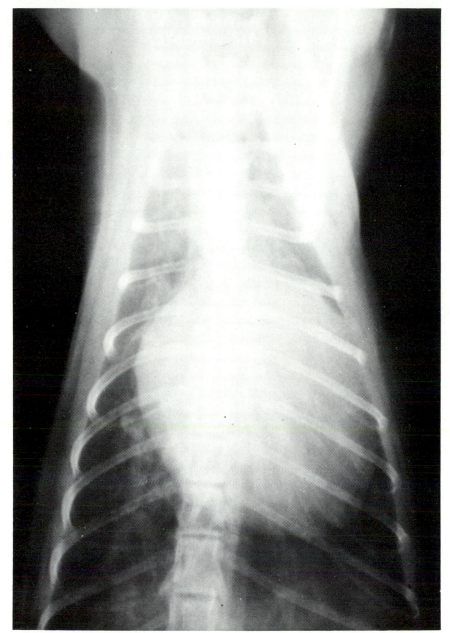

Figure 44–4 Lateral view of Figure 44–3 shows severe cardiomegaly with the left heart margin against the chest wall. Diagnosis: heart changes consistent with cardiomyopathy. Sonography confirmed congestive cardiomyopathy.

45

HEARTWORM IN THE DOG

General Considerations

Dirofilariasis or heartworm disease is caused by the obstructive effects of the adult dirofilaria in the right heart and associated pulmonary arteries, and by the presence of their highly antigenic microfilaria in the lung. It is the vascular lesions of the lung that ultimately produce pulmonary hypertension and signs of right heart failure. This form of secondary right heart disease is referred to as *pulmonary heart disease* or *cor pulmonale*. Acute heart failure may occur following treatment of the adult filariae, secondary to acute, widespread pulmonary thromboembolism of the dead worms. Acute failure may also be precipitated when large numbers of adults accumulate in the right ventricle and cranial and/or caudal vena cava. This condition is called the *vena caval syndrome*. Diagnosis is usually made radiologically and confirmed with the microscopic identification of microfilaria in the peripheral blood, or by immunodiagnostic tests such as indirect fluorescent antibody (IFA) and enzyme-linked immunosorbent assay (ELISA).

Major Radiographic Observations

Radiographic abnormalities are contingent on the severity of the disease and may include cardiomegaly with right-sided emphasis; enlargement of the main pulmonary arterial segment; enlargement, distortion, and abbreviation of the pulmonary arteries; and increased lung density (Figs. 45–1 to 45–5).

Diagnostic Strategy

As with any serious cardiovascular condition, undue patient stress must be avoided. A dorsoventral projection provides the best view of the large caudal pulmonary arteries as they project above the liver. A 10-percent increase in kilovolt peak (penetrated view) further improves the definition of these structures. The lateral view should be centered directly over the heart and confined to the thorax. If the vena caval syndrome is suspected, a lateral view of the abdomen is advisable to evaluate liver size and possible ascites. This view should be made using abdominal technique, determined by measuring the cranial abdomen, and it should include the entire diaphragm.

Pitfalls

A dorsoventral oblique view of the thorax accentuates the aorta and main pulmonary arterial segment, thus mimicking heartworm disease. A lateral projection of the heart made during systole often shows a normal (physiologic) enlargement of the main pulmonary arterial segment, which may resemble early heartworm disease.

Alternative Diagnosis

Chronic ventricular septal defect with pulmonary hypertension and reversed blood flow (Eisenmenger's syndrome).

Suggested Reading

Calvert CA, Rawlings CA. Therapy of canine heart worm disease. In: Kirk RW, ed. Current veterinary therapy IX. Philadelphia: WB Saunders, 1986:406.

Cantwell HD. Heartworm disease. In: Farrow CS, ed. Decision making in small animal radiology. Toronto: BC Decker, 1987:152.

Holmberg DL. Canine heartworm. In: Binnington AG, Cockshutt JR, eds. Decision making in small animal soft tissue surgery. Toronto: BC Decker 1988: 102.

Losonsky JM. The pulmonary vasculature. In: Thrall DE, ed. Textbook of veterinary diagnostic radiology. Philadelphia: WB Saunders, 1986:294.

Suter PF. Cardiac diseases. In: Suter PF, ed. Thoracic radiography. Davis, CA: Stonegate Publishing, 1984:439.

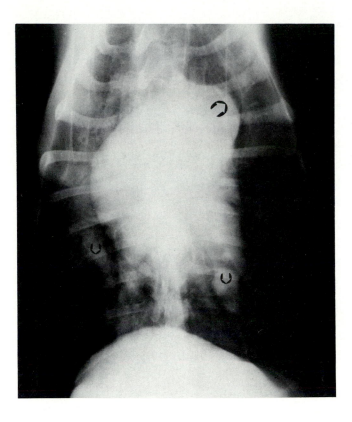

Figure 45–1 Dorsoventral view of canine thorax shows cardiomegaly with right-sided emphasis, as well as enlargement of the pulmonary trunk (*large arrow*) and central pulmonary arteries (*small arrows*). Diagnosis: heartworm disease.

Figure 45–2 Dorsoventral view of canine thorax shows cardiomegaly with right-sided emphasis, enlargement of the pulmonary trunk (*large arrow*) and central pulmonary arteries, and two large areas of pulmonary consolidation (*small arrows*). Diagnosis: heartworm disease with secondary lung infarcts.

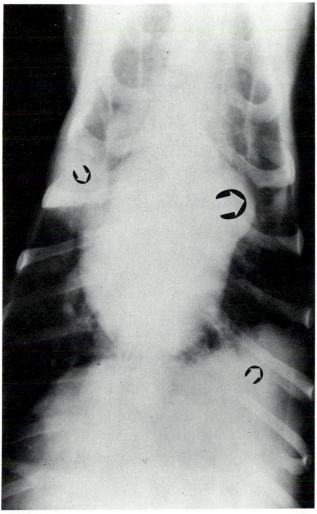

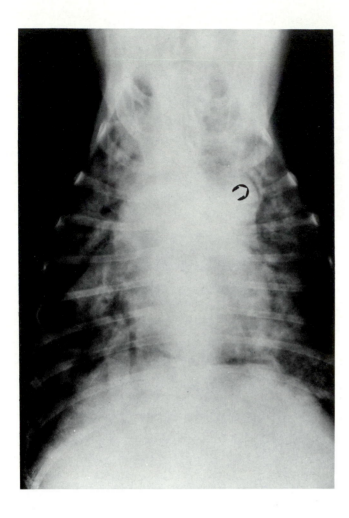

Figure 45–3 Dorsoventral view of canine thorax shows cardiomegaly with right-sided emphasis, enlargement of the pulmonary trunk (*arrow*) and main pulmonary arteries, and patchy lung consolidation. Diagnosis: congestive heart failure secondary to heartworm disease.

Figure 45–4 Dorsoventral view of canine thorax shows little of the heart because of a large pleural effusion and partial lung collapse; nevertheless, two enlarged pulmonary arteries are visible (*arrows*). Diagnosis: congestive heart failure secondary to heartworm disease.

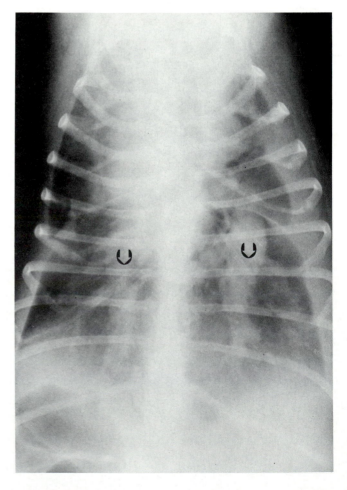

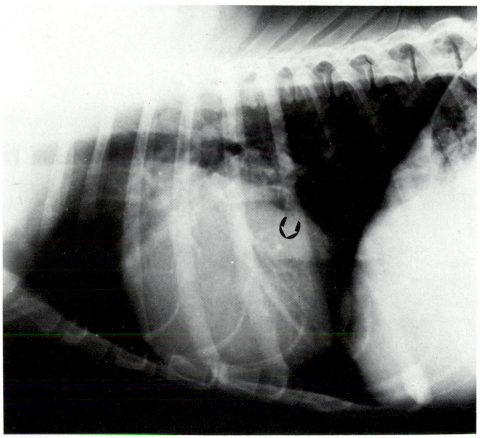

Figure 45–5 Lateral view of canine thorax shows cardiomegaly with right-sided emphasis and enlargement of the caudal vena cava (*arrow*). Diagnosis: caudal vena caval syndrome secondary to heartworm disease.

46

HEARTWORM IN THE CAT

General Considerations

Heartworm disease in cats, once believed rare, is now seen regularly in endemic areas, although not with the frequency of dirofilariasis in the dog. The pathologic condition in the cat is identical to that in the dog: immunoarteritis producing pulmonary hypertension, cor pulmonale, and, eventually, right-sided heart failure. Acute and chronic forms of the disease occur. The former is associated with a wide range of clinical signs, including vomiting and diarrhea, tachycardia, dyspnea, collapse, convulsions, and blindness. Because of reduced awareness (and in some cases, misconceptions about feline dirofilariasis), heartworms is often diagnosed incidentally, usually from thoracic radiographs made in an attempt to confirm suspected cardiomyopathy or pulmonary disease. Diagnostic confirmation is usually made with the Knott indirect fluorescent antibody (IFA), or enzyme-linked immunosorbent assay (ELISA) test.

Major Radiographic Observations

Pulmonary arterial enlargement is the most reliable indication of heartworms in the cat (Figs. 46–1 and 46–2). Mild to moderate cardiomegaly with right-sided emphasis is usually present but is not nearly as obvious as in the dog. Lung densities are often increased but are usually of a nonspecific nature and are difficult to separate from the additional lung density resulting from vascular enlargement.

Diagnostic Strategy

Contrary to some previously published reports, the dorsoventral view of the thorax provides the optimal view of the heart and associated pulmonary arteries. The lateral view best shows vascular tortuosity when this is present.

Pitfalls

All else being equal, feline dirofilariasis shows fewer and less pronounced radiographic abnormalities than the canine version. This becomes a problem in mild infections, which may appear normal (especially to the untrained eye). Thus, early cases of suspected feline heartworms should be evaluated serologically.

Alternative Diagnoses

Cardiomyopathy, chronic ventricular septal defect.

Suggested Reading

Dillon R. Feline heartworm disease. In: Kirk RW, ed. Current veterinary therapy IX. Philadelphia: WB Saunders, 1986: 420.

Losonsky JM. The pulmonary vasculature. In: Thrall DE, ed. Textbook of veterinary diagnostic radiology. Philadelphia: WB Saunders, 1986: 294.

Suter PF. Cardiac diseases. In: Suter PF, ed. Thoracic radiography. Davis, CA: Stonegate Publishing, 1984: 447.

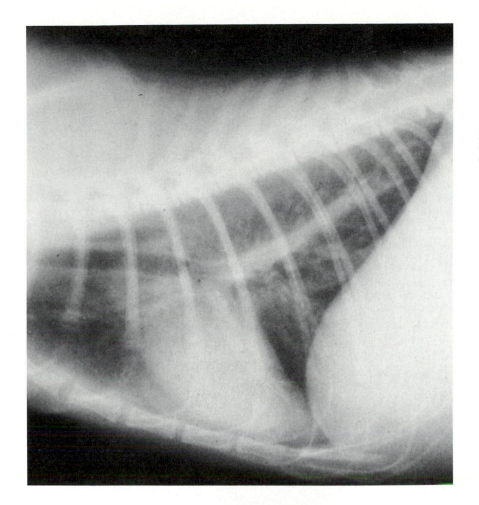

Figure 46-1 Lateral view of feline thorax shows a generalized increase in lung vascularity.

Figure 46-2 Ventrodorsal view of cat shown in Figure 46-1 shows marked enlargement of right caudal lobe artery (*arrows*). Diagnosis: heartworms. (Figures 46-1 and 46-2 are provided courtesy of Dr. L. Turner, Small Animal Internist, Texas Veterinary Medical Center, Texas A&M University).

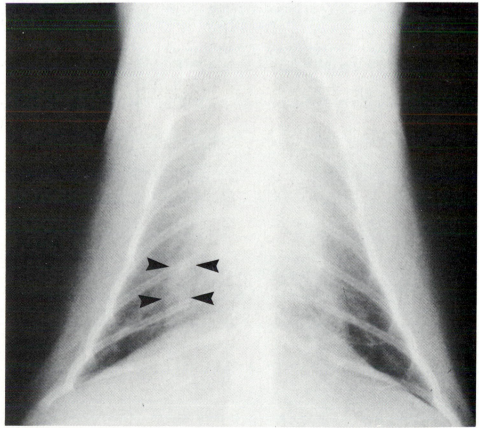

47

BENIGN PERICARDIAL EFFUSION: TAMPONADE

General Considerations

Pericardial effusion is a disorder of large, middle-aged dogs, particularly German Shepherds. The condition is rare in cats. Effusions are traditionally classified according to their cytologic characteristics as transudative, exudative, or hemorrhagic. They may also be described as malignant or benign, with the latter being further divided into infectious and non-infectious subcategories. Circulatory disturbances result from the compressive effects of the pericardial fluid on the heart chambers, which in turn reduce cardiac filling. Decreased left ventricular output and systemic venous hypertension result. Clinically, these cardiovascular alterations produce muffled heart sounds, venous engorgement, and a weak pulse. Affected animals may range from subclinical to acutely ill, depending on the size of the effusion and its rate of formation.

Major Radiographic Observations

Survey radiographs typically show globular cardiomegaly if moderate to large pericardial effusions are present (Figs. 47–1 and 47–2). Small effusions are usually not recognized or are mistaken for mild cardiomegaly. *Nonselective angiography* shows increased distance between the opacified heart chambers and the edge of the cardiac silhouette, suggesting pericardial effusion. *Pneumopericardiography* shows pericardial alterations such as thickening, as well as changes in the heart margin, particularly protruding masses. *Echocardiography*, when it is available, shows both pericardial fluid and intracardiac masses. *Fluoroscopy* reveals either an absence of contractility or a shimmering of the heart margin.

Diagnostic Strategy

Both lateral and dorsoventral-ventrodorsal films are recommended for the assessment of pericardial fluid. This is especially true of smaller effusions in which cardiac rounding usually is not pronounced. Sonography is the safest and most definitive of the listed special procedures.

Pitfalls

Varying degrees of cardiac rounding are present in most heart diseases, especially on the right side. For this reason, a diagnosis of pericardial effusion should not be based on radiography alone.

Alternative Diagnoses

Cardiac dilatation-hypertrophy secondary to congenital or acquired heart disease, right atrial hemangiosarcoma, heart base tumor.

Suggested Reading

Holmberg DL. Pericardial effusion tamponade. In: Binnington AG, Cockshutt JR, eds. Decision making in small animal soft tissue surgery. Toronto: BC Decker, 1988: 96.
Suter PF. Cardiac diseases. In: Suter PF, ed. Thoracic radiography. Davis, CA: Stonegate Publishing, 1984:407.

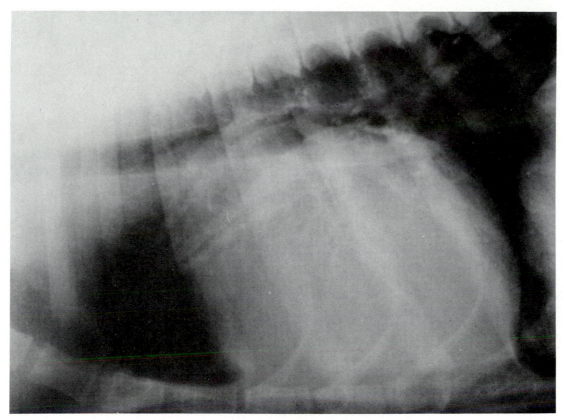

Figure 47-1 Lateral view of canine thorax shows marked, generalized cardiomegaly.

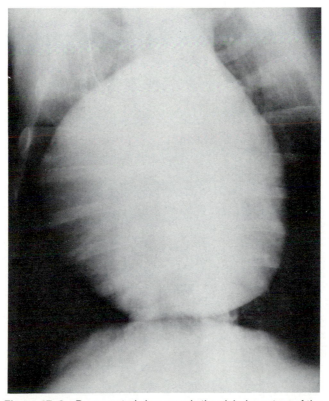

Figure 47-2 Dorsoventral view reveals the globular nature of the cardiomegaly seen in Figure 47-1. Diagnosis: benign (noninfectious) pericardial effusion.

48

HEMANGIOSARCOMA OF RIGHT ATRIUM PRODUCING PERICARDIAL EFFUSION

General Considerations

Pericardial hemangiosarcoma is a relatively rare tumor, occurring primarily in older, male German Shepherds and Boxers. Associated clinical signs are most often of a secondary nature, such as pericardial effusion, right heart failure, or pulmonary metastasis. Malignant mesothelioma and chemodectoma (heart-base and aortic-body tumors) may produce similar signs. Sudden death may result from cardiac tamponade induced by acute pericardial bleeding following right atrial perforation. Alternatively, the pericardial effusion may develop gradually, allowing cardiac compensation and thereby a delayed onset of clinical signs. In older animals with heart murmurs, the signs of pericardial hemangiosarcoma may be misinterpreted as those of valvular disease, which is far more common.

Major Radiographic Observations

Large pericardial effusions secondary to pericardial hemangiosarcomas are typically associated with a globular cardiomegaly (Figs. 48–1 and 48–2). Smaller effusions are less obvious, although they may be inferred by rounding of the heart shadow and dorsal displacement of the terminal trachea. An atrial mass is also suggested by signs of right heart failure, although the tumor mass is usually impossible to see without the aid of special procedures.

Diagnostic Strategy

Survey radiographs typically show indirect signs only. *Nonselective angiocardiography* is often effective in demonstrating right atrial masses. *Pneumopericardiography* is less specific but usually shows masses that project away from the normal heart margin. *Pleurography* has never lived up to its clinical promise and is only recommended for the experienced. *Cardiac ultrasound* when available, is very effective in detecting intra-atrial masses.

Pitfalls

The first step in diagnosing pericardial neoplasms is to keep them in mind, which may be difficult since they are comparatively rare.

Alternative Diagnoses

Congestive right or right-left heart failure, benign pericardial effusion, heart base tumor.

Suggested Reading

Suter PF. Cardiac diseases. In: Suter PF, ed. Thoracic radiography. Davis, CA: Stonegate Publishing, 1984:416, 430.
Thomas WP, Reed JR. Pericardial disease. In: Kirk RW, ed. Current veterinary therapy 1X. Philadelphia: WB Saunders, 1986:364.

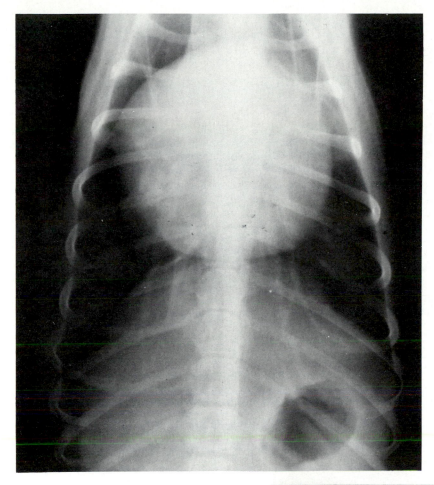

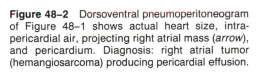

Figure 48–1 Dorsoventral view of canine thorax shows globular cardiomegaly.

Figure 48–2 Dorsoventral pneumoperitoneogram of Figure 48–1 shows actual heart size, intrapericardial air, projecting right atrial mass (*arrow*), and pericardium. Diagnosis: right atrial tumor (hemangiosarcoma) producing pericardial effusion.

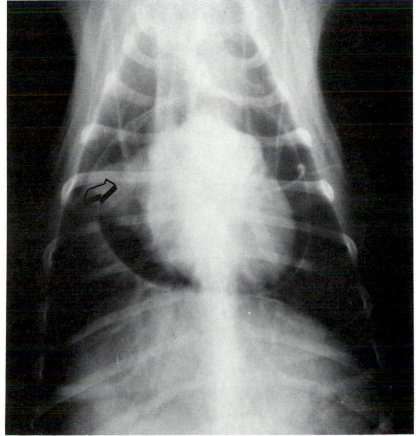

49

HEART BASE TUMOR PRODUCING HEART FAILURE

General Considerations

Most heart base tumors or chemodectomas arise from chemoreceptors located between the aortic arch and the pulmonary artery or right atrium. Their growth is slow and they rarely metastasize, although they may be locally invasive. They are most common in older brachiocephalic breeds, especially Boston Terriers. Although relatively discrete masses, they are difficult to see radiographically because they blend into the surrounding soft tissues, and as such often resemble individual variations. Clinically, the tumor may produce a wide variety of signs relating to the organs affected. Pericardial effusion and right heart failure often result in emergency presentation.

Major Radiographic Observations

Survey radiographs may show localized tracheal elevation over the cranial heart base in lateral projection, and localized right lateral tracheal displacement in the dorsoventral or ventrodorsal view. The cranial heart base may appear increased in density and widened, depending on the size of the mass (Fig. 49–1). *Contrast studies* of the regional vasculature may provide indirect information in the form of displacement or distortion of the involved structure. Pleurography, although capable of outlining a heart base tumor, requires considerable technical skill and diagnostic experience (Fig. 49–2). *Echocardiography* may also be useful.

Diagnostic Strategy

Penetrated views (high kilovolt-peak technique) may improve lesion detail of areas of suspicion seen on survey radiographs. Pleurography may outline the mass, but can be confusing or equivocal without a normal comparison film and knowledge of normal variations common to this area.

Pitfalls

Normal rounding of the brachiocephalic heart, combined with a relatively large cardiac-thoracic ratio, may result in a false positive diagnosis of heart base tumor. End-on projections of the pulmonary artery may mimic a hilar mass.

Alternative Diagnoses

Regional adenopathy or other hilar-perihilar masses or mass effects, right atrial hemangiosarcoma, and other causes of right atrial enlargement, benign or malignant pericardial effusions.

Suggested Reading

Holmberg DL. Pericardial effusion tamponade. In: Binnington AG, Cockshutt JR, eds. Decision making in small animal soft tissue surgery. Toronto: BC Decker, 1988: 96.

Suter PF. Cardiac diseases. In Suter PF, ed. Thoracic radiography. Davis, CA: Stonegate Publishing, 1984:428.

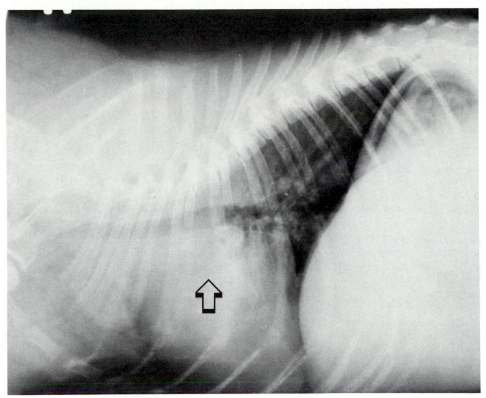

Figure 49–1 Lateral view of canine thorax shows generalized cardiomegaly (particularly in the vertical dimension) with increased density over the cranial half of the heart (*arrow*).

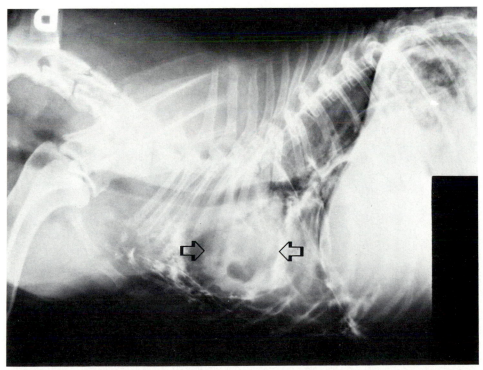

Figure 49–2 Lateral pleurogram of Figure 49-1 shows a large mass superimposed on the cranial half of the heart (*arrows*). Diagnosis: heart base tumor (chemodectoma).

50

TRAUMATIC PNEUMOPERICARDIUM

General Considerations

Little has been written about traumatic pneumopericardium in animals. In human beings traumatic pneumopericardium is usually associated with blunt chest trauma, and often with pneumothorax. The origin of pericardial air is conjectural, as is its effect. I have encountered this condition twice in dogs that were hit by cars. In neither case was there a pneumothorax or pneumomediastinum, although there were pulmonary contusions. Electrocardiography suggested myocardial injury in one dog and was normal in the other. Both animals recovered, with the pericardial air lasting about 3 days.

Major Radiographic Observations

Survey radiographs show air surrounding the heart, particularly its base (Fig. 50–1). This gives the heart base a distinctive lobular appearance as the air dissects around the atria and their appendages.

Diagnostic Strategy

If uncertainty exists about the presence of pericardial air, make a postural radiograph with the dog in the standing position, using a horizontal x-ray beam. This allows any pericardial air to rise to the heart base where it may be more easily identified as it outlines the atria.

Pitfalls

Concomitant pneumothorax or pneumomediastinum may mimic or obscure pericardial air.

Alternative Diagnoses

See "Pitfalls" above.

Suggested Reading

Suter PF. Cardiac diseases. In: Thoracic radiography. Davis, CA: Stonegate Publishing, 1984:148.

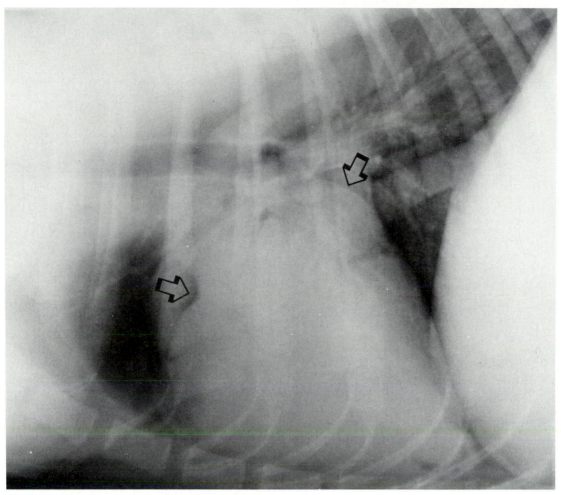

Figure 50-1   Lateral view of canine thorax shows intrapericardial air dissecting around the atria and base of the great vessels (*arrows*). Diagnosis: traumatic pneumopericardium.

II
The Abdomen

ABDOMINAL WALL

51

LATERAL ABDOMINAL HERNIA PRODUCING INTESTINAL HERNIATION

General Considerations

This combination of injuries typically results from trauma. In cats, they are often produced by dog bites, sometimes without any evidence of external injury other than localized swelling. Contained bowel is often not palpable or is of questionable nature. Pain is variable, as are constitutional signs. Signs of peritonitis may not develop for 24 hours or more.

Major Radiographic Observations

Survey radiographs may show a focal or regional convexity in the margin of the abdominal wall, as seen in ventrodorsal projection (Fig. 51–1). Contained intestine may or may not have sufficient air for identification. If surrounding soft-tissue inflammation of infection is present, underlying gas may be obscured. Fluid-filled loops usually blend imperceptibly into adjacent soft-tissue shadows and therefore cannot be recognized as individual structures.

Diagnostic Strategy

The examination should begin with standard abdominal films to evaluate the entire abdomen. If the area of suspected hernia is equivocal, make an additional ventrodorsal view centered on the lesion. When a perforated intestinal content is suspected, an iodine contrast study should be performed.

Films should be made at 20-minute intervals until the question is resolved.

Pitfalls

Intestinal atony (paralytic ileus) sometimes results from peritonitis. In such cases, the contrast may pass very slowly or remain in the stomach. This functional disturbance may be mistaken for mechanical obstruction.

Alternative Diagnoses

Torn abdominal wall (without visceral herniation), hematoma, abscessation, lipoma.

Suggested Reading

Barber DL, Mahaffey MB. The peritoneal space. In: Thrall DE, ed. Textbook of veterinary diagnostic radiology. Philadelphia: WB Saunders, 1986:390.

O'Brien TR. Normal radiographic anatomy of the abdomen. In: O'Brien TR, ed. Radiographic diagnosis of abdominal disorders in the dog and the cat. Philadelphia: WB Saunders, 1978:24.

Olsson S-E, ed. The radiological diagnosis in canine and feline emergencies. Philadelphia: Lea & Febiger, 1973:148.

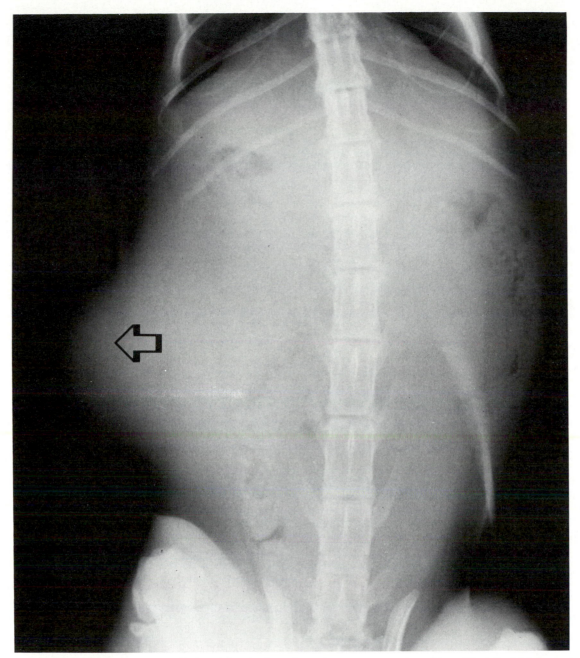

Figure 51–1 Ventrodorsal view of feline abdomen shows large, homogeneous outpouching of the left midabdominal wall (*arrow*) and poor visceral detail. Diagnosis: lateral abdominal-wall hernia with intestinal prolapse (the herniated intestine cannot be identified since it contains fluid and therefore is radiographically indistinguishable from the surrounding tissues), intestinal perforation, and secondary peritonitis.

52

INGUINAL HERNIA PRODUCING INTESTINAL HERNIATION

General Considerations

Inguinal hernias involving bowel most frequently result from car accidents. Some are not associated with trauma and are termed *spontaneous*. Most are readily identifiable on physical examination, although it is not always obvious that they contain intestine. Early recognition of herniated bowel is important in the event that there is incarceration or torsion. Occasionally, herniated loops are severely contused or otherwise partially or wholly devitalized. This may in turn result in subsequent leakage and the development of a regional infection or abscess. The development of a partial or complete obstruction is dependent on both the size of the inguinal opening and the configuration of the contained intestine. Some animals exhibit extreme pain; others show little discomfort. Generally, the more pain, the more serious the injury.

Major Radiographic Observations

Survey radiographs typically show a soft-tissue mass ventral to, or partially superimposed on, the caudoventral aspect of the abdominal wall. Contained bowel is best identified by its gas content (Fig. 52–1). A *barium contrast* study may show opacified intestine within the hernia, depending on the amount of barium given, the timing of the radiograph(s), and the presence of any intestinal obstruction.

Diagnostic Strategy

Initially make standard projections of the abdomen to evaluate the hernia and the remaining abdomen, including the spine and pelvis. When there is a question about hernia content, make both lateral and ventrodorsal views centered on the hernia. If uncertainty persists regarding bowel involvement, give one-third the normal dose of barium and make films at 20-minute intervals until diagnosis is confirmed or denied. If intestinal trauma is suspected, use an iodinated contrast medium instead of barium.

Pitfalls

Administering barium, and making one or more randomly timed films, does not constitute a legitimate radiographic rule-out.

Alternative Diagnoses

Inguinal hernia with herniation of the urinary bladder or the uterus, (Fig. 52–2) regional inguinal contusion, hematoma, cellulitis or abscessation, peri-inguinal tumor.

Suggested Reading

Barber DL, Mahaffey MB. The peritoneal space. In: Thrall DE, ed. Textbook of veterinary diagnostic radiology. Philadelphia: WB Saunders, 1986:389.

Feeney DA, Johnston GR. The ovaries and testes. In: Thrall DE, ed. Textbook of veterinary diagnostic radiology. Philadelphia: WB Saunders, 1986:471.

Feeney DA, Johnston GR. The uterus. In: Thrall DE, ed. Textbook of veterinary diagnostic radiology. Philadelphia: WB Saunders, 1986:463.

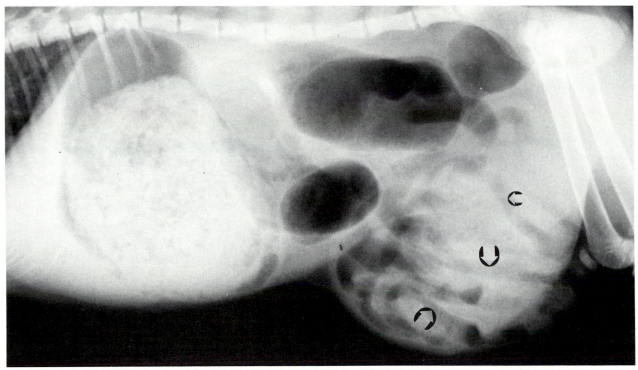

Figure 52–1 Lateral view of feline abdomen shows a large soft-tissue mass projecting from the caudoventral abdomen; the mass contains multiple cylindrical gas shadows (*arrows*). Diagnosis: inguinal hernia with intestinal prolapse.

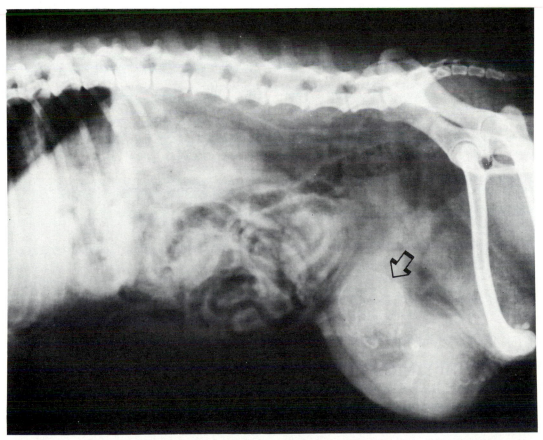

Figure 52–2 Lateral view of canine abdomen shows large mass or mass effect caudoventrally containing a mineralized fetus, which appears dead based on overlapping cranial bones (*arrow*). Diagnosis: inguinal hernia with uterine prolapse and late-term fetal death.

53

BITE WOUND PRODUCING PERITONITIS

General Considerations

Abdominal bite wounds often penetrate the peritoneal cavity, producing peritonitis and, occasionally, intestinal puncture. Frequently, there are no clinical signs referable to peritonitis, or such signs are masked by shock associated with the attack. There is often poor correlation between the location of surface wounds and underlying punctures in the abdominal wall. This is because of the highly mobile nature of dog and cat skin and the tearing nature of the injury. Accordingly, probing is often inaccurate and cannot be relied upon to rule out peritoneal involvement consistently.

Major Radiographic Observations

Survey radiographs vary according to whether or not peritonitis has had sufficient time to become radiographically apparent. If peritonitis is well underway, the associated signs are typical: increased abdominal density, decreased visceral clarity, and, in advanced cases, increased abdominal girth, secondary to peritoneal fluid accumulation. In less advanced cases, there may only be a slight increase in overall abdominal density, often a mottled nature (Fig. 53–1). Early or delayed peritonitis may show nothing. In such instances, inferential findings such as localized deep cutaneous gas, loss of deep fascial planes, or disruption of the associated abdominal musculature suggest the possibility of peritoneal penetration.

Diagnostic Strategy

The radiographic findings of peritonitis require no adjustments in technique. However, the less obvious changes of deep fascial and abdominal-wall trauma are best shown by reducing the normal abdominal exposure by half and centering on the surface lesions, in the ventrodorsal position.

Pitfalls

Puppies and kittens normally lack the abdominal contrast of adult dogs and cats because of a relatively smaller amount of intra-abdominal fat. Thin animals and animals that have lost weight because of illness also lack visceral detail for the same reason.

Alternative Diagnoses

Peritonitis secondary to pancreatitis; ruptured stomach, intestine, gallbladder, ureter, urinary bladder, proximal urethra, uterus, or prostate. See "Pitfalls" above.

Suggested Reading

Barber DL, Mahaffey MB. The peritoneal space. In: Thrall DE, ed. Textbook of veterinary diagnostic radiology. Philadelphia: WB Saunders, 1986:380.

Mathews KA. Septic peritonitis. In: Binnington AG, Cockshutt JR, eds. Decision making in small animal soft tissue surgery. Toronto: BC Decker, 1988:210

O'Brien TR. Density and structure in interpreting radiographs. In: O'Brien TR, ed. Radiographic diagnosis of abdominal disorders in the dog and the cat. Philadelphia: WB Saunders, 1978:62.

Olsson S-E, ed. The radiological diagnosis in canine and feline emergencies. Philadelphia: Lea & Febiger, 1973:121, 123, 128.

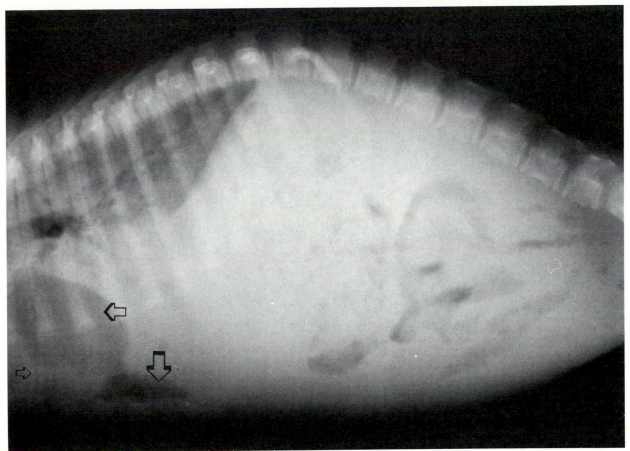

Figure 53–1   Lateral view of canine abdomen (puppy) shows abdominal distention and decreased visceral detail, pleural fluid (*small arrow*), partially collapsed lung lobe (*medium arrow*), and a cranioventral gas pocket (*large arrow*). Diagnosis: peritonitis and pyothorax secondary to multiple abdominal and thoracic bite wounds.

PERITONEAL CAVITY

54

RUPTURED GALLBLADDER AND BILE DUCT PRODUCING PERITONITIS

General Considerations

Rupture of the gallbladder or common bile duct typically results from trauma and is particularly insidious because it often requires as much as a week to become clinically evident (or at least distinguishable from other injuries sustained at the time of the original accident). Added to the diagnostic difficulty is the nonspecificity of the early clinical signs: vomiting, anorexia, and abdominal pain. However, with time a generalized peritonitis develops, usually with sufficient intra-abdominal bile to be recovered on abdominocentesis. Unfortunately, the patient's condition is usually very poor by this point, making recovery difficult.

Major Radiographic Observations

Survey radiographs often appear normal initially, but later films typically reveal the classic signs of peritonitis: increased abdominal density and decreased visceral detail (Fig. 54–1). Sonographically, the repeated absence of a gallbladder in the context of abdominal fluid suggests rupture.

Diagnostic Strategy

Make standard abdominal radiographs (lateral and ventrodorsal views) centered over the liver. Be certain to set the radiographic technique according to the measurement of the cranial abdomen, otherwise the region of interest will be underpenetrated. Localized liver hemorrhage suggests the possibility of injury to contiguous organs such as the gallbladder. If it is available, ultrasound should be used to locate the gallbladder. If this attempt is unsuccessful, repeat the ultrasound examination later to be certain that the bladder was not simply empty at the time of the initial study (as opposed to being ruptured).

Pitfalls

Many ruptured gallbladder-bile-duct injuries are initially associated with a normal radiographic examination.

Alternative Diagnoses

Traumatic pancreatitis, ruptured urinary-tract component, and other sources of peritonitis.

Suggested Reading

Mathews KA. Biliary tract trauma. In: Binnington AG, Cockshutt JR, eds. Decision making in small animal soft tissue surgery. Toronto: BC Decker, 1988:56.

Olsson S-E, ed. The radiological diagnosis in canine and feline emergencies. Philadelphia: Lea & Febiger, 1973:153.

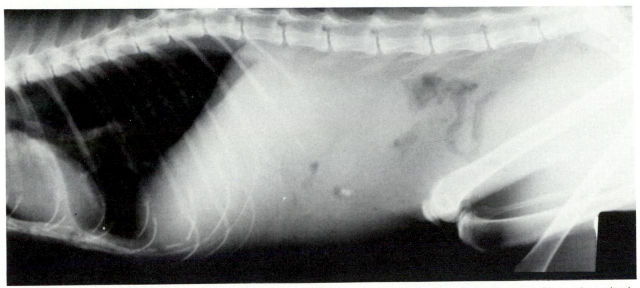

Figure 54–1 Lateral view of feline abdomen shows increased density, poor visceral detail, and mild distention. Diagnosis: peritonitis secondary to ruptured gallbladder (sustained in a three-storey fall 6 days earlier).

55

ABDOMINAL GUNSHOT WOUND

General Considerations

The extent of an abdominal gunshot injury, based on the entrance or exit wounds, is very difficult to determine. The damage to involved organs is a function of multiple factors, including the speed, size and composition of the missile, as well as the density of the encountered tissues or organs. The apparent well-being of the patient at the time of examination does not rule out internal injury, nor does negative abdominal palpation. Alternatively, organ-specific clinical signs may be masked by pain and shock. Diagnostic peritoneal lavage or abdominocentesis is often equivocal or negative. Even exploratory surgery, unless scrupulously thorough, may miss small intestinal punctures.

Major Radiographic Observations

Survey films show the missile (bullet, air gun, or shotgun pellet) at its point of deepest penetration. Fragments may indicate the missile's abdominal pathway and, therefore, the organs that have been potentially injured. When both entry and exit wounds are found, a missile is not, although fragments may be present. If advanced peritonitis exists, there is an overall increase in abdominal density accompanied by a reduction in organ detail (Fig. 55–1). If gastrointestinal perforation is present, circumstantial evidence in the form of free abdominal air may be seen. Hemorrhage resembles peritonitis.

Diagnostic Strategy

Two views are needed to determine accurately the position of the missile. The entire abdomen and associated skele-tal structures should be included, since there are often injuries distant from the missile. Postural radiography (standing and lateral positions, using a horizontal x-ray beam) may be necessary to identify free abdominal air or blood. If follow-up films are required, the same radiographic technique must be used, to allow an accurate comparison.

Pitfalls

High-velocity bullets may pass through the abdomen, leaving no trace.

Alternative Diagnoses

Peritonitis from other causes; a bullet is an *incidental* radiographic finding.

Suggested Reading

Barber DL, Mahaffey MB. The peritoneal space. In: Thrall DE, ed. Textbook of veterinary diagnostic radiology. Philadelphia: WB Saunders, 1986:389.

O'Brien TR. Density and structure in interpreting radiographs. In: O'Brien TR, ed. Radiographic diagnosis of the abdominal disorders in the dog and the cat. Philadelphia: WB Saunders, 1978:73.

Seim HB III. Intestinal perforation. In: Binnington AG, Cockshutt JR, eds. Decision making in small animal soft tissue surgery. Toronto: BC Decker, 1988:32.

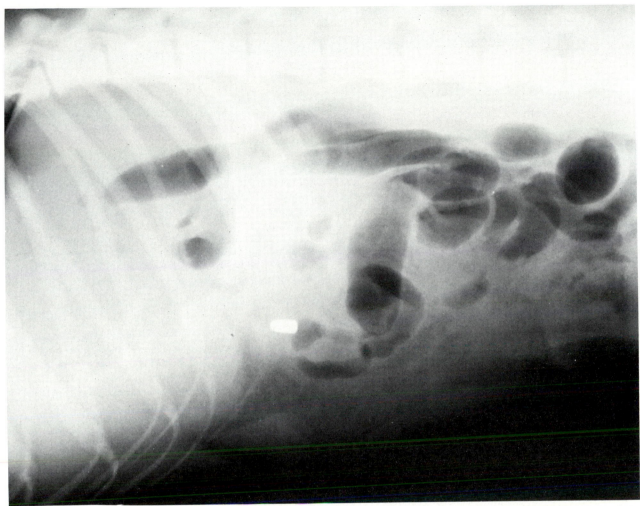

Figure 55–1 Lateral view of canine thorax shows bullet, increased abdominal density and decreased detail, and gas-distended bowel. Diagnosis: abdominal gunshot wound with intestinal perforation causing hemorrhage, functional ileus, and peritonitis.

56

SPONTANEOUS PNEUMOPERITONEUM

General Considerations

The term *spontaneous* is often used as a synonym for unknown cause; therefore, the term *spontaneous pneumoperitoneum* means free abdominal air of unknown origin. Free abdominal air is either of extrinsic or intrinsic origin. Large, penetrating abdominal wounds are the most common cause of extrinsic air; perforation of the abdominal esophagus or stomach are the leading causes of intrinsic gas. Esophageal perforation is most often iatrogenic, secondary to attempted intubation of the stomach. Gastric rupture may occur after dilation or torsion. Less commonly, perforation follows ulceration. Intestinal rupture typically produces little or no detectable peritoneal gas. Once pneumoperitoneum is detected, the primary task becomes the identification of its origin. By inference, the clinical significance of pneumoperitoneum (with an intact abdominal wall) is that the stomach or abdominal esophagus are perforated and leaking their contents into the abdominal cavity—a situation that rapidly produces peritonitis.

Major Radiographic Observations

Survey radiographs show greatly improved organ margins. Normally invisible structures, such as the diaphragm, cranial liver margins, and the inner surface of the abdominal wall, are visible (Fig. 56–1). *Contrast* studies may show leakage, depending on the size and site of the perforation.

Diagnostic Strategy

If pneumoperitoneum is clinically or radiographically suspected, reduce the measured kilovolt peak by 10 percent to improve the chances of detecting free abdominal air. If uncertainty continues after making standard views, make postural views (standing lateral patient position using a horizontal x-ray beam, or left lateral recumbent patient position using a horizontal x-ray beam). Again, reduce radiographic technique by at least 10 percent. If contrast studies are performed, iodinated contrast media should be used instead of barium, because the latter is harmful to the peritoneum. The examination should be conducted according to the suspected location of the lesion and the time required for the contrast to reach this point (patient-tailored examination). For example, if the lesion is suspected in the stomach, then the majority of films should be made in the first 10 minutes following contrast administration.

Pitfalls

An air-distended stomach may mimic pneumoperioneum. Abdominal surgical drains may allow retrograde air flow, producing pneumoperitoneum. Varying amounts of air remain in the abdomen following abdominal surgery. These gas accumulations may persist for a week or longer and can be difficult to separate from visceral leakage, especially if gastrointestinal surgery has been performed.

Alternative Diagnoses

See "Pitfalls" above.

Suggested Reading

Olsson S-E, ed. The radiological diagnosis in canine and feline emergencies. Philadelphia: Lea & Febiger, 1973:75, 121.

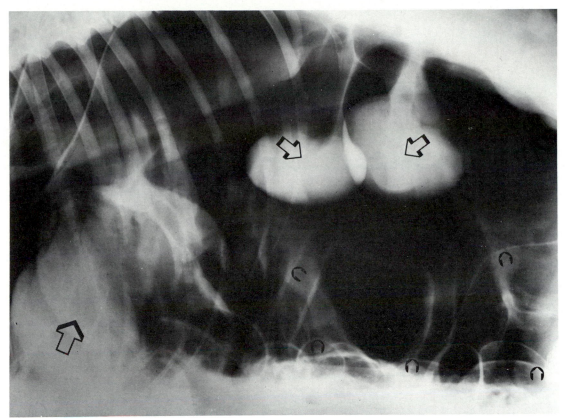

Figure 56-1 Lateral view of canine central abdomen shows a large accumulation of free air that outlines the liver (*large arrow*), kidneys (*medium arrows*), and intestine (*small arrows*). Diagnosis: pneumoperitoneum secondary to perforation of the abdominal esophagus.

57

PERITONEAL FOREIGN BODY SECONDARY TO GASTROESOPHAGEAL PERFORATION

General Considerations

Occasionally, pets swallow unbelievably large objects. In my opinion, this possibility should not be discounted, especially if the owner has seen the dog with a missing object in its mouth, or otherwise believes it has been swallowed. Because most of these large objects provide some radiographic evidence of their presence, a radiographic examination is the most rapid and effective means of assessment. Clinical signs vary from pronounced (in the case of pharyngeal or esophageal foreign bodies), to relatively mild or nonexistent (with intestinal objects). Some foreign bodies penetrate the esophagus or gastrointestinal tract and present as peritonitis. Others become embedded in paraintestinal organs, often producing organ-specific signs. Some penetrate the gut without causing peritonitis and are encapsulated in the omentum, mesentery, or peritoneal cavity. However, most such outsized foreign bodies require surgical removal.

Major Radiographic Observations

Metallic, mineral, or bony foreign bodies show readily on survey radiograph (Fig. 57–1). Lightweight foil, wood, fabric, paper, and plastic do not, but these may be associated with trapped or backed-up air or fluid that serves as indirect evidence of a foreign body. Contrast examination typically reveals a large filling defect, often accompanied by delayed or nontranset, depending on the size, shape, composition, and location of the object.

Diagnostic Strategy

High-density foreign bodies pose no diagnostic difficulty. Medium- or low-opacity objects may be hard to detect, especially in the intestine. In the latter case, a gastrointestinal contrast examination should be performed using barium, or an iodinated contrast agent if perforation is suspected. If the foreign body is thought to be esophageal, a barium swallow is advisable. A double-contrast gastrogram (a small amount of barium or Gastrografin, followed by a medium to large volume of air) is optimal when a gastric foreign body is sought.

Pitfalls

When coughing or gagging are not present, esophageal foreign bodies may be overlooked. Subcutaneous or intramuscular foreign bodies superimposed on the peritoneal cavity may mimic intraperitoneal foreign bodies.

Alternative Diagnoses

See "Pitfalls" above.

Suggested Reading

McNeel SV. Gastrointestinal perforation. In: Farrow CS, ed. Decision making in small animal radiology. Toronto: BC Decker, 1987:172.
O'Brien TR. Density and structure in interpreting radiography. In O'Brien TR, ed. Radiographic diagnosis of abdominal disorders in the dog and cat. Philadelphia: WB Saunders, 1978:62.

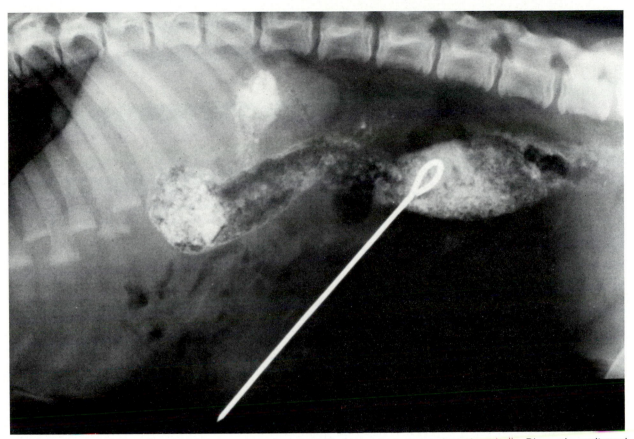

Figure 57–1 Lateral view of canine abdomen shows large metallic foreign body (meat skewer) centrally. Diagnosis: peritoneal foreign body (at surgery the eye of the skewer was within the duodenum; the point was embedded in a fibrous mass on the right abdominal floor).

58

FOREIGN BODY GRANULOMA INDUCED
BY SURGICAL SPONGE

General Considerations

A surgical sponge, inadvertently left in the abdomen following laparotomy, may produce acute, subacute, or chronic effects. Early signs are associated with a foreign-body reaction and may remain localized to the sponge. With time, the condition may progress to a sterile peritonitis. Later, with or without an intervening peritonitis, a granuloma may form around the sponge. Associated clinical signs, if any, are variable.

Major Radiographic Observations

Early on, a so-called *textile pattern* (mottled, localized density) may be seen. Once a granuloma has formed (weeks to months later), lesion visibility may be improved, depending on its size and location (Fig. 58–1). Early peritonitis may be undetectable or may appear as a subtle increase in abdominal density with a corresponding loss in organ detail. These findings are usually localized or at most regional. If unchecked, peritonitis eventually results in a generalized increase in abdominal density and loss of visceral detail.

Diagnostic Strategy

Sponge granulomas are usually found in the caudal half of the abdomen. Most are round and are about the size of a kidney. They are sometimes mistaken for the urinary bladder or for overlapping bowel loops. When uncertainty exists, compression radiography often can isolate a questionable shadow to the extent it can be identified.

Alternative Diagnoses

Uterine-stump granuloma, paraprostatic cyst, displaced urinary bladder, unilateral uterine enlargement.

Suggested Reading

Olsson S-E, ed. The radiological diagnosis in canine and feline emergencies. Philadelphia: Lea & Febiger, 1973:208.

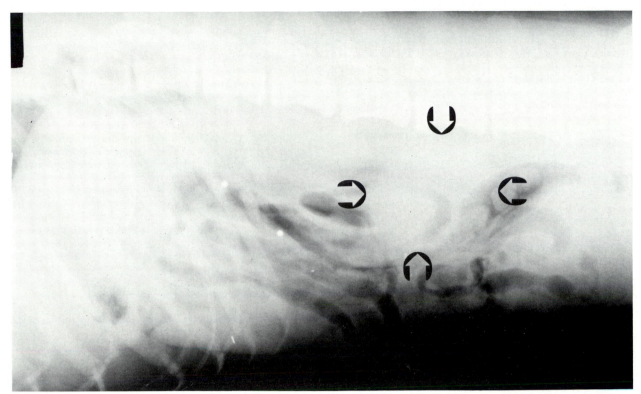

Figure 58–1   Lateral view of canine abdomen shows circular midabdominal mass (*arrows*). Diagnosis: foreign-body (surgical-sponge) granuloma.

59

FELINE INFECTIOUS PERITONITIS LEADING TO INTUSSUSCEPTION

General Considerations

Currently, feline infectious peritonitis (FIP) is believed to be caused by an opportunistic virus that infects immuno-deficient cats. Although both thorax and abdomen may be affected, the most typical presentation is that of a cat with abdominal fluid and frequently organomegaly. The intestine may also be involved, often seen as a midabdominal mass, secondary to multiple adhesions. Sometimes intussusception occurs. Much or all of this pathology may be obscured by fluid. Abdominocentesis is usually diagnostic.

Major Radiographic Observations

When medium or large volumes of fluid are present, there is a generalized increase in abdominal density, with a decrease or loss in abdominal detail. The abdomen is often distended. With less fluid, other patterns may emerge, such as regional organomegaly (liver, spleen, and kidneys) or a central bunching of the bowel, made evident by a relative increase in density and peripheralization of surrounding air-filled intestine (Fig. 59–1). The so-called *dry form* of FIP leaves little radiographic evidence, in my experience.

Diagnostic Strategy

Standard abdominal films are adequate. When fluid is present, withdraw it for laboratory assessment. When film results are equivocal, remake and reassess radiographs for organ enlargement and an abnormal bowel-distribution pattern.

Pitfalls

Most intussusceptions cannot be directly identified on a radiograph.

Alternative Diagnoses

Lymphoma, right heart failure, hemorrhage, ruptured bladder.

Suggested Reading

O'Brien TR. Density and structure in interpreting radiographs. In: O'Brien TR, ed. Radiographic diagnosis of abdominal disorders in the dog and the cat. Philadelphia: WB Saunders, 1978:106.

Seim HB III. Intussusception. In: Binnington AG, Cockshutt JR, eds. Decision making in small animal soft tissue surgery. Toronto: BC Decker, 1988:28.

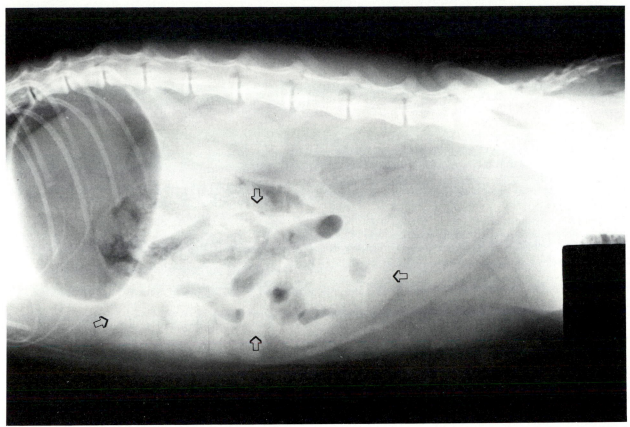

Figure 59–1 Lateral view of feline abdomen shows clustered small-bowel loops in the midventral abdomen (*arrows*) associated with an interrupted intestinal gas pattern and a small volume of pleural fluid. Diagnosis: feline infectious peritonitis with intussusception.

60

DISSEMINATED PERITONEAL FIBROSARCOMA

General Considerations

The suffix, -matosis, may be added to those malignancies that originate and spread within the abdomen, particularly along the peritoneal surface. Although carcinomatosis has been described most frequently, sarcomas may also disseminate in this fashion. Involvement of the liver, and especially the peritoneum, often results in fluid formation. Splenic involvement may produce hemorrhage, which is sometimes fatal. Clinical signs, when present, usually reflect the organs involved, unless there is a large hemorrhage, in which case shock predominates. The latter case is the typical emergency presentation.

Major Radiographic Observations

Unfortunately, survey radiographs are highly variable. Possible observations include single or multiple organ enlargement, fluid, or a slight increase in abdominal density (Fig. 60–1). When organ enlargement is minimal or obscured, or when peritoneal metastases are small, the radiographic appearance may be normal.

Diagnostic Strategy

Survey radiographs should be searched for the findings described. If fluid is present, it should be sampled and re-moved as indicated. Additional abdominal films may then be made, in an attempt to identify previously hidden organs.

Pitfalls

Lack of a grid in larger dogs may result in abdominal indistinctness resembling peritoneal disease.

Alternative Diagnoses

Peritonitis, abdominal hemorrhage, ascites, feline infectious peritonitis, steatitis.

Suggested Reading

McNeel SV. Abdominal metastasis. In: Farrow CS, ed. Decision making in small animal radiology. Toronto: BC Decker, 1987:180.
O'Brien TR. Density and structure in interpreting radiographs. In: O'Brien TR, ed. Radiographic diagnosis of abdominal disorders in the dog and the cat. Philadelphia: WB Saunders, 1978:62.

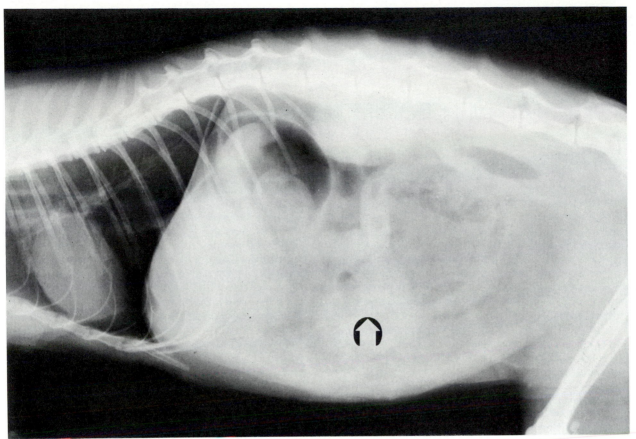

Figure 60–1 Lateral view of feline abdomen shows increased abdominal volume and density, decreased visceral detail, and at least one mass (*arrow*); free air around kidneys and diaphragm is from a previous abdominal drain. Diagnosis: disseminated peritoneal fibrosarcomatosis with fluid.

THE STOMACH

61

GASTRIC FOREIGN BODIES

General Considerations

A great variety of objects are eaten by dogs. The cat appears somewhat more discriminating but is prone to playing with and often eating string. Although a majority of these objects pass harmlessly through the gastrointestinal tract, some do not; these usually lodge in the stomach and small intestine. In the case of linear foreign bodies, both the stomach and small bowel may be jointly involved. Vomiting is the most common clinical sign, sometimes with the dog appearing otherwise normal. With time, the animal becomes weak from fluid and electrolyte loss, exacerbated by an inability to retain food. Occasionally, vomiting is intermittent, suggesting that the foreign body is having a ball-valve effect on the pylorus. The fact that an object is sharp does not necessarily mean it will engage the rugae and become entrapped. Most bone fragments pass without delay; some fishing lures do so as well. Flat, smooth objects such as stones and larger coins often encounter difficulty in passage, even when supported by a high-bulk meal. Large-volume foreign bodies, such as carpeting, fabrics, or newspaper, are difficult to differentiate from food in both survey and contrast examinations.

Major Radiographic Observations

Survey films may reveal a foreign body, often accompanied by enlargement of the stomach, especially if the animal has not vomited recently (Figs. 61–1 and 61–3). *Contrast* studies are more likely to show a filling defect, because most swallowed objects are relatively less dense than opaque contrast media (Fig. 61–2).

Diagnostic Strategy

At least two films should be made, centered on the stomach, using an appropriate radiographic technique (measure at the eleventh intercostal space). The left lateral view allows air into the pylorus, potentially enhancing small- to medium-sized foreign bodies in this location. Larger foreign bodies, which require more space and are therefore more apt to be located in the body-fundus, are best detected in the right lateral projection. Ventrodorsal or dorsoventral views are most useful in cats and small- to medium-sized dogs. If nothing is seen on plane films, a contrast examination is indicated, usually with barium. Generally, the smaller the volume of contrast, the less likely the dog is to vomit; therefore, one-half the normal dose is recommended, given by a small-caliber feeding tube. Films should be made immediately and on a patient-tailored basis thereafter, until the diagnosis is confirmed or denied. Air is an effective contrast medium, especially in demonstrating low-density foreign bodies; however, it is often passed into the intestine before radiographs can be made. If the stomach contains a large volume of fluid, the fluid should be removed before beginning a contrast study. When large amounts of air or fluid are present, a postural radiograph should be made, using a horizontal x-ray beam with the dog in a standing position. This technique is especially effective in demonstrating large masses such as carpeting as it extends above the fluid line.

Pitfalls

Barium, when given in large volume and high concentration, often hides a foreign body. Most foreign bodies, including fabrics, do not absorb sufficient contrast medium to improve their radiographic detectability.

Alternative Diagnoses

Gastritis, pancreatitis, gastric tumor.

Suggested Reading

Barber DL, Mahaffey MB. The peritoneal space. In: Thrall DE, ed. Textbook of veterinary diagnostic radiology. Philadelphia: WB Saunders, 1986:481.

McNeel SV. Gastric foreign object. In: Farrow, CS, ed. Decision making in small animal radiology. Toronto: BC Decker, 1987:160

O'Brien TR. Stomach. In: O'Brien TR, ed. Radiographic diagnosis of abdominal disorders in the dog and the cat. Philadelphia: WB Saunders, 1978:216.

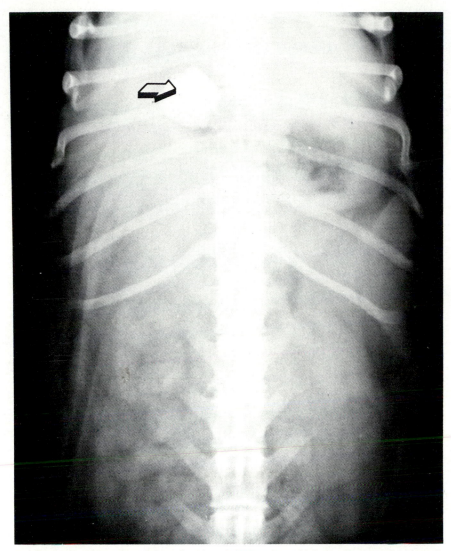

Figure 61–1 Ventrodorsal view of canine abdomen shows high-density object in stomach (*arrow*). Diagnosis: gastric foreign body (rock).

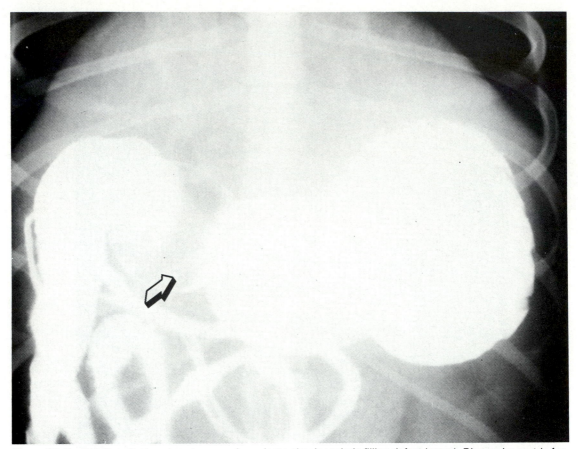

Figure 61–2   Detail ventrodorsal gastrogram shows large circular pyloric filling defect (*arrow*). Diagnosis: gastric foreign body (rubber ball).

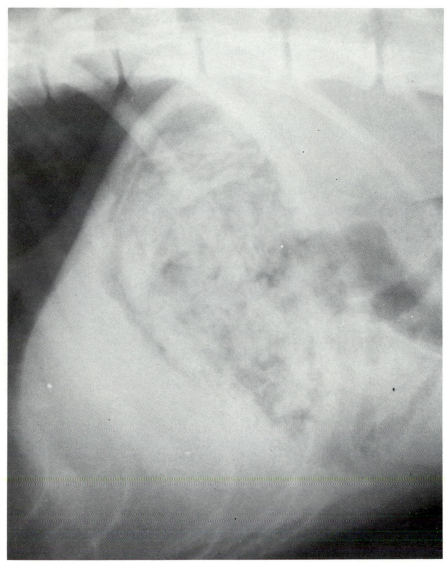

Figure 61–3 Detail lateral view of canine stomach shows mixed luminal densities, which appear linear dorsally and nonstructured ventrally. Diagnosis: gastric foreign body (fresh newspaper—sports page).

62

GASTROINTESTINAL FOREIGN BODY

General Considerations

Combined gastrointestinal foreign bodies are typically linear in shape and are often composed of two parts, one of which is frequently fixed in the stomach. Because of this anchorage, the proximal small intestine "climbs" the contained object, resulting in a distinctive serpentine or bunched appearance. For the same reason, the small intestine may be penetrated by the foreign body, resulting in peritonitis. Vomiting and colic are usual presenting signs; sudden worsening often accompanies the development of peritonitis. Massed bowel loops are often palpable.

Major Radiographic Observations

An abnormal bowel distribution pattern (small intestine coiled or bunched in the right cranial abdomen) is often accompanied by an interrupted gas pattern. The latter radiographic feature may allow for plane-film recognition; the former usually requires contrast examination (Figs. 62–1 and 62–2).

Diagnostic Strategy

Most linear foreign bodies are radiographically invisible; accordingly, they must be inferred from circumstantial evidence, e.g., an abnormal bowel distribution pattern. Therefore, it is best to accumulate as much radiographic information as is reasonable under the given clinical circum-stances. Contrast examinations are best in this regard. As with any condition associated with vomiting, the volume of contrast is best reduced by at least a half. Gastric emptying is usually delayed because of partial pyloric obstruction as well as pyloric irritation and spasm, in some instances for an hour or more. If peritonitis is suspected, then an iodinated contrast medium should be used. Gentle abdominal compression radiography is useful in isolating suspicious bowel segments.

Pitfalls

It is easy to mistake a normal variation (location, configuration, or gas content) of the proximal small bowel for evidence of linear foreign body.

Alternative Diagnoses

Gastritis, obstruction of small intestine, pancreatitis.

Suggested Reading

McNeel SV. The small bowel. In: Thrall DE, ed. Textbook of veterinary diagnostic radiology. Philadelphia: WB Saunders, 1986:504.
O'Brien TR. Small intestine. In: O'Brien TR, ed. Radiographic diagnosis of abdominal disorders in the dog and the cat. Philadelphia: WB Saunders, 1978:300.

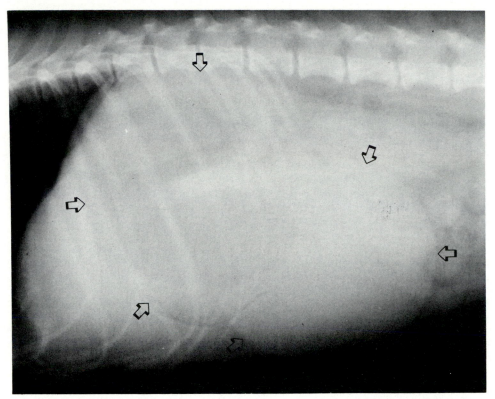

Figure 62–1 Lateral view of canine abdomen shows large, dilated, and predominantly fluid-filled stomach (*arrows*).

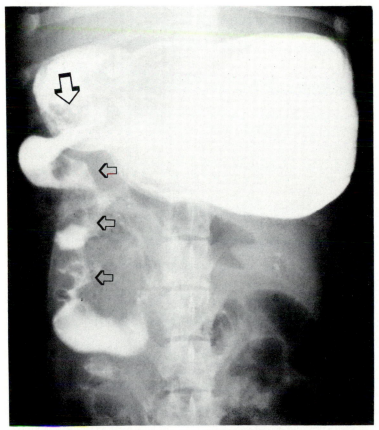

Figure 62–2 Ventrodorsal gastrogram of Figure 62–1 shows nonstructured filling defects in pyloric part of stomach (*large arrow*) and bunching of duodenum (*small arrows*). Diagnosis: gastrointestinal foreign body (ball of cassette tape within stomach passing into proximal small intestine).

63

GASTRIC DILATATION

General Considerations

Severe gastric dilatation may be clinically indistinguishable from gastric torsion, although typically the signs of torsion are more severe. A majority of torsions are probably preceded by dilatations, with the specific cause(s) remaining conjectural. Intubation does not consistently separate the two, because both may allow or prohibit the passage of a stomach tube, depending on the type and size of tube, the relative positions of the esophagus and stomach, and the experience of the operator. Other conditions, although relatively less common, may mimic gastric dilatation or torsion, specifically those that result in abdominal distention and affect the cardiovascular system. Conventional wisdom dictates that animals suspected of having these disorders first be given emergency medical or surgical treatment, and then be radiographed. However, given the speed and simplicity of radiographic examination, I believe this recommended priority to be questionable.

Major Radiographic Observations

Survey films typically show a large, relatively noncompartmentalized stomach, often containing excessive air. Fluid and food are usually present in lesser amounts (Figs. 63–1 and 63–2). *Contrast* studies are generally uninformative or confusing, especially for the inexperienced.

Diagnostic Strategy

A single postural radiograph, made with the dog in the standing position and using a horizontal x-ray beam, is the quickest and least stressful means of making the diagnosis. If the dog is not able to stand, a right lateral recumbent view is best. Ventrodorsal or dorsoventral projections are often difficult to make in larger dogs, and once obtained, they are hard to read. Thus, they are best omitted or used on a selected basis.

Pitfalls

A dilated, fluid-filled stomach may mimic a large cranial abdominal mass.

Alternative Diagnoses

Gastric torsion, normal food- or fluid-distended stomach.

Suggested Reading

Barber DL, Mahaffey MB. The peritoneal space. In: Thrall DE, ed. Textbook of veterinary diagnostic radiology. Philadelphia: WB Saunders, 1986:483.

McNeel SV. Gastric dilatation or volvulus? In: Farrow CS, ed. Decision making in small animal radiology. Toronto: BC Decker 1987:162.

O'Brien TR. Stomach. In: O'Brien TR, ed. Radiographic diagnosis of abdominal disorders in the dog and the cat. Philadelphia: WB Saunders, 1978:231.

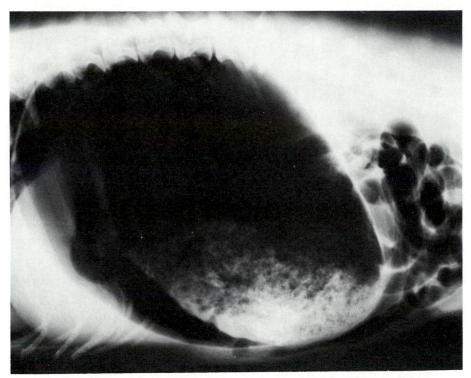

Figure 63–1 Lateral view of canine abdomen shows an air-distended, partially food-filled stomach.

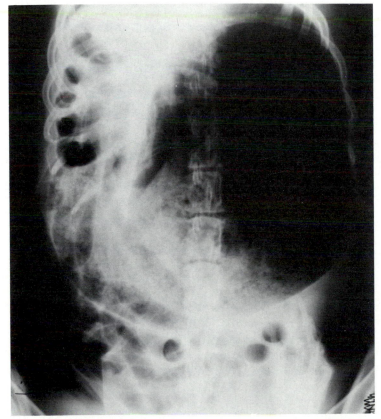

Figure 63–2 Dorsoventral view of Figure 63–1 shows an enlarged but normally positioned stomach. Diagnosis: gastric dilatation without torsion.

64

GASTRIC TORSION: VOLVULUS

General Considerations

Gastric torsion usually follows acute dilatation and results in varying degrees of inlet and outlet obstruction, depending on the degree of stomach displacement. Associated clinical signs, such as attempted vomiting, abdominal distention, and shock, develop rapidly, reflecting the ischemic as well as the obstructive nature of this disorder. Giant breeds are most prone to this often fatal condition. Anatomic predilection, diet, and exercise have all been incriminated in what many currently term the *gastric dilatation volvulus syndrome* (GDVS). Quick, effective surgical and medical treatment is necessary for survival.

Major Radiographic Observations

Standard abdominal radiographs typically show a greatly enlarged stomach filled with food, fluid, and air, usually producing a mottled gray appearance as opposed to distinct air-fluid shadows. Air-fluid levels are only seen in postural radiographs. The pylorus is displaced dorsally and to the left, often accompanied by some degree of splenic dislocation (Fig. 64–1). The stomach often appears divided in two by a horizontally oriented soft-tissue line extending across the central stomach in lateral view; this is referred to as *compartmentalization*. Contrast examinations are often confusing as well as time-consuming. In my experience, they are rarely required.

Diagnostic Strategy

Contrary to most published reports, the radiographic differentiation of gastric torsion from gastric dilatation is often difficult or impossible. This uncertainty probably stems from a combination of factors, including stomach content, patient positioning, radiographic technique, and viewer ability. I have found postural radiography (standing lateral patient position with a horizontal x-ray beam) to be the most diagnostic, as well as the least uncomfortable for the dog. Often it is possible to confirm the clinical diagnosis using only this single view.

Pitfalls

Not all large, fluid-filled stomachs that are radiographically identified in large-breed dogs are associated with obstruction, even though there may be some patient distress. Beware of guilt by association!

Alternative Diagnoses

Normal fluid- or food-distended stomach (potentially an incidental radiographic finding), acute gastric dilatation (without or before torsion).

Suggested Reading

Barber DL, Mahaffey MB. The stomach. In: Thrall DE, ed. Textbook of veterinary diagnostic radiology. Philadelphia: WB Saunders, 1986:483.

McNeel SV. Gastric dilatation or volvulus? In: Farrow CS, ed. Decision making in small animal radiology. Toronto: BC Decker, 1987:162.

O'Brien TR. Stomach. In: O'Brien TR, ed. Radiographic diagnosis of abdominal disorders in the dog and the cat. Philadelphia: WB Saunders, 1978:224.

Orton EC. Gastric dilatation-volvulus. In: Kirk RW, ed. Current veterinary therapy IX. Philadelphia: WB Saunders, 1986:856.

Seim HB III. Gastric dilatation-volvulus. In: Binnington AG, Cockshutt JR, eds. Decision making in small animal soft tissue surgery. Toronto: BC Decker, 1988:24.

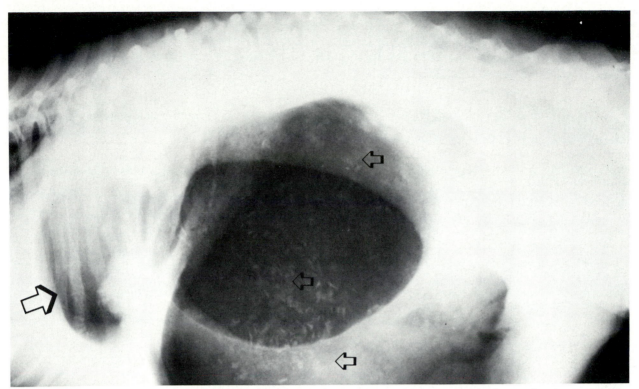

Figure 64–1 Right lateral view of canine stomach shows compartmentalization of the stomach (*small arrows*) and a cranially displaced, air-filled pylorus (*large arrow*). Diagnosis: gastric torsion (volvulus).

65

HEMORRHAGIC GASTROENTERITIS

General Considerations

Hemorrhagic gastritis is an acute disorder of uncertain etiology and is often fatal. Hematemesis and melena are the primary clinical signs, usually accompanied by diarrhea, weakness, and collapse.

Major Radiographic Observations

Plane films are usually not revealing. A gastrogram may show a roughened, spiculated mucosal margin. Rugal folds may be enlarged if intrarugal hemorrhage is great. Barium-coated surfaces may appear smudged because of the mixing of blood and contrast (Fig. 65–1).

Diagnostic Strategy

Use one-half the normal barium dose and administer with a small feeding tube; avoid mechanical irritation of the stomach wall by premeasuring the required tube length against the distance from the mouth to the eleventh inter-

costal space. Center on the stomach and make films (right lateral and ventrodorsal) immediately, and thereafter depending on what was seen in the previous radiographs. (A patient-tailored examination is superior to a standard protocol study as long as you are present to monitor its progress.)

Pitfalls

Some cases of hemorrhagic gastritis are associated with a normal or near-normal gastrogram.

Alternative Diagnoses

Acute corrosive gastritis, bleeding gastric ulcer, or tumor.

Suggested Reading

Carbone JV, Brandborg LL, Silverman S. Alimentary tract and liver. In: Krupp MA, Chatton MJ, eds. Current medical diagnosis and treatment. Los Altos: Lange, 1982:353.

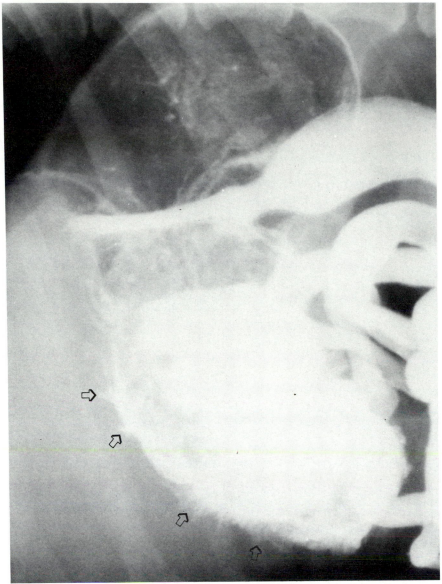

Figure 65–1 Lateral canine gastrogram (detail view) shows roughened, spiculated mucosal margin (*arrows*). Diagnosis: hemorrhagic gastritis.

66

PENETRATING GASTRIC ULCER

General Considerations

Gastric bleeding is typically associated with hematemesis and melena, and may or may not be painful. If major blood loss has occurred, weakness or shock is usually present. Ulceration may result from some infections, poisons, corrosives, and drugs such as aspirin. Hemorrhage may also develop from ulcerated gastric tumors, or secondarily from distant tumors that produce ulcerogenic substances such as histamine or gastrin. Perforation is the most serious complication of gastric ulceration; it leads to intraperitoneal hemorrhage and peritonitis.

Major Radiographic Observations

Plane films usually show nothing specific. A *gastrogram* may reveal contrast leakage at the ulcer site, or delayed emptying if the lesion is within or close to the pylorus (Fig. 66–1).

Diagnostic Strategy

Expect little confirmatory information from abdominal survey radiographs. Large or prominent rugal folds are not diagnostic and are often incidental. Air content is more a function of distress than of disease. Increased fluid volume may suggest obstruction; usually in the pyloric region this is secondary to inflammatory swelling of ulcerated tissue. Because perforation is suspected, an iodinated medium (Gastrografin) is recommended if a contrast examination is performed. Barium leads to granulomatous peritonitis if leaked to the abdominal cavity, and is difficult to remove surgically. If contrast leakage secondary to perforation is present, it would be most evident during the first few minutes of the study when it was in the greatest concentration and closest to the site of leakage. The lesion is best demonstrated when the film is centered over the stomach, in contrast to a standard abdominal field. Four views are optimal: right and left lateral, ventrodorsal, and dorsoventral views. If vomiting is frequent, an injectable antiemetic should be given to effect, and the contrast dose should be reduced by half. If vomiting persists, then further contrast studies should be postponed until the animal has stabilized. Barium, even with its attendant risks, may be substituted if the iodinated contrast continues to be poorly tolerated.

Pitfalls

Demonstration of penetrated ulcers is inconstant, owing to variations in size, shape, and location of the lesion, as well as in the methods of radiographic examination.

Alternative Diagnoses

Systemic bleeding disorders, hemorrhagic gastroenteritis, bleeding gastric tumor.

Suggested Reading

Barber DL, Mahaffey MB. The stomach. In: Thrall DE, ed. Textbook of veterinary diagnostic radiology. Philadelphia: WB Saunders, 1986:489.

Farrow CS. Exercise in diagnostic radiology. Can Vet J 1982; 23:67–69.

O'Brien TR. Stomach. In: O'Brien TR, ed. Radiographic diagnosis of abdominal disorders in the dog and cat. Philadelphia: WB Saunders, 1978:245, 264.

Urs G, Gorman NT. Gastrointestinal emergencies. In: Kirk RW, ed. Current veterinary therapy IX. Philadelphia: WB Saunders, 1986:454.

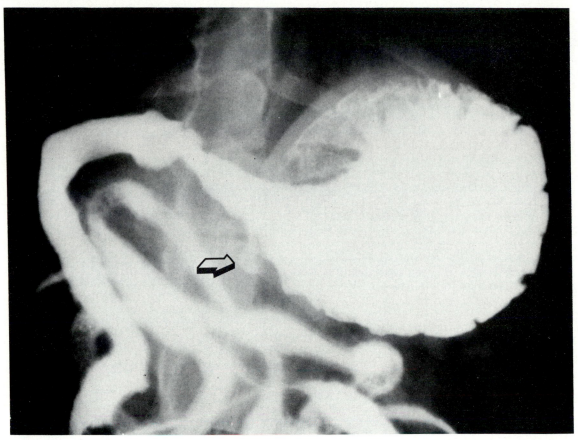

Figure 66-1 Ventrodorsal canine gastrogram (detail view) shows localized pyloric antral leakage (*arrow*). Diagnosis: penetrating gastric ulcer.

67

INCARCERATED HIATAL HERNIA

General Considerations

There are two types of hiatal hernia: *axial* and *paraesophageal*. Paraesophageal hiatal hernia is distinguished from axial hiatal hernia by the location of the gastroesophageal junction. In the paraesophageal form, the gastroesophageal junction remains caudal to the diaphragm, and the stomach is displaced into the caudal mediastinum. Both the gastroesophageal junction and the stomach are displaced into the caudal mediastinum in the axial variety. Intermittent axial hiatal hernia is occasionally seen in older cats, but rarely in dogs. Occasionally such displacements become incarcerated, and as such are associated with more overt clinical signs, including dysphagia, dyspnea, and esophageal bleeding.

Major Radiographic Observations

A semicircular mass is present in the dorsal aspect of the caudal mediastinum. A contrast examination typically shows a shortened esophagus and permanent displacement of the stomach into the thorax (Fig. 67–1). Varying degrees of obstruction may be present depending on the magnitude of gastric entrapment.

Diagnostic Strategy

Place the animal in the left lateral position with the x-ray beam centered as nearly as possible over the dorsal diaphragm (tenth intercostal space). Expose the film on expiration using thoracic technique. Expiration relatively increases lesional density, and thoracic technique avoids potential overpenetration associated with abdominal exposure. Dorsoventral or ventrodorsal views should also be made but are not as informative. A barium swallow should also be performed to confirm the survey-film diagnosis and to differentiate the axial from the paraesophageal forms of hiatal hernia.

Pitfalls

In many older cats, intermittent hiatal hernia appears to be an age-associated, incidental finding.

Alternative Diagnoses

Transient hiatal hernia, gastroesophageal hernia, esophageal foreign body, *Spirocerca sanguinolenta* lesion or tumor.

Suggested Reading

O'Brien TR. Esophagus. In: O'Brien TR, ed. Radiographic diagnosis of abdominal disorders in the dog and the cat. Philadelphia: WB Saunders, 1978:193.

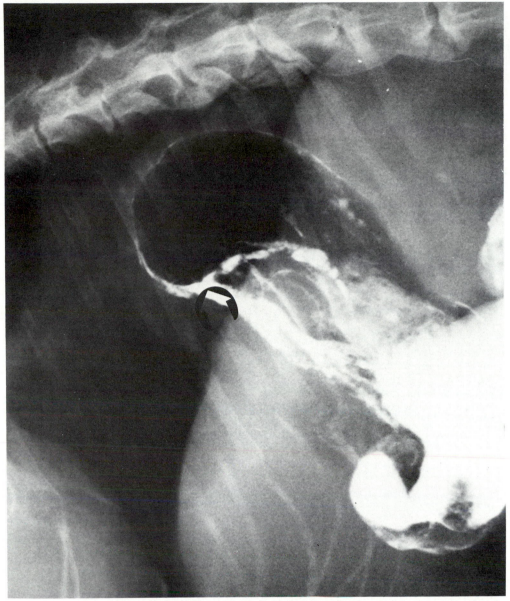

Figure 67–1 Lateral canine gastrogram (detail view) shows the proximal part of the stomach within the thorax (*arrow*), as did subsequent films and fluoroscopy. Diagnosis: hiatal hernia.

68

PYLORIC TUMOR

General Considerations

Most pyloric tumors produce a gradual onset of clinical signs, usually vomiting and weight loss. However, some may present as acute collapse, probably as a result of secondary metabolic dysfunction.

Major Radiographic Observations

Overall enlargement of the stomach, with disproportionate increase in the pyloric part, is seen. Contrast studies often show a pyloric filling defect.

Diagnostic Strategy

Survey films rarely show a lesion (Fig. 68–1). Consequently, *contrast* examination is required. It is best to start the examination when the animal has an empty stomach. Use a full dose of contrast, center the film over the stomach, and begin filming immediately. Delayed emptying or vomiting should be anticipated owing to the location and obstructive nature of the lesion (Fig. 68–2).

Pitfalls

Excessive contrast concentration and/or poor radiographic technique may hide the lesion.

Alternative Diagnoses

Foreign body, large inflamed ulcer, luminal abscess, trapped gas.

Suggested Reading

Barber DL, Mahaffey MB. The stomach. In: Thrall DE, ed. Textbook of veterinary diagnostic radiology. Philadelphia: WB Saunders, 1986:490.

McNeel SV. Chronic pyloric outflow obstruction. In: Farrow CS, ed. Decision making in small animal radiology. Toronto: BC Decker, 1987:164.

O'Brien TR. Stomach. In: O'Brien TR, ed. Radiographic diagnosis of abdominal disorders in the dog and the cat. Philadelphia: WB Saunders, 1978:242.

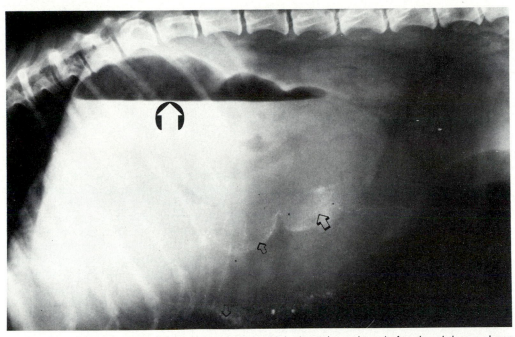

Figure 68–1 Postural view (standing patient position with horizontal x-ray beam) of canine abdomen shows large, fluid-filled, gas-capped stomach (*large arrow*) containing high-density sediment (*small arrows*). Diagnosis: pyloric tumor (adenocarcinoma).

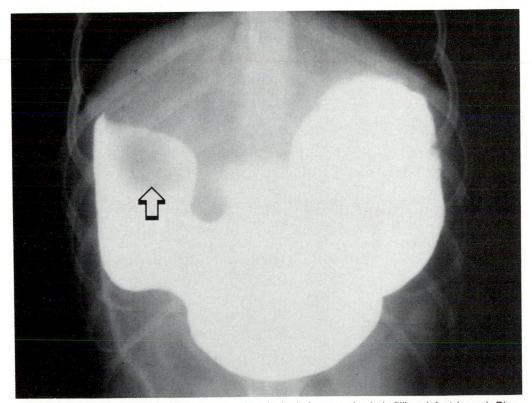

Figure 68–2 Ventrodorsal canine gastrogram (detail view) shows oval pyloric filling defect (*arrow*). Diagnosis: pyloric tumor (leiomyoma).

THE INTESTINE

69

LINEAR INTESTINAL FOREIGN BODY

General Considerations

Linear intestinal foreign bodies can be classified as *free* or *fixed*. The latter are more common in cats which are prone to playing with and eating string or thread. These materials may wrap around the base of the tongue, thus fixing the proximal end of the foreign body while the remainder trails into the gastrointestinal tract. If the string is long enough, it may pass into the intestine where it serves as a kind of trellis upon which surrounding gut can move proximally. It is this retrograde displacement that results in the coiled appearance of the involved bowel. A similar mechanism accounts for an associated interrupted (segmented) intestinal-gas pattern. Peritonitis results if the bowel is lacerated by the foreign body. A free linear foreign body behaves in a traditional manner: stopping or passing according to its size, shape, and composition.

Major Radiographic Observations

Survey-film detection of linear foreign bodies is dependent on high radiographic density. Fixed linear foreign bodies may be inferred from characteristic intestinal coiling or segmented gas pattern. *Contrast* examination usually confirms either diagnosis and should be performed when diagnostic doubt exists (Fig. 69–1).

Diagnostic Strategy

A coiled intestine is not easily seen on a survey radiograph; an interrupted gas pattern may be identified if it is pronounced. Accordingly, a contrast examination should be done when doubt exists. A half-dose of barium is best, un-less there are radiographic signs of peritonitis, in which case an iodinated contrast medium is indicated. Delayed gastric emptying is typical; therefore, allow at least 2 hours before diagnosing gastric obstruction. When only a small amount of barium enters the proximal intestine, detection is enhanced greatly with compression radiography of the right cranial abdomen with the patient in the ventrodorsal position.

Pitfalls

Sole reliance on an interrupted gas pattern to diagnose linear intestinal foreign body is hazardous, because a similar pattern may be seen with some types of enteritis, as well as with a normal intestinal variation.

Alternative Diagnoses

Enteritis, intussusception, tumor, functional ileus.

Suggested Reading

McNeel SV. Linear intestinal foreign object. In: Farrow CS, ed. Decision making in small animal radiology. Toronto: BC Decker, 1987:170.

McNeel SV. The small bowel. In: Thrall DE, ed. Textbook of veterinary diagnostic radiology. Philadelphia: WB Saunders, 1986:504.

O'Brien TR. Small intestine. In: O'Brien TR, ed. Radiographic diagnosis of abdominal disorders in the dog and the cat. Philadelphia: WB Saunders, 1978:300.

Seim HB III. Linear intestinal foreign body. In: Binnington AG, Cockshutt JR, eds. Decision making in small animal soft tissue surgery. Toronto: BC Decker, 1988:30

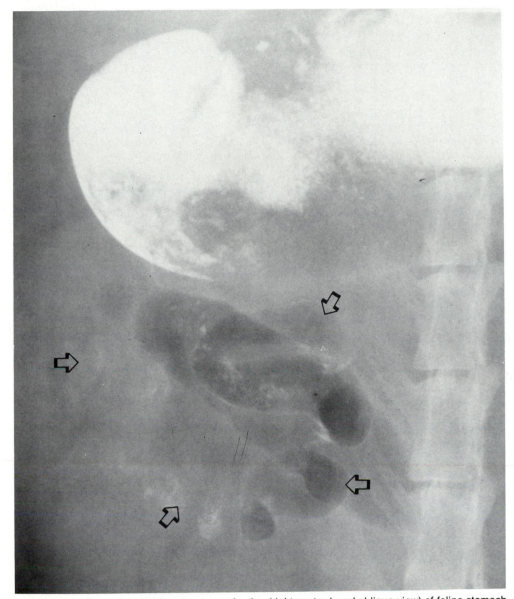

Figure 69–1 Gastrointestinal contrast examination (right ventrodorsal oblique view) of feline stomach and proximal intestine shows bunching of the duodenum with minimal filling (*arrows*). Diagnosis: linear foreign body.

70

NONLINEAR, INTESTINAL FOREIGN BODY

General Considerations

Intestinal foreign bodies, like their gastric counterparts, may be opaque or transparent, thus determining their radiographic detectability. Most are associated with vomiting. Although it is generally believed that younger animals are more prone to eating foreign bodies than older (more experienced, wiser ?) animals, age should not be a basis for diagnostic exclusion.

Major Radiographic Observations

Survey films show one or more high-density shadows in the intestinal field (Fig. 70–1). Lucent objects are suggested by excessive intestinal gas or fluid proximally. *Contrast* examinations show a filling defect, with or without obstruction (Fig. 70–2).

Diagnostic Strategy

Opaque foreign bodies are identified readily, although their specific location may be uncertain. Radiolucent foreign bodies may only be identified indirectly or by using barium. Compression radiography is useful in isolating a suspicious area from surrounding shadows (remember to reduce the radiographic technique by an amount equivalent to the animal's abdominal measurement *after* it is compressed).

Pitfalls

Some foreign bodies are merely incidental radiographic findings, unrelated to the animal's illness. When uncertainty exists, follow-up films resolve the question.

Alternative Diagnoses

Gastroenteritis, intussusception, tumor, functional ileus.

Suggested Reading

McNeel SV. Intestinal obstruction. In: Farrow CS, ed. Decision making in small animal radiology. Toronto: BC Decker, 1987:166.

McNeel SV. The small bowel. In: Thrall DE, ed. Textbook of veterinary diagnostic radiology. Philadelphia: WB Saunders, 1986.

O'Brien TR. Small intestine. In: O'Brien TR, ed. Radiographic diagnosis of abdominal disorders in the dog and the cat. Philadelphia: WB Saunders, 1978:295.

Olsson S-E, ed. The radiological diagnosis in canine and feline emergencies. Philadelphia: Lea & Febiger, 1973:78, 83, 87, 92, 95, 99, 102.

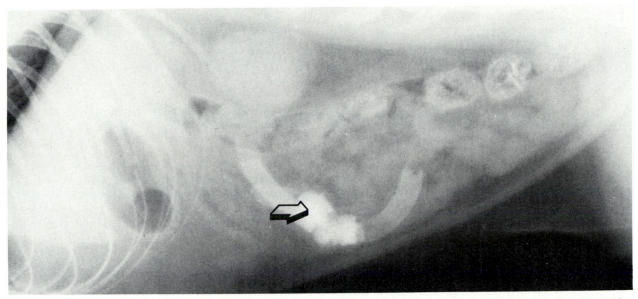

Figure 70–1 Lateral view of feline abdomen shows high-density object in midventral abdomen (*arrows*). Diagnosis: intestinal foreign body (knotted, canning sealer ring).

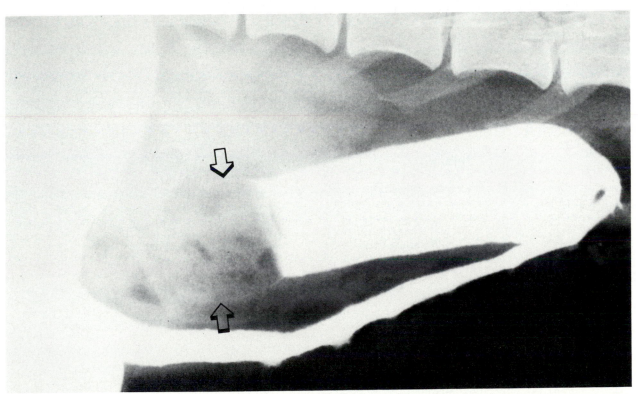

Figure 70–2 Lateral detail view of canine gastrointestinal contrast examination shows a circular filling defect (*arrows*) in the ascending duodenum with marked distention proximally. Diagnosis: intestinal foreign body (rubber ball).

71

INTUSSUSCEPTION

General Considerations

The telescoping of the intestine into itself (from proximal to distal) is termed *intussusception*. Although the specific mechanism of this condition is unknown, an etiologic classification used in human beings has been adopted for the dog. In this scheme, lesions with no apparent organic cause are termed *functional*; those in which structural abnormality is present are termed *organic*. Most of the intussusceptions reported in companion animals are of the functional variety and tend to occur in the midportion of the small intestine. Disagreement exists about whether or not younger animals are more susceptible. A triad of clinical signs is classically present: vomiting, abdominal pain, and a bloody, mucoid, rectal discharge. An abdominal mass may or may not be palpable.

Major Radiographic Observations

Survey films typically show a cranioventral or central abdominal mass surrounded by gas or fluid-dilated bowel loops (Fig. 71–1). Contrast examinations (upper-gastrointestinal—UGI—or barium enema) are highly variable but are usually sufficiently abnormal to allow detection of the lesion, provided a film is made at or near the time the contrast reaches the intussusception.

Diagnostic Strategy

Survey radiographs are often confusing because of the accumulated gas and fluid secondary to the obstructive nature of the lesion. If a mass can be palpated, it should be compressed and radiographed, since this greatly enhances lesion visibility. A postural radiograph (standing lateral with a horizontal x-ray beam) often provides the best view of both the intussusception (mass) and the surrounding distended bowel loops. Contrast examination should begin with a barium enema, because it requires much less time than a UGI, and in most cases it identifies an ileocolic or cecocolic intussusception. If these possibilities are ruled out, a UGI should be done using one-half the normal dose of barium. Films (lateral and ventrodorsal views) must be made at frequent intervals until the diagnosis is confirmed or denied.

Pitfalls

Not all intussusceptions cause complete intestinal obstruction; consequently a UGI conducted with long radiographic intervals may miss the lesion and result in a false-negative diagnosis.

Alternative Diagnoses

Functional ileus, intestinal volvulus, intestinal incarceration.

Suggested Reading

Biery DN. The large bowel. In: Thrall DE, ed. Textbook of veterinary diagnostic radiology. Philadelphia: WB Saunders, 1986:518.

McNeel SV. Intestinal obstruction. In: Farrow CS, ed. Decision making in small animal radiology. Toronto: BC Decker, 1987:166.

Seim HB III. Intussusception. In: Binnington AG, Cockshutt JR, eds. Decision making in small animal soft tissue surgery. Toronto: BC Decker, 1988:28.

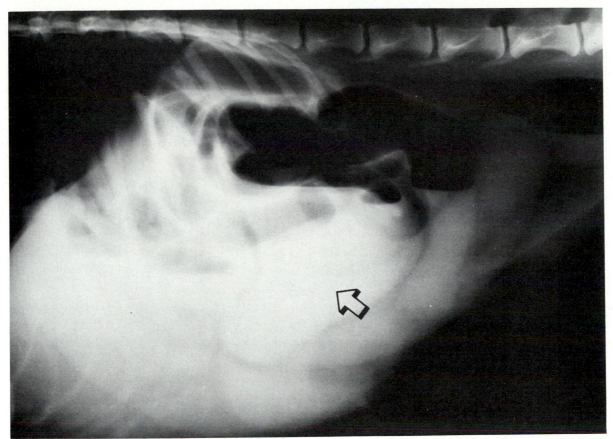

Figure 71–1 Lateral view of canine abdomen shows dilated, fluid-filled, and air-filled intestinal segments. A mass effect appears ventrally (*arrow*). Diagnosis: intussusception.

72

INTESTINAL INCARCERATION

General Considerations

Incarceration (strangulation, entrapment) of the small intestine occurs when a part of the bowel passes through a natural or unnatural body opening (herniation) and becomes fixed, or relatively fixed, in position. Potential entrapment sites include tears in the body wall, diaphragm, intra-abdominal ligaments, and mesentery. Other less common locations include the inguinal rings, mesenteric foramina, and a congenital opening between the peritoneum and pericardium. Most incarcerations develop acutely and are associated with complete intestinal-vascular obstruction. The resulting ischemia rapidly produces intestinal necrosis, leading to peritonitis. Affected animals may show severe abdominal colic, vomiting, and later shock. Accompanying abdominal distention resembles gastric dilation-torsion. The condition frequently is fatal.

Major Radiographic Observations

Typically, an incarcerated small bowel shows as multiple, air-distended small bowel segments. Because of space limitations, these distended intestinal loops are forced to fold over one another, appearing stacked or layered. Postural views show multiple air-fluid levels (Fig. 72–1).

Diagnostic Strategy

Because incarcerations usually involve most of the small intestine, affected animals rapidly become very ill. Accordingly, they must be diagnosed and operated on as quickly as possible. To this end, the radiographic examination may be expedited by making a single sternal or standing lateral view using a horizonatal x-ray beam, in place of conventional recumbent projections.

Pitfalls

Intestinal atony or standstill (functional ileus) often results in gas accumulation and dilatation, which may resemble incarceration of the small intestine.

Alternative Diagnoses

Intestinal obstruction due to other causes, such as foreign body, intussusception, tumor, or volvulus. See "Pitfalls" above.

Suggested Reading

Farrow CS. Known case conference (incarcerated small intestine: case 5). Vet Rad 1983; 24:149.

McNeel SV. Intestinal obstruction. In: Farrow CS, ed. Decision making in small animal radiology. Toronto: BC Decker, 1987:166.

McNeel SV. The small bowel. In: Thrall DE, ed. Textbook of veterinary diagnostic radiology. Philadelphia: WB Saunders, 1986:499.

O'Brien TR. Small intestine. In: O'Brien TR, ed. Radiographic diagnosis of abdominal disorders in the dog and the cat. Philadelphia: WB Saunders, 1978:311.

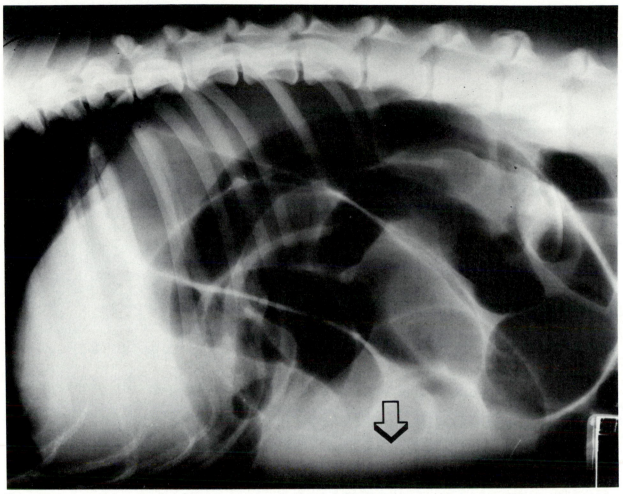

Figure 72–1 Lateral view of canine abdomen shows greatly dilated, air-filled bowel loops which, because of their longitudinal orientation, appear "stacked." An engorged spleen lies ventrally (*arrow*). Diagnosis: intestinal incarceration.

73

INTESTINAL VOLVULUS

General Considerations

Volvulus of the small bowel is typically an acute event in which the small intestine is twisted about its mesentery. The resulting obstruction, usually complete, produces a closed bowel loop and, frequently, ischemia. In people, the intestine may be partially or completely affected; in my clinical experience, the majority of the small bowel is usually involved. The condition is often fatal, even when recognized early.

Major Radiographic Observations

Multiple, dilated (often larger than the colon), gas- or fluid-filled small bowel loops are seen, frequently lying parallel to one another (stacked) (Fig. 73–1).

Diagnostic Strategy

Because of the extreme seriousness of this condition, it is imperative that the radiographic examination be as rapid and as nonstressful as possible. To this end, a postural radiograph, made with the dog in the standing position and using a horizontal x-ray beam, is most effective. If the dog cannot stand, then make a right lateral projection centered over the midabdomen. If abdominal distention is present, decrease the radiographic technique by one-half, anticipating excess intestinal gas. Contrast studies should be reserved for those animals able to bear the stress. If in doubt, omit special procedures in this type of patient.

Pitfalls

Splenomegaly, usually present in this condition, often mimics an intussusception. However, the two conditions may often be separated on the basis of patient condition, which is typically much worse with intestinal volvulus.

Alternative Diagnoses

Functional ileus, intestinal incarceration, foreign body, tumor, intussusception.

Suggested Reading

McNeel SV. Intestinal obstruction. In: Farrow CS, ed. Decision making in small animal radiology. Toronto: BC Decker, 1987:166.

O'Brien TR. Small intestine. In: O'Brien TR, ed. Radiographic diagnosis of abdominal disorders in the dog and the cat. Philadelphia: WB Saunders, 1978:288.

Reinhold RB. The small intestine. In: Reinhold RB, ed. Consultation in general surgery. Toronto: BC Decker, 1985:73.

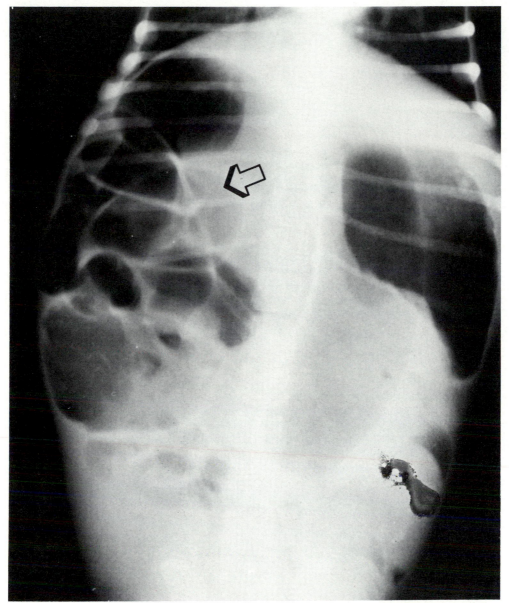

Figure 73–1 Ventrodorsal view of canine abdomen shows multiple dilated, air-filled, small-bowel loops bunched in the right cranial abdomen (*arrow*). The surrounding abdomen is abnormally dense, obscuring organ detail. Diagnosis: subtotal volvulus of small intestine.

74

TUMOR OF THE SMALL INTESTINE

General Considerations

Tumors of the small intestine, particularly those that are proximally located, often cause vomiting. Although onset is usually gradual, occasionally it is sudden. The reasons for this atypical presentation are uncertain but are probably related to some form of intestinal decompensation. As with other tumors, intestinal tumors affect old animals most frequently.

Major Radiographic Observations

Survey films typically show nothing. *Contrast* radiographs may show narrowing, widening, or distortion of the intestinal lumen, with or without a filling defect (Figs. 74–1 and 74–2).

Diagnostic Strategy

Unless they are very large, most intestinal tumors go undetected on *survey* radiographs. Even when detected, the mass is not anatomically specific and may only be inferred to be intestinal, based upon indirect radiographic evidence. Consequently, diagnosis requires a *contrast* examination. As with any upper-gastrointestinal (UGI) study, the examination should be patient tailored, with the majority of films made in the first 2 hours when visualization of the small intestine is optimal. When a suspected lesion is obscured by one or more overlying bowel loops, compression radiography should be used for relative isolation of the questionable part.

Pitfalls

Because not all intestinal tumors are completely obstructive and, therefore, cannot be expected to prevent the passage of contrast indefinitely, lesions may be missed if UGI film intervals are too great.

Alternative Diagnoses

Gastric or intestinal foreign body.

Suggested Reading

McNeel SV. Intestinal neoplasia. In: Farrow CS, ed. Decision making in small animal radiology. Toronto: BC Decker, 1987:168.

McNeel SV. The small bowel. In: Thrall DE, ed. Textbook of veterinary diagnostic radiology. Philadelphia: WB Saunders, 1986.

O'Brien TR. Small intestine. In: O'Brien TR, ed. Radiographic diagnosis of abdominal disorders in the dog and the cat. Philadelphia: WB Saunders, 1978:307.

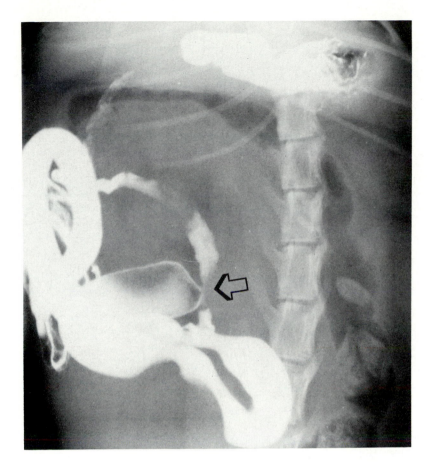

Figure 74–1 Upper gastrointestinal examination, ventrodorsal oblique view of canine abdomen, shows focal narrowing of midjejunum (*arrow*) with proximal luminal distention. Diagnosis: small intestinal tumor (annular carcinoma).

Figure 74–2 Upper gastrointestinal examination, ventrodorsal view of canine abdomen, shows localized dilatation and deformity of the midjejunum (*arrows*). Diagnosis: small intestinal tumor (undifferentiated sarcoma).

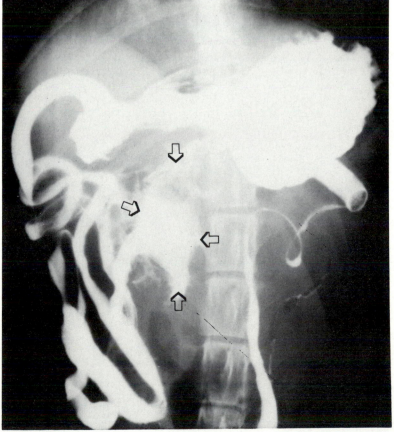

75

CANINE PARVOVIRAL ENTERITIS

General Considerations

Canine parvoviral enteritis (CPE) causes extensive mucosal injury to the small intestine; there are no direct effects on the stomach. Immature dogs are most commonly affected; however, older animals are not exempt from infection. Intussusception may occur secondary to serosal edema. Radiographic recognition of this obstructive complication is made difficult by the generalized fluid and gas distention of the bowel usually seen with this disease.

Major Radiographic Observations

Early in the disease, *survey* films are normal. As the disease progresses, gas and fluid distention of the small bowel become evident (Fig. 75–1). *Contrast* radiographic findings are also normal early in the disease. Later the bowel often shows a highly distinctive scalloplike or cobblestone pattern.

Diagnostic Strategy

The important factor in CPE is not to mistake its radiographic abnormalities for those of intestinal obstruction. The most reliable, distinguishing radiographic feature is the *generalized nature* of the intestinal abnormalities in CPE.

Although low-bowel obstructions can be associated with a great deal of fluid distention, this is the exception rather than the rule. Extensive intestinal fluid accumulation may also be used to exclude most cases of functional ileus, in which the bowel, although distended by air, rarely contains much fluid. When obstruction is suspected, barium may be used, although it is apt to be vomited shortly after being given. Alternatively, a retrograde small-intestine examination may be performed, although this is imprecise and time-consuming without a fluoroscope.

Pitfalls

Coexisting CPE and intussusception may be impossible to differentiate on either a clinical or a radiographic basis.

Alternative Diagnoses

Enteritis, small-bowel obstruction.

Suggested Reading

Farrow CS. Radiographic appearance of canine parvovirus enteritis. JAVMA 1982; 180:43–47.

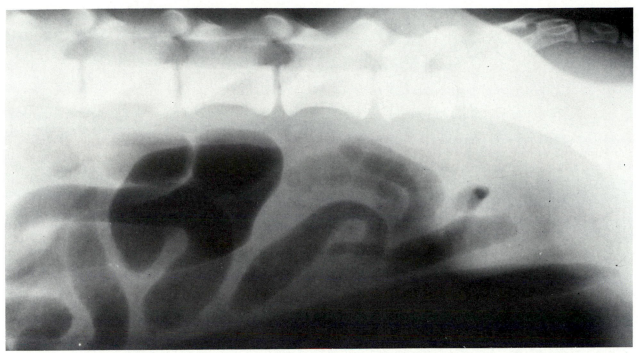

Figure 75–1 Lateral view of canine abdomen shows multiple, distended, air-filled bowel loops. Reduced abdominal detail is a function of the dog's age, breed, and illness. Diagnosis: canine parvovirus enteritis (8-month-old Saluki, ill for 2 weeks).

76

RUPTURED COLON

General Considerations

Colonic rupture may occur secondary to an enema, over inflation of a catheter cuff, excessive distention during a barium enema, or a penetrating ulcer; it may also occur following biopsy or surgery. Most such ruptures result in the rapid formation of peritonitis. Pneumoperitoneum is variable.

Major Radiographic Observations

Radiographic evidence is indirect: peritonitis and/or pneumoperitoneum (Figs. 76–1 to 76–3).

Diagnostic Strategy

Make standard abdominal radiographs (lateral and ventrodorsal views). If they are normal but perforation is strongly suspected, make a postural radiograph (patient on left side with horizontal x-ray beam centered over the sternum at the level of the midabdomen). Reduce the measured kilovolt peak by 20 percent because you are looking for a small amount of air lying beneath the uppermost peritoneal surface. If perforation is believed to have occurred during a barium enema, make lateral and ventrodorsal views and search for extra-colonic barium. If the perforation occurred under other circumstances, a diagnostic enema may be performed using an iodinated contrast medium, *not barium.* However, be aware that iodinated compounds are osmotically very active and draw water into the bowel. This not only dehydrates the animal further but may also result in more leakage of bowel content into the peritoneum.

Pitfalls

With contrast studies performed to show intestinal leakage, iodinated compounds may be absorbed by the circulation and eliminated through the urinary tract. This may lead to the false conclusion that the contrast has leaked from the colon.

Alternative Diagnoses

Gunshot and other penetrating abdominal wounds. For pneumoperitoneum: ruptured rectum or other hollow, gas-containing organs. For peritonitis: perforated component of gastrointestinal or urinary tracts; ruptured gallbladder, prostate, or uterus.

Suggested Reading

Biery DN. The large bowel. In: Thrall DE, ed. Textbook of veterinary diagnostic radiology. Philadelphia: WB Saunders, 1986:514.

Olsson S-E, ed. The radiological diagnosis in canine and feline emergencies. Philadelphia: Lea & Febiger, 1973:122.

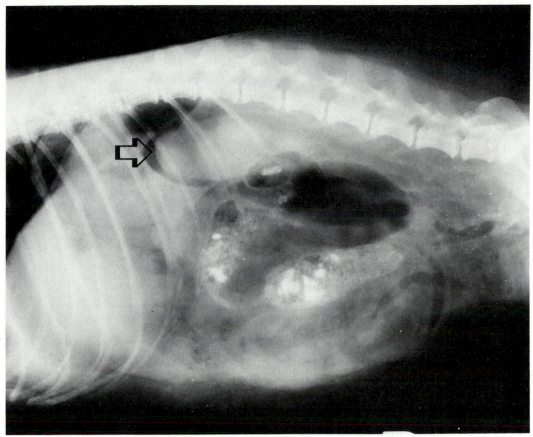

Figure 76–1   Lateral view of canine abdomen shows increased abdominal density, decreased organ detail, and free abdominal air around the kidneys (*arrow*).

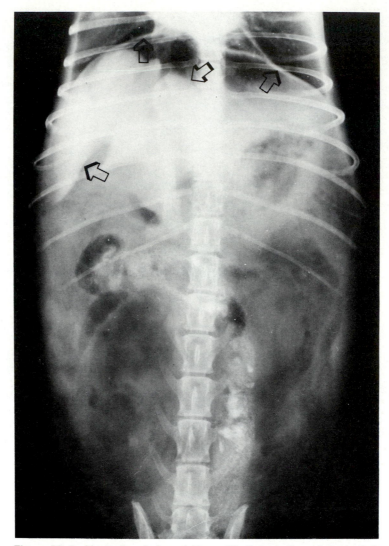

Figure 76–2 Ventrodorsal view of Figure 76–1 shows free abdominal air around the liver and diaphragm (*arrows*), increased abdominal density, and decreased visceral detail. Diagnosis: perforated colon secondary to fecal impaction and associated bowel necrosis.

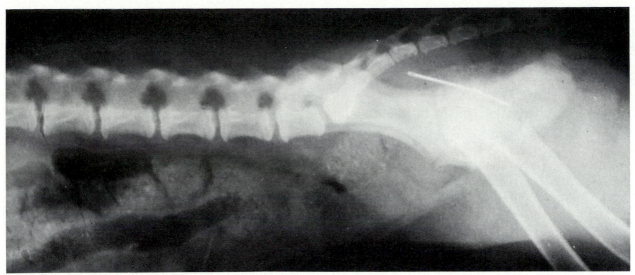

Figure 76–3   Lateral view of feline abdomen shows rectal foreign body, apparently penetrating dorsal rectal wall. Diagnosis: needle penetrating rectal wall causing intrapelvic abscess.

77

POST - TRAUMATIC MEGACOLON

General Considerations

Megacolon is a radiologic term describing colonic enlargement, and it is not etiospecific. Causes of megacolon include the following: the congenital absence, or reduced number, of myenteric plexuses; denervation secondary to congenital spinal defects or trauma; intrinsic or extrinsic mechanical obstruction; and pain associated with defecation. Regardless of cause, the accumulated feces tends to become hard and abrasive, resulting in straining and possible rectal bleeding, bloody stools, or both. These last signs constitute the emergency, because they may be seen with more serious conditions.

Major Radiographic Observations

Typically, the colon is three or more times its normal diameter and contains high-density feces (Fig. 77–1). Megacolon creates a caudal abdominal-mass effect, resulting in cranial displacement of the adjacent abdominal organs.

Diagnostic Strategy

A single lateral radiograph is sufficient to make a diagnosis of megacolon, although it often does not establish the cause.

Pitfalls

The normal colon is capable of considerable enlargement; consequently, increased colonic size may be an incidental finding.

Alternative Diagnoses

Normal anatomic variation.

Suggested Reading

Biery DN. The large bowel. In: Thrall DE, ed. Textbook of veterinary diagnostic radiology. Philadelphia: WB Saunders, 1986:516.

O'Brien TR. Large intestine. In: O'Brien TR, ed. Radiographic diagnosis of abdominal disorders in the dog and the cat. Philadelphia: WB Saunders, 1978:360.

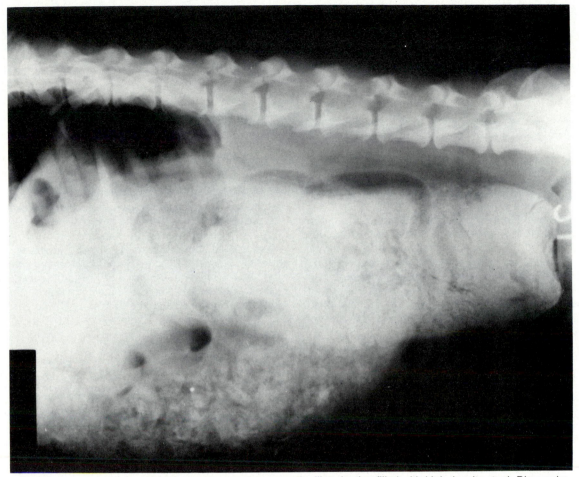

Figure 77-1 Lateral view of canine abdomen shows greatly dilated colon filled with high-density stool. Diagnosis: megacolon (secondary to pelvic deformity caused by earlier fractures).

Urinary Tract

78

RUPTURED KIDNEY PRODUCING RETROPERITONEAL HEMORRHAGE

General Considerations

Renal fracture typically occurs following a car accident and is often associated with injury to the surrounding rib cage, lung, and liver. Additionally, the kidney may be torn from its vascular or ureteral moorings, producing serious and sometimes fatal consequences. Fracture of the renal parenchyma results in hemorrhage, which initially accumulates around the kidney and eventually extends into the retroperitoneal space. Tearing of the renal collecting system allows urine to locate in the same areas.

Major Radiographic Observations

Perirenal bleeding eliminates the normally sharp renal shadow and leaves in its place an enlarged, roughly marginated facsimile. Perirenal urine leakage is less distinct. Either blood or urine in the retroperitoneal space, especially in large volume, eliminates the associated renal shadow but produces a large, distinctive, convex density in the dorsal abdomen as viewed in lateral projection (Fig. 78–1). Urography shows contrast medium accumulating outside the kidney or within the retroperitoneal space. Sonography shows fluid around the kidney and abnormal renal echogenicity.

Diagnostic Strategy

Make paired abdominal radiographs centered over the kidneys, being certain to set the exposure according to the measurement of the cranial abdomen. If one or both kidneys are not seen, make a ventrodorsal compression over the suspected lesion, remembering to reduce the radiographic technique in accordance with the amount of compression obtained. If a question remains, perform urography using an intravenous, organic iodine compound (1 ml per pound), making films at 10, 20, and 30 minutes or until leakage is established. Be aware that iodinated contrast media have anticoagulation properties and may aggravate hemorrhage.

Pitfalls

Avoid using abdominal compression to enhance renal opacification, because it may obstruct venous return and promote or aggravate existing shock.

Alternative Diagnoses

Ruptured ureter, retroperitoneal abscess.

Suggested Reading

Biery DN. Upper urinary tract. In: O'Brien TR, ed. Radiographic diagnosis of abdominal disorders in the dog and the cat. Philadelphia: WB Saunders, 1986:523.

McNeel SV. Renal or ureteral rupture. In: Farrow CS, ed. Decision making in small animal radiology. Toronto: BC Decker, 1987:192.

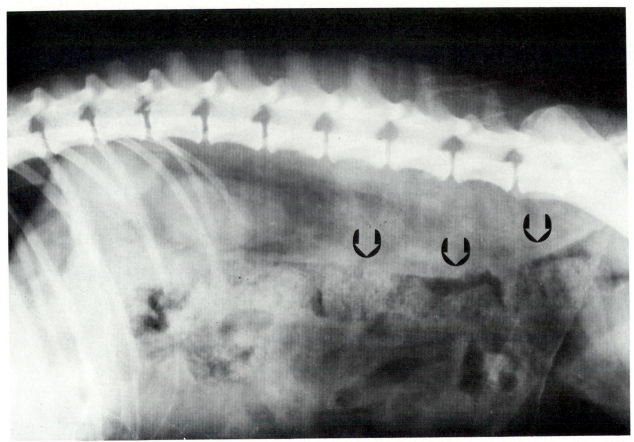

Figure 78–1 Lateral view of feline abdomen shows enlarged, fluid-filled retroperitoneal space (*arrows*). Diagnosis: ruptured kidney with retroperitoneal hemorrhage.

79

RENAL ABSCESS

General Considerations

Renal infection occasionally produces renal abscessation. Often there is paralumbar pain and a distinctive arching of the back, accompanied by a short-strided gait similar to that seen in lumbar spondylitis. Gross hematuria is often present. Abscessation may be difficult or impossible to detect using survey radiography. The diagnosis may need to be made by inference.

Major Radiographic Observations

The affected kidney is usually enlarged and sometimes mineralized. Urography typically shows multiple filling defects, often with poor opacification overall.

Diagnostic Strategy

Survey films should be centered over the kidneys using an appropriate technique (Fig. 79–1). When overlying feces obscures one or both kidneys, *compression* films should be made. This also greatly improves renal detail. *Urography* should focus on the kidneys first, followed by the lower urinary tract as necessary (Fig. 79–2). Compression films are use-

ful in this context as well. Radiographs should be made at 5, 10, and 20 minutes. *Sonography* (ultrasound) can be used to separate solid from fluid lesions and to evaluate dilated renal diverticula, the renal pelvis, and the ureters.

Pitfalls

Renal enlargement, whether generalized or regional, may be due to compensatory hypertrophy, as opposed to disease.

Alternative Diagnoses

Compensatory hypertrophy, tumor, nephritis.

Suggested Reading

O'Brien TR. Abdominal mass. In: O'Brien TR, ed. Radiographic diagnosis of abdominal disorders in the dog and the cat. Philadelphia: WB Saunders, 1978:100.

Biery DN, Upper urinary tract. In: O'Brien TR, ed. Radiographic diagnosis of abdominal disorders in the dog and the cat. Philadelphia: WB Saunders, 1978:492, 520.

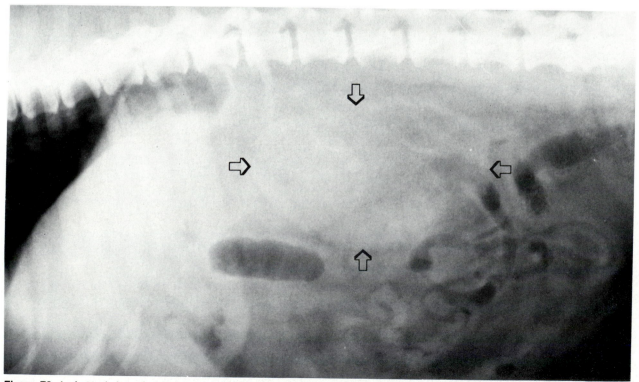

Figure 79–1 Lateral view of canine abdomen shows enlarged, misshapen left kidney (*arrows*) overlapping normal right kidney.

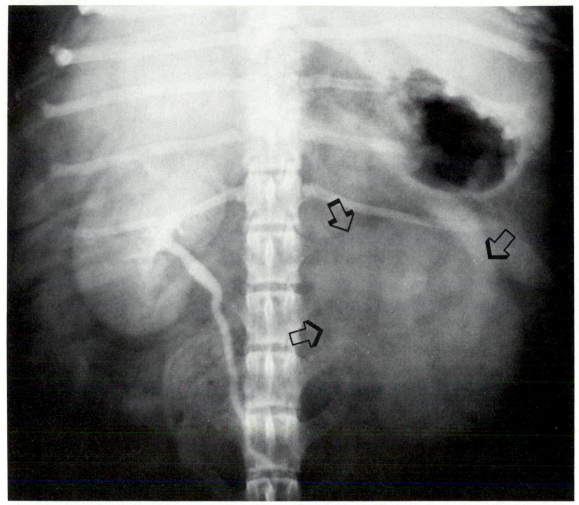

Figure 79–2 Ventrodorsal urogram (detail view) of Figure 79–1 shows no opacification of the left kidney (*arrows*) or ureter; the right kidney and associated collecting system opacify normally. Diagnosis: left renal abscess.

80

RUPTURED URINARY BLADDER PRODUCING PERITONITIS

General Considerations

Rupture of the urinary bladder usually results from abdominal or pelvic trauma and is most common in male dogs after road accidents. Clinical signs may be masked by shock or missed because of more obvious injuries. Often the injury is not suspected until urinary peritonitis has produced abdominal pain and swelling. The fact that the animal does not urinate can suggest serious bladder injury, but urination does not conclusively rule out rupture.

Major Radiographic Observations

Survey films typically show little, unless there is associated edema, hemorrhage, or peritonitis. The presence of such changes results in varying degrees of indistinctness involving the urinary bladder and surrounding tissues (Fig. 80–1). Positive *contrast* studies are usually conclusive, showing contrast leakage in the region of the bladder (Fig. 80–2).

Diagnostic Strategy

Begin with abdominal survey films in order to evaluate the entire abdomen, including the pelvis. If the bladder is suspicious, make an additional lateral film centered over the caudal abdomen. If suspicion persists, perform a positive-contrast cystogram, and make lateral abdominal films immediately and at 5-minute intervals as necessary. If films are negative and abdominocentesis is positive for urine, do positive-contrast, retrograde urethrogram.

Pitfalls

Negative-contrast studies are inferior to iodine examinations, because leakage of gas into the peritoneum is difficult to detect in the context of normal intestinal gas content.

Alternative Diagnoses

Urethral rupture as indicated by leakage of contrast medium into the soft tissues of the pelvic cavity; bladder herniation or torsion.

Suggested Reading

McNeel SV. Traumatic urinary bladder and urethral rupture. In: Farrow CS, ed. Decision making in small animal radiology. Toronto: BC Decker, 1987:194.

Olsson S-E, ed. The radiological diagnosis in canine and feline emergencies. Philadelphia: Lea & Febiger, 1973:182.

Park RD. Radiology of the urinary bladder and urethra. In: O'Brien TR, ed. Radiographic diagnosis of abdominal disorders in the dog and the cat. Philadelphia: WB Saunders, 1978:594.

Park RD. The urinary bladder. In: Thrall DE, ed. Textbook of veterinary diagnostic radiology. Philadelphia: WB Saunders, 1986:436.

Stone EA. Uroperitoneum. In: Binnington AG, Cockshutt JR, eds. Decision making in small animal soft tissue surgery. Toronto: BC Decker, 1988:114.

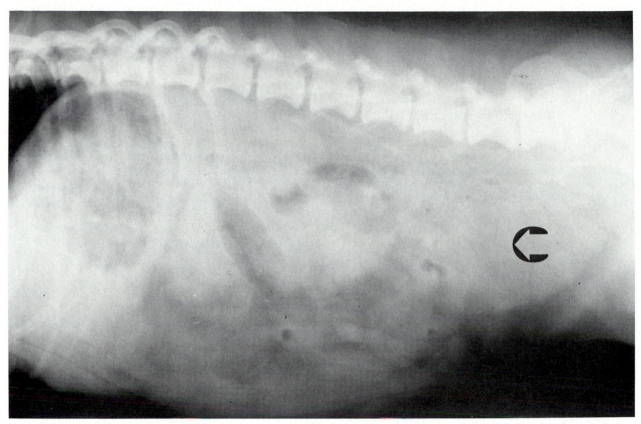

Figure 80–1   Lateral view of canine abdomen shows increased abdominal density and poor organ detail. Note that most of the urinary bladder shadow *is visible* (*arrow*).

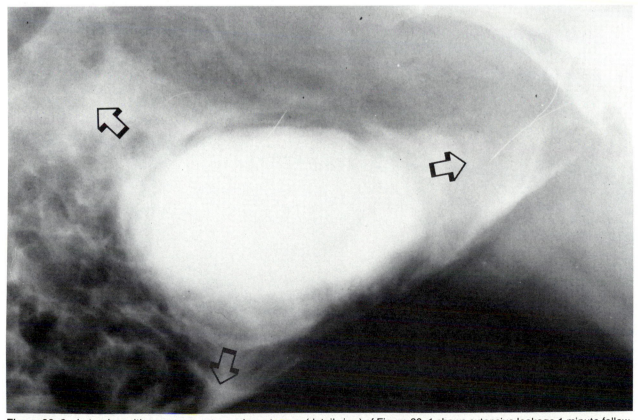

Figure 80–2   Lateral, positive-contrast, retrograde cystogram (detail view) of Figure 80–1 shows extensive leakage 1 minute following injection of contrast medium (*arrows*). Diagnosis: ruptured urinary bladder (three small tears were found in the bladder neck).

81

BLADDER DISLOCATION: RETROFLEXION

General Considerations

Typically, retroflexion of the urinary bladder occurs in animals with a preexisting perineal hernia. Displacement is probably related to the increased intra-abdominal pressure normally associated with defecation (Valsalva's maneuver). Diagnostic keys include a sudden enlargement in the size of the hernia and, most importantly, an inability to urinate.

Major Radiographic Observations

Survey films fail to show a bladder shadow. When a visible hernia exists, it is enlarged but otherwise unchanged radiographically. *Contrast* examination (positive-contrast, retrograde cystography) shows the bladder (by virtue of its opacification) displaced into the perineal region (Fig. 81–1).

Diagnostic Strategy

Bladder retroflexion requires cystographic proof. This is most simply obtained by passing a small-caliber catheter into the bladder and injecting a small volume of iodinated contrast. The object is to identify the location of the bladder (marking study), and not to perform a complete cystographic analysis, unless it appears to be called for diagnostically. Al-ternatively, a Foley catheter may be inserted into the distal urethra, using the technique described. If catheterization fails and the location of the bladder is known, contrast medium may be injected transabdominally into the bladder or its suspected location. If the contrast does not reach the intended target, it will cause no side effects other than possibly to obscure the actual location of the bladder on a subsequent injection. A lateral view establishes the diagnosis, but not its laterality (right versus left). If none of these methods is successful, a low-dose urogram (1 ml per kilogram) should be done with similar objectives.

Pitfalls

Absence of a bladder shadow does not prove retroflexion.

Alternative Diagnoses

Bladder torsion.

Suggested Reading

Olsson S-E, ed. The radiological diagnosis in canine and feline emergencies. Philadelphia: Lea & Febiger, 1973:191.

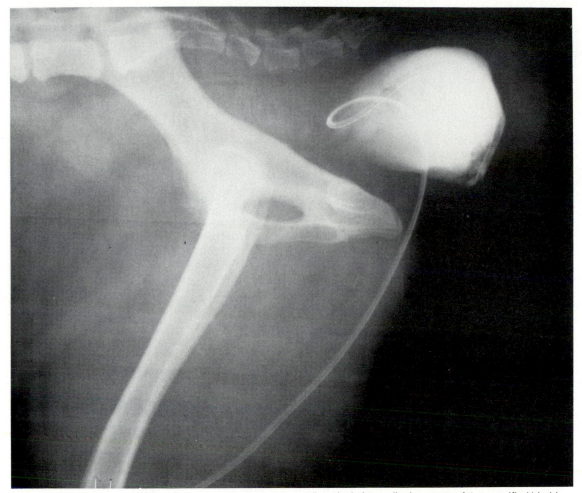

Figure 81–1 Lateral, positive-contrast, retrograde cystogram (in a dog) shows displacement of the opacified bladder and associated catheter to the perineal region. Diagnosis: retroflexion of the urinary bladder into a perineal hernia.

82

BLADDER STONES LEADING TO OBSTRUCTION

General Considerations

Bladder stones are an emergency when they obstruct the bladder or, more usually, the mid- or distal urethra. In the case of the midurethra, the obstruction is often functional, resulting from inflammatory hypertrophy of the bladder mucosa and/or proximal urethra. Straining and hemorrhage often accompany multiple large stones.

Major Radiographic Observations

Most *survey* films clearly show medium- to large-sized, radiodense urinary bladder stones (Fig. 82–1). Clustered small calculi are also readily detectable. Radiodense and radiolucent stones typically show as filling defects with cystography.

Diagnostic Strategy

Usually, standard abdominal films are sufficient, provided they include the entire caudal abdomen. When the bladder is obscured by a stool-filled colon, a lateral compression film made over the urinary tract clears the bladder field. Sand-like calculi, commonly found in cats, often are impossible to see. Postural radiographs (standing lateral patient position using a horizontal x-ray beam) are often useful in such cases.

Pitfalls

A urethral stone is more apt to cause obstruction than a bladder stone. Consequently, be certain to radiograph the entire urethra, especially the penile urethra in a male dog, even when multiple, large bladder stones are seen. Air bubbles often mimic calculi in cystograms; blood clots do so less often.

Alternative Diagnoses

Distal ureteral or proximal urethral stones, dystrophic calcification of the bladder wall.

Suggested Reading

McNeel SV. Urethral obstruction. In: Farrow CS, ed. Decision making in small animal radiology. Toronto: BC Decker, 1987:200.

Park RD. Radiology of the urinary bladder and urethra. In: O'Brien TR, ed. Radiographic diagnosis of abdominal disorders in the dog and the cat. Philadelphia: WB Saunders, 1978:610.

Park RD. The urinary bladder. In: Thrall DE, ed. Textbook of veterinary diagnostic radiology. Philadelphia: WB Saunders, 1986:435.

Stone EA. Canine urethral obstruction. In: Binnington AG, Cockshutt JR, eds. Decision making in small animal soft tissue surgery. Toronto: BC Decker, 1988:110.

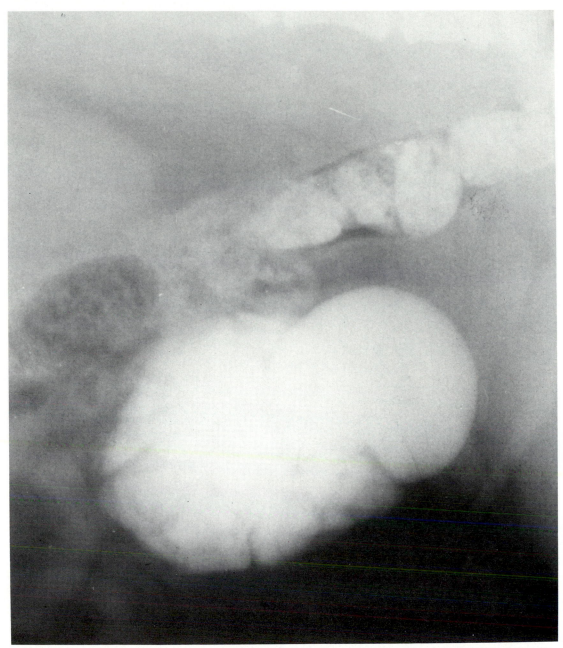

Figure 82–1 Lateral detail view of canine caudoventral abdomen shows multiple, large, closely packed densities in the bladder field. High-density stool is seen in the overlying colon. Diagnosis: bladder stones (this dog was completely obstructed when presented).

83

EMPHYSEMATOUS CYSTITIS

General Considerations

Although emphysematous cystitis has been reported as a side effect of diabetes mellitus, this has not been my experience. Rather, I have found the condition to be associated with isolated bacterial cystitis, often *Escherichia coli.* Because of the dissecting nature of the condition, complications such as mucosal slough and perforation may develop. Prevention of these possible problems constitutes the emergency nature of this condition.

Major Radiographic Observations

Survey films show varying amounts of gas in the urinary bladder, often arranged in a cylindrical fashion (Fig. 83–1).

Diagnostic Strategy

Emphysematous cystitis is not usually anticipated but is readily identified when gas is present in large volume. If there is a question about the presence of gas, remake the lateral view, centered over the bladder. Contrast studies are of little help and may do harm by irritating already damaged tissue, as well as by potentiating rupture by further distention.

Pitfalls

One or more overlying, gas-filled bowel loops may mimic bladder gas.

Alternative Diagnoses

Overlying bowel loops, previous catheterization, or cystography. Luminal involution of the bladder mucosa following air-contrast cystography.

Suggested Reading

Farrow CS. Intimal dissection and luminal involution secondary to double contrast cystography. Can Vet J 1981; 22:260–261.
Park RD. Radiology of the urinary bladder and urethra. In: O'Brien TR, ed. Radiographic diagnosis of abdominal disorders in the dog and the cat. Philadelphia: WB Saunders, 1978:583.

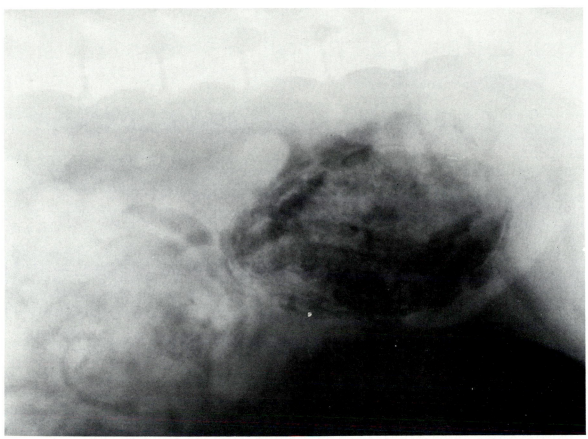

Figure 83–1   Lateral detail view of canine caudoventral abdomen shows horizontally oriented gas shadows in the bladder field. Diagnosis: emphysematous cystitis.

84

OBSTRUCTIVE BLADDER TUMOR

General Considerations

Most bladder tumors clinically resemble cystitis because of their associated hematuria, and they may be misdiagnosed accordingly. Some bladder-neck tumors may produce acute urinary-tract obstruction, often incorrectly attributed to urethral calculi. Both urethral calculi and trigonal neoplasia may prevent passage of a retrograde urethral catheter into the bladder, making differentiation on this basis impossible. Some calculi are not sufficiently dense to be detected radiographically, rendering a negative radiographic examination equivocal. When doubt exists about the cause of the obstruction, retrograde cystourethrography should be done.

Major Radiographic Observations

Survey films usually show nothing and are only of worth in ruling out conditions such as radiodense calculi. *Contrast* examination typically reveals a filling defect at or near the bladder neck (Fig. 84–1).

Diagnostic Strategy

Perform a retrograde cystourethrogram with the catheter as close to the bladder neck as possible; the approximate distance may be estimated by positioning the catheter above the animal prior to catheterization. Inject nondiluted, iodinated contrast medium (6 ml, plus whatever is required to fill the catheter), making the exposure *as the last milliliter of contrast is being injected*. Be especially sensitive to abnormally high injection pressure. If the pressure is excessive, reduce the force of injection and make the exposure, regardless of whether the entire dose has been given or not. Do not remove the catheter until the films have been checked. When there is doubt concerning validity of the radiographic findings, repeat the questionable view. Do not remove the catheter until the films have been checked for adequate quality.

Pitfalls

Cystourethrograms of bladder-neck tumors or other obstructive conditions made *following* injection of contrast medium are often less informative than films made *during* injection. This is because the contrast medium accumulates in the area of lowest pressure, usually away from the lesion.

Alternative Diagnoses

Urethral calculi or neoplasm, cystic calculi, severe prostatic disease.

Suggested Reading

McNeel SV. Urinary bladder neoplasia. In: Farrow CS, ed. Decision making in small animal radiology. Toronto: BC Decker, 1987:198.

Park RD. Radiology of the urinary bladder and urethra. In: O'Brien TR, ed. Radiographic diagnosis of abdominal disorders in the dog and the cat. Philadelphia: WB Saunders, 1978:585.

Park RD. The urinary bladder. In: Thrall DE, ed. Textbook of veterinary diagnostic radiology. Philadelphia: WB Saunders, 1986:435.

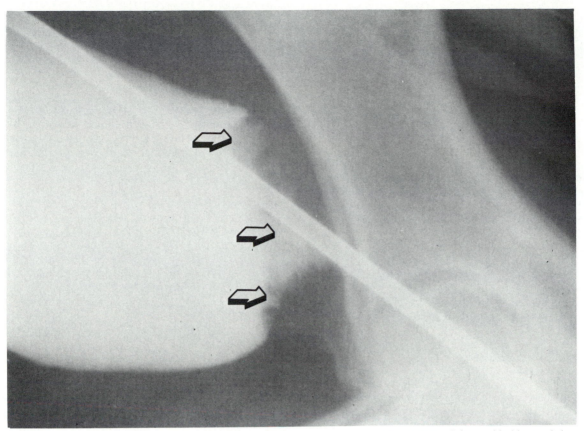

Figure 84–1 Lateral, positive-contrast, retrograde cystogram (in a dog) shows large filling defect at bladder neck (*arrows*). Diagnosis: bladder tumor (rhabdomyosarcoma).

85

UREMIA SECONDARY TO RENAL INSUFFICIENCY

General Considerations

Uremia may develop at different levels in the urinary tract and from assorted causes, some of which (such as small, misshapen kidneys) may be diagnosed or inferred radiographically. Although typically a chronic process, renal insufficiency may present as a variety of seemingly acute conditions such as heart failure, seizures, pancreatitis, or enteritis, based on the associated clinical signs of pulmonary edema, vomiting, and diarrhea.

Major Radiographic Observations

Variable, but usually bilaterally small, kidneys, often irregularly marginated (scarred) (Fig. 85–1).

Diagnostic Strategy

Survey films may reveal small kidneys, especially in the ventrodorsal view. If substantial weight loss exists, the appearance of perirenal fat can be reduced with a corresponding reduction in renal definition. Renal compression radiography usually overcomes this problem. A diagnostic view of the kidneys may be difficult to obtain in deep-chested, large- and giant-breed dogs. A *renal marking study* should be done in such cases, using high-dose urography (1,200 mg of iodine per kilogram). Ventrodorsal views, centered over the kidneys, with compression if possible, should be made at 10, 20, and 30 minutes or until the kidney has been visualized. If it is not seen within an hour, the study should be terminated.

Pitfalls

Renal scarring as determined radiographically by an irregular renal margin is typically underestimated.

Alternative Diagnoses

Pre- or postrenal uremia.

Suggested Reading

Biery DN. Upper urinary tract. In: O'Brien TR, ed. Radiographic diagnosis of abdominal disorders in the dog and the cat. Philadelphia: WB Saunders, 1978:481.

Feeney DA, Johnston GR. The kidneys and ureters. In: Thrall DE, ed. Textbook of veterinary diagnostic radiology. Philadelphia: WB Saunders, 1986:408.

McNeel SV. Small kidney. In: Farrow CS, ed. Decision making in small animal radiology. Toronto: BC Decker, 1987:190.

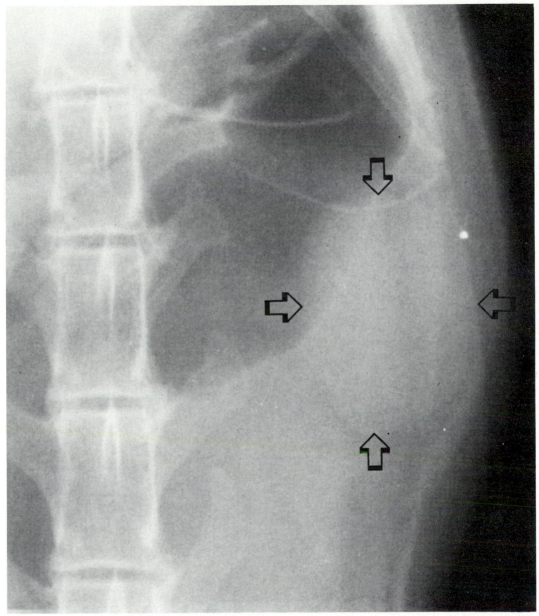

Figure 85–1 Ventrodorsal compression study of feline left cranial abdomen shows small kidney (*arrows*). Diagnosis: chronic nephritis (resulting in renal failure and uremia).

THE PROSTATE

86

PROSTATIC ABSCESS

General Considerations

Prostatitis often follows cystic hypertrophy, in some instances leading to abscessation. Large abscesses may compress the colon and/or the urethra, resulting in the animal's reluctance to defecate or urinate. Prostatitis is often very painful and may affect the animal's posture and gait, which are typically hump-backed and short strided. Many, but not all, patients show marked discomfort when palpated rectally. Owners often present such individuals because of difficulty, pain, and bleeding when urinating. Occasionally, prostatic abscesses may rupture into the abdomen causing peritonitis.

Major Radiographic Observations

Survey radiographs usually show marked prostatomegaly. Cystourethrography typically reveals a cranially displaced urinary bladder associated with a narrowed, stretched urethra (Fig. 86–1).

Diagnostic Strategy

A lateral abdominal survey film usually shows an obviously large prostate, increased density in the prostatic field, or indirect evidence of prostatomegaly such as dorsal displacement of the colon. Presumptive evidence of prostatic enlargement, in the form of a double-bladder sign, is frequently seen. A lateral compression view of the prostatic field is also useful. When uncertainty exists, retrograde cystourethrography should be done. The catheter should be placed as close to the anticipated location of the prostate as pos-

sible, then 6 ml of iodinated contrast medium should be injected. The radiographic exposure should be made during the final part of the injection. A lateral projection is best, with other views as necessary.

Pitfalls

A large prostatic abscess may be mistaken for a normal urinary bladder. When a double-bladder sign is observed, it cannot be assumed that the cranialmost shadow represents the urinary bladder, because large prostatic cysts and occasional abscesses may locate cranial to the bladder.

Alternative Diagnoses

Advanced cystic hyperplasia, prostatic cancer, paraprostatic cyst.

Suggested Reading

Bartels JE. Radiology of the genital tract. In: O'Brien TR, ed. Radiographic diagnosis of abdominal disorders in the dog and the cat. Philadelphia: WB Saunders, 1978:647.

Buckrell BC. Prostatic disease. In: Binnington AG, Cockshutt JR, eds. Decision making in small animal soft tissue surgery. Toronto: BC Decker, 1988:134.

Lattimer JC. The prostate. In: Thrall DE, ed. Textbook of veterinary diagnostic radiology. Philadelphia: WB Saunders, 1986:446.

McNeel SV. Enlarged prostate. In: Farrow CS, ed. Decision making in small animal radiology. Toronto: BC Decker, 1987:202.

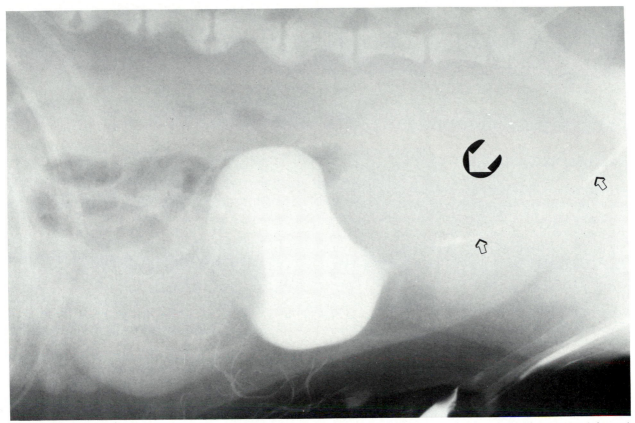

Figure 86–1 Lateral retrograde cystogram (detail view) shows enlarged prostate (*large arrow*); cranially displaced or deformed urinary bladder; and elongated, narrowed urethra (*small arrows*). The mass cranial to the bladder is an unrelated granuloma. Diagnosis: prostatic abscess.

87

RUPTURED PROSTATE PRODUCING PERITONITIS

General Considerations

Occasionally, prostatic abscesses rupture, leading to peritonitis. Little is known about why some abscesses rupture and others do not. Because few are associated with observed trauma, it is assumed that necrosis and internal pressure are the principal causes. Theoretically, the larger the abscess, the more likely it is to perforate. Affected individuals show signs typical of peritonitis: obvious illness, abdominal pain, and various positions of protection such as an arched back or tucked-up abdomen. The condition is often fatal.

Major Radiographic Observations

Survey radiographs are usually dominated by the signs of peritonitis: reduced visceral detail and a generalized increase in abdominal density. In spite of poor organ visibility, it is sometimes possible to detect increased density in the prostatic field, suggesting prostatic involvement (Fig. 87–1). Retrograde cystourethrography is usually unsuccessful in detecting the leakage site, although it may incriminate the prostate.

Diagnostic Strategy

Rely on high-quality survey radiographs and clinical acumen. Abdominocentesis is helpful, but it is often equivocal in early cases.

Pitfalls

A large urinary bladder may be mistaken for prostatomegaly.

Alternative Diagnoses

Other causes of peritonitis.

Suggested Reading

Bartels JE. Radiology of the genital tract. In: O'Brien TR, ed. Radiographic diagnosis of abdominal disorders in the dog and the cat. Philadelphia: WB Saunders, 1978:647.

Lattimer JC. The prostate. In: Thrall DE, ed. Textbook of veterinary diagnostic radiology. Philadelphia: WB Saunders, 1986:446.

Mathews KA. Septic peritonitis. In: Binnington AG, Cockshutt JR, eds. Decision making in small animal soft tissue surgery. Toronto: BC Decker, 1988:210.

Olsson S-E, ed. The radiological diagnosis in canine and feline emergencies. Philadelphia: Lea & Febiger, 1973:179.

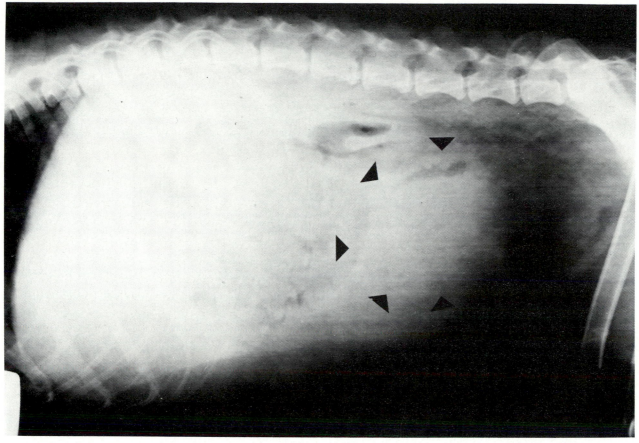

Figure 87–1 Lateral view of canine abdomen shows ill-defined caudoventral abdominal mass (arrows) against a background of increased abdominal density and decreased visceral detail. Diagnosis: prostatic abscess leading to peritonitis.

88

PROSTATIC TUMOR

General Considerations

Prostatic tumors that cause clinical signs are relatively rare compared with prostatitis, cystic hyperplasia, and paraprostatic cysts. Most such tumors are discovered incidentally during postmortem examination. Occasionally, prostatic tumors become large enough to constrict or stretch the contained urethra, producing partial or complete obstruction. The prostate is usually incriminated on the basis of a palpable enlargement found on physical examination, although it is not possible to confirm an etiology on this basis.

Major Radiographic Observations

Survey radiographs often show prostatomegaly: however, this is a nonspecific finding with regard to both etiology and urethral influence. Retrograde cystourethrography typically reveals cranial displacement of the urinary bladder with narrowing and elongation of the associated urethra (Fig. 88–1).

Diagnostic Strategy

Urethral narrowing, to the extent that it may explain lower urinary-tract obstruction, is best demonstrated by retrograde cystourethrography. The catheter should be advanced as far into the urethra as possible without excessive force. Iodinated contrast should then be injected, with the exposure made just before completion of the injection. A lateral view usually is sufficient.

Pitfalls

Reflux of the contrast medium is a nonspecific finding, indicating only enlargement of the prostatic ducts.

Alternative Diagnoses

Advanced cystic hyperplasia, prostatic cancer, paraprostatic cyst.

Suggested Reading

Bartels JE. Radiology of the genital tract. In: O'Brien TR, ed. Radiographic diagnosis of abdominal disorders in the dog and the cat. Philadelphia: WB Saunders, 1978:647.

Lattimer JC. The prostate. In: Thrall DE, ed. Textbook of veterinary diagnostic radiology. Philadelphia: WB Saunders, 1986:447.

McNeel SV. Enlarged prostate. In: Farrow CS, ed. Decision making in small animal radiology. Toronto: BC Decker, 1987:202.

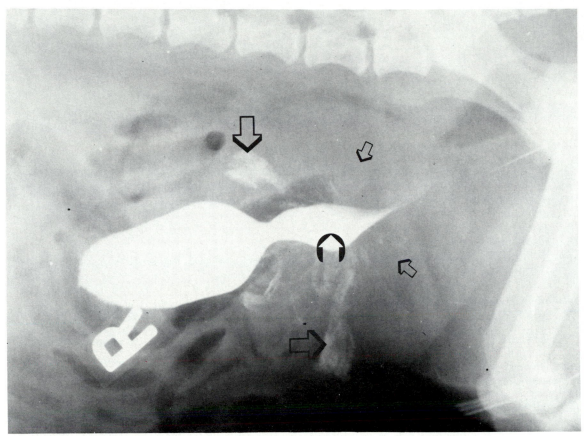

Figure 88–1   Lateral retrograde cystogram (detail view) shows enlarged prostate (*small arrows*), dilated central prostatic urethra (*medium arrow*), contrast medium within dilated-distorted prostatic ducts (*large arrows*), and cranial displacement of the urinary bladder. Diagnosis: prostatic tumor (adenocarcinoma).

THE UTERUS

89
DYSTOCIA

General Considerations

Dystocia may be classified as mechanical or functional. In *mechanical* dystocia, the fetus may be abnormally positioned so that passage through the birth canal is impossible. Alternatively, the fetus may be oversized and simply too large to pass through the pelvic inlet. Extrinsic obstruction may result from a previous pelvic fracture that secondarily has narrowed the birth canal. *Functional* dystocia is caused by a physiologic disturbance in the birthing mechanism.

Major Radiographic Observations

A mature fetus is seen malpositioned or malpresented at or near the pelvic inlet, or within the pelvic canal (Fig. 89–1). Alternatively, a disproportionately large fetus is seen at or partially within the birth canal. In the latter instance, the diameter of the fetal skull is larger than the diameter of the maternal pelvis. A deformed pelvis may be present as a result of prior injury or nutritional or metabolic disease (Fig. 89–2).

Diagnostic Strategy

Obtain lateral and ventrodorsal views of the entire abdomen, *including the entire pelvis*. Compare the transverse diameter of the fetal skull to the transverse diameter of the maternal pelvic canal centrally; the later should be larger. If not, dystocia is likely.

Pitfalls

Oblique views of the pelvis may simulate narrowing of the pelvic canal.

Alternative Diagnoses

Functional dystocia, fetal death.

Suggested Reading

Bartels JE. Radiology of the genital tract. In: O'Brien TR, ed. Radiographic diagnosis of abdominal disorders in the dog and the cat. Philadelphia: WB Saunders, 1978:637.

Buckrell BC. Canine dystocia. In: Binnington AG, Cockshutt JR, eds. Decision making in small animal soft tissue surgery. Toronto: BC Decker, 1988:126.

Farrow CS. Maternal-fetal evaluation in suspected canine dystocia. Can Vet J 1978; 19:24–26.

Feeney DA, Johnston GR. The uterus. In: Thrall DE, ed. Textbook of veterinary diagnostic radiology. Philadelphia: WB Saunders, 1986:458.

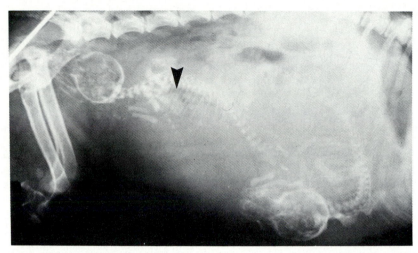

Figure 89-1 Lateral view of canine abdomen shows two fetuses, the more caudal of which is in an abnormal birth position (anterior presentation, dorsopubic position); the skull is located in the proximal part of the birth canal (*arrow*). Diagnosis: mechanical dystocia.

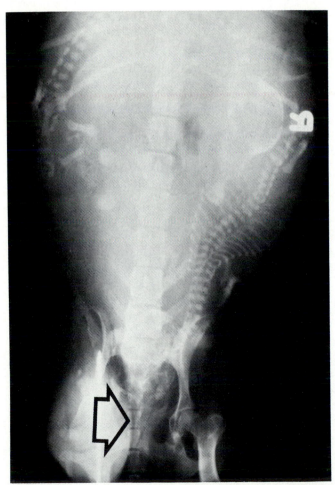

Figure 89-2 Ventrodorsal view of feline abdomen shows four fetuses; the head of one (*arrow*) is lodged in the cranial part of the pelvis, unable to pass further because of pelvic narrowing secondary to previous fractures. Diagnosis: mechanical dystocia.

90

LATE-TERM FETAL DEATH

General Considerations

Fetal death may be classified as early- or late-term, depending on the time of fetal death relative to the gestation period. In *early-term* fetal death, the fetus is in various stages of decomposition, depending on when death occurred and when the mother is radiographed. The radiographic alterations are usually obvious. Often the dog is very ill. Conversely, *late-term* fetal death is associated with relatively subtle radiographic and clinical signs.

Major Radiographic Observations

Early-term fetal death, depending on the length of time between its occurrence and presentation, may be associated with cranial collapse, skeletal deformity/disarticulation or mummification, and large volumes of intrafetal/extrafetal gas. *Late-term* fetal death, also depending on duration relative to presentation may show overlapping cranial bones, abnormal (often curled), fetal position and small volumes of intrafetal gas (Fig. 90–1).

Diagnostic Strategy

Establishing fetal viability requires high-quality radiographs, ideally centered over the fetus(es) in question. When fetal visibility is poor owing to suboptimal position, overlying tissues, other fetuses, or stool, compression radiography should be performed. Late-term fetal death requires compression in a majority of cases. If sonography is available, it may be used to identify whether or not a fetal heartbeat is present.

Pitfalls

The fetal skull normally molds as it passes through the birth canal; however, although the frontal and parietal bones may become more closely approximated, they should not overlap.

Alternative Diagnoses

Functional or mechanical dystocia.

Suggested Reading

Farrow CS. Late-term fetal death in the dog. Early radiographic diagnosis. Vet Rad 1976; 17:11–17.

Feeney DA, Johnston GR. The uterus. In: Thrall DE, ed. Textbook of veterinary diagnostic radiology. Philadelphia: WB Saunders, 1986:461.

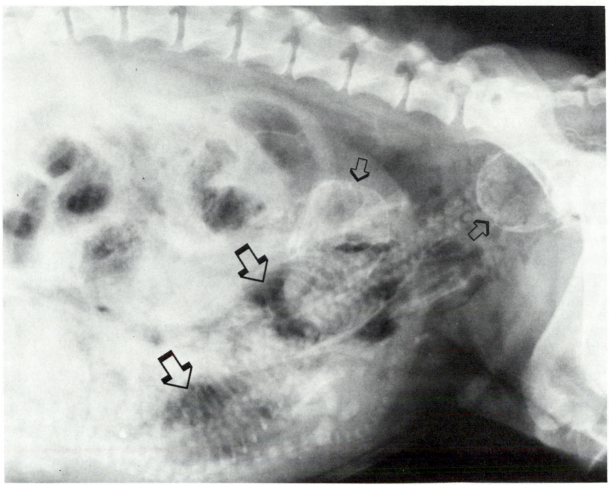

Figure 90–1   Lateral view of caudal canine abdomen shows multiple term fetuses, intrafetal gas (*large arrows*), and overlapping cranial bones (*small arrows*). Diagnosis: late-term fetal death.

91

PYOMETRA

General Considerations

Advanced pyometra typically produces gross uterine enlargement with variable degrees of associated illness. Early pyometra may be clinically occult. Hematologic and biochemical data are often equivocal. Consequently, the presumptive clinical diagnosis is often made on circumstantial evidence, followed by radiologic confirmation.

Major Radiographic Observations

Multiple tubular or spherical shadows located in the caudal and midabdomen create mass effect(s) that displace the adjacent bowel into the cranial abdomen, thereby resulting in an abnormal bowel-distribution pattern (Fig. 91–1). Less advanced cases may only show a tubular, bowel-like shadow midway between the colon and bladder, on the lateral view made with compression.

Diagnostic Strategy

The mass effect created by an advanced pyometra and the resulting abnormal bowel-distribution pattern usually provide a clear-cut diagnosis. Less advanced cases are more difficult to confirm because of smaller uterine size; these often require compression radiography. This is best done with the patient in the lateral position and the x-ray beam centered over the midcaudal abdomen just in front of the hindlimb (which is drawn, without tension, caudally). Remember to remeasure the caudal abdomen with the compression paddle in place and to reset the radiographic technique accordingly. Sonography is diagnostic in most cases.

Caution: Although compression radiography has been shown to be a very safe procedure when performed by an experienced person, it must be done gently to avoid rupturing a turgid uterus or any other sensitive structure. Fortunately, such potentially vulnerable organs are usually obvious on noncompression films.

Pitfalls

A gravid uterus without fetal mineralization is impossible to distinguish from pyometra or any other condition resulting in uterine enlargement.

Alternative Diagnoses

Pregnancy, hydro-, muco-, and hemometra.

Suggested Reading

Bartels JE. Radiology of the genital tract. In: O'Brien TR, ed. Radiographic diagnosis of abdominal disorders in the dog and the cat. Philadelphia: WB Saunders, 1978:621.

Buckrell BC. Pyometra. In: Binnington AG, Cockshutt JR, eds. Decision making in small animal soft tissue surgery. Toronto: BC Decker, 1988:132.

Farrow CS. Abdominal compression radiography in the dog and the cat. JAAHA 1978; 14:337–342.

Feeney DA, Johnston GR. The uterus. In: Thrall DE, ed. Textbook of veterinary diagnostic radiology. Philadelphia: WB Saunders, 1986:458.

Root CR. Abdominal masses. In: Thrall DE, ed. Textbook of veterinary diagnostic radiology. Philadelphia: WB Saunders, 1986:458.

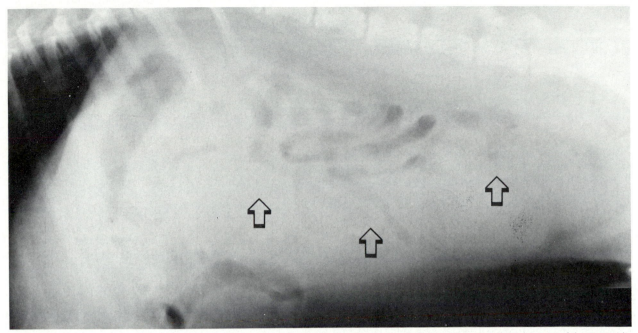

Figure 91-1　Lateral view of canine abdomen shows an abnormal bowel-distribution pattern and cranial displacement of the stomach as a result of a large caudal ventral mass effect (*arrows*). Diagnosis: pyometra.

92

NECROTIC PYOMETRITIS

General Considerations

Draining pyometra is usually treated by immediate ovario-hysterectomy, especially if the animal is quite ill. However, in some cases there is need to preserve reproductive capacity. Although the success of medical treatment is based on multiple factors, none is more important than the pretreatment condition of the uterus. Hysterography (contrast examination of the uterus), may be used in such instances to evaluate the inner surface of the uterus.

Major Radiographic Observations

Contrast examination shows a roughened, irregular endometrial lining with uneven density and luminal filling defects. Marginal scalloping is usually present (Fig. 92–1). *Survey* films are of no use in evaluating the uterine lining.

Diagnostic Strategy

A hysterogram may be made in two ways. The simplest method is to place a Foley catheter in the vagina, inflate the cuff, and inject a sufficient volume of contrast to fill the anticipated size of the uterus, or inject contrast until injection pressure becomes excessive. Alternatively, the uterus may be selectively catheterized by passing a rigid catheter through the cervix into the uterus, and proceeding as described.

Pitfalls

Marginal scalloping may occasionally be seen in the normal uterus, particularly post partum.

Alternative Diagnoses

Normal postpartum uterus, mucometria, hemometra.

Suggested Reading

Bartels JE. Radiology of the genital tract. In: O'Brien TR, ed. Radiographic diagnosis of abdominal disorders in the dog and the cat. Philadelphia: WB Saunders, 1978:628.

Feeney DA, Johnston GR. The uterus. In: Thrall DE, ed. Textbook of veterinary diagnostic radiology. Philadelphia: WB Saunders, 1986:459.

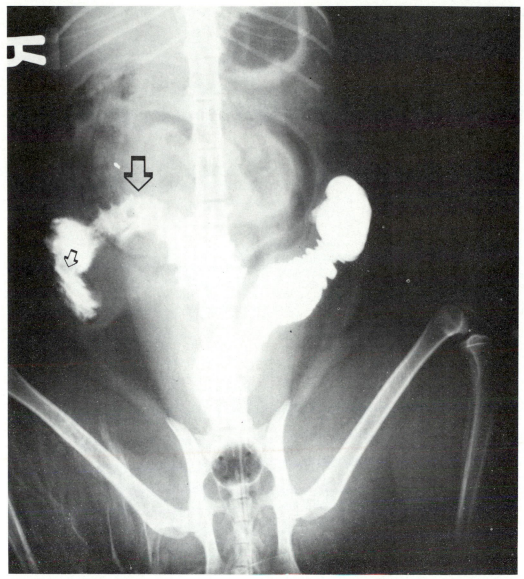

Figure 92–1 Positive-contrast hysterogram (ventrodorsal view in a cat) shows scalloped uterine margin (*large arrow*) and multiple filling defects (*small arrow*) in the right uterine horn. Diagnosis: necrotic pyometritis.

MISCELLANEOUS PROBLEMS

93

HEMORRHAGING LIVER TUMOR

General Considerations

The most common cause of generalized liver enlargement is probably fatty infiltration followed by neoplasia. Hemangiomas, hemangioendotheliomas, and hemangiosarcomas may hemorrhage, producing hypovolemic shock. This condition is usually the reason for emergency presentation. When the biliary system is obstructed, the resulting illness develops more gradually and is typically associated with icterus, depression, and anorexia. Lymphoid tumors of the liver are often associated with bilateral renomegaly.

Major Radiographic Observations

Generalized hepatomegaly is most evident by the associated caudal displacement of adjacent organs, including stomach, intestines, and spleen (Fig. 93–1). The liver margins may or may not be abnormally rounded. Extension of the liver beyond the ribs is variable, being influenced by the animal's age (older animals often have abdominal laxity that results in a relatively caudal liver position), and respiratory phase (liver is more caudally positioned in inspiration). When localized bleeding is present, the liver margins may be indistinct; a large-volume hemorrhage results in an increase in abdominal density with a corresponding reduction in organ visibility (Fig. 93–2).

Diagnostic Strategy

Measure the animal at the level of the caudal rib cage, thus assuring optimal penetration. Center the x-ray beam just behind the last rib, being certain to include the diaphragm. If there is a question of stomach displacement, give 10 ml of barium to mark its location (barium marking study).

Pitfalls

A predominantly fluid-filled stomach may mimic generalized hepatomegaly. An enlarged spleen that is closely approximated to the caudoventral border of the liver can resemble liver enlargement.

Alternative Diagnoses

Hepatic edema (congestion) secondary to right or combined right-left heart failure, ruptured hepatic abscess, liver–lobe torsion, traumatic liver fracture.

Suggested Reading

McNeel SV. Hepatomegaly. In: Farrow CS, ed. Decision making in small animal radiology. Toronto: BC Decker, 1987:176.

O'Brien TR, ed. Radiographic diagnosis of abdominal disorders in the dog and the cat. Philadelphia: WB Saunders, 1978:405.

Pechman RD. The liver and the spleen. In: Thrall DE, ed. Textbook of veterinary diagnostic radiology. Philadelphia: WB Saunders, 1986:392.

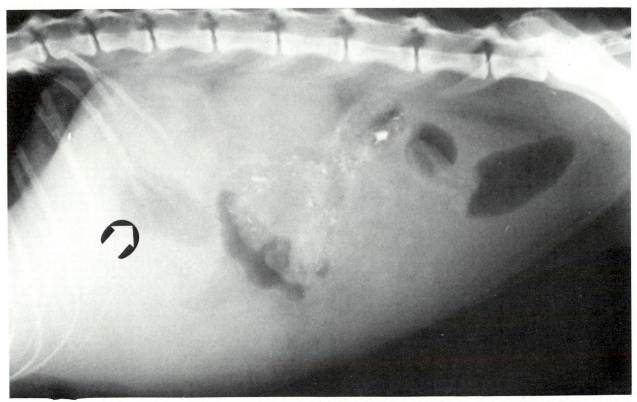

Figure 93–1 Lateral view of feline abdomen shows caudally displaced stomach, suggesting hepatomegaly (*arrow*); increased abdominal density; and decreased organ detail. Diagnosis: hemorrhaging liver tumor.

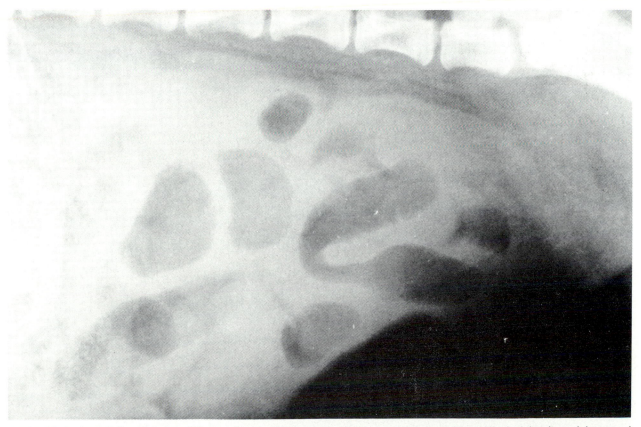

Figure 93–2 Lateral view of canine abdomen shows multiple gas filled bowel segments, increased abdominal density and decreased visceral detail. Diagnosis: massive abdominal hemorrhage secondary to multiple liver lobe fractures (following car accident).

HEMORRHAGING SPLENIC TUMOR

General Considerations

Splenic tumors are prone to rupture, with resulting hemorrhage. If blood loss is substantial it may produce collapse, which is often the reason for emergency presentation. In such cases, the animal shows signs of hemorrhagic shock, often with a readily palpable abdominal mass. Liver tumors may also bleed, but this is not as common.

Major Radiographic Observations

Splenic tumors typically appear as large circular masses in the midventral abdomen, as seen in lateral view (Fig. 94–1). The intestine is peripheralized by the mass, producing an abnormal bowel-distribution pattern. Then ventrodorsal appearance of a splenic mass varies according to its location. Enlargement of the splenic head produces right lateral displacement of the adjacent intestine; enlargement of the splenic tail produces right lateral displacement. Generalized splenic enlargement usually results in a proportionate increase in the size of the spleen, so that it appears more outstanding. Associated intestinal displacement is not as pronounced as with regional enlargement. Splenic bleeding results in an overall loss of visceral detail and a commensurate increase in abdominal density.

Diagnostic Strategy

The lateral view best demonstrates splenic lesions in large- and giant-breed dogs and is also less stressful on the animal, an important consideration when there is associated bleeding. Once the spleen has been identified as abnormal in lateral projection, a ventrodorsal view may be added as required.

Pitfalls

Older dogs often show splenic prominence in the lateral view, which is largely due to laxity of the abdominal musculature and the resulting caudoventral displacement (and therefore enhanced visibility) of the splenic shadow.

Alternative Diagnoses

Hemorrhage from a nonsplenic source (e.g., liver) with concomitant but unrelated splenomegaly, splenic torsion with hemorrhagic transudate, traumatic splenic fracture or avulsion.

Suggested Reading

McNeel SV. Generalized splenomegaly. In: Farrow CS, ed. Decision making in small animal radiology. Toronto: BC Decker, 1987:154.

McNeel SV. Focal splenic enlargement: radiologic identification. In: Farrow CS, ed. Decision making in small animal radiology. Toronto: BC Decker, 1987:156.

McNeel SV. Focal splenic enlargement: differential diagnosis. In: Farrow CS, ed. Decision making in small animal radiology. Toronto: BC Decker, 1987:158.

Olsson S-E, ed. The radiological diagnosis in canine and feline emergencies. Philadelphia: Lea & Febiger, 1973:134.

Root CR. Abdominal masses. In: Thrall DE, ed. Textbook of veterinary diagnostic radiology. Philadelphia: WB Saunders, 1986:363.

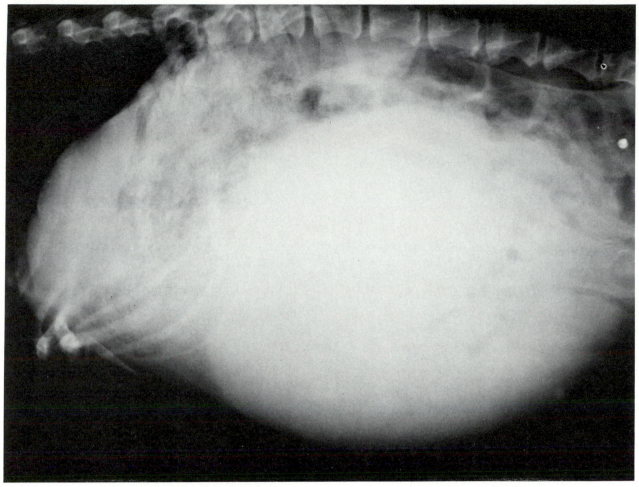

Figure 94–1 Lateral view of canine abdomen shows large central mass and poor abdominal detail. Diagnosis: hemorrhaging splenic tumor.

PANCREATITIS SECONDARY TO PENETRATING FOREIGN BODY

General Considerations

Small gastric or intestinal foreign bodies are often considered incidental findings when identified on abdominal radiographs. This is especially true in dogs, in which asymptomatic intestinal foreign bodies are not unusual. Occasionally such objects, although in proximity to the intestine, actually lie in an adjacent abdominal organ such as the liver, spleen, or pancreas, with or without regional or generalized peritonitis. Localizing signs are often absent except in the pancreas, which frequently shows signs and chemistries typical of acute pancreatitis.

Major Radiographic Observations

Typically, a lateral abdominal radiograph shows a needle superimposed upon, or immediately caudal to, the ventral half of the stomach (Fig. 95–1). Ventrodorsal films are quite variable, largely due to differences in centering the beam. A barium marking study shows contrast within the stomach; the foreign body appears extraluminal, and therefore is not gastric.

Diagnostic Strategy

Rarities like pancreatic foreign bodies are not usually considered in routine differentials unless they have been recently encountered. Consequently, they are most apt to be found on survey abdominal radiography. Precise anatomic localization may be difficult or impossible. Compression radiography, centered over the suspect foreign body, often clarifies a questionable location. A postural film (standing lateral position, made with a horizontal x-ray beam) usually separates gastric from other surrounding locations. A gastric marking study (small-volume barium study used to identify the location of an organ) separates gastric from nongastric locations.

Pitfalls

The observed foreign body may be superimposed on but not actually within the pancreas.

Alternative Diagnoses

Pancreatic disease is unrelated to the observed foreign body.

Suggested Reading

Olsson S-E, ed. The radiological diagnosis in canine and feline emergencies. Philadelphia: Lea & Febiger, 1973:144, 147.
Seim HB III. Pancreatitis. In: Binnington AG, Cockshutt JR, eds. Decision making in small animal soft tissue surgery. Toronto: BC Decker, 1988:60.

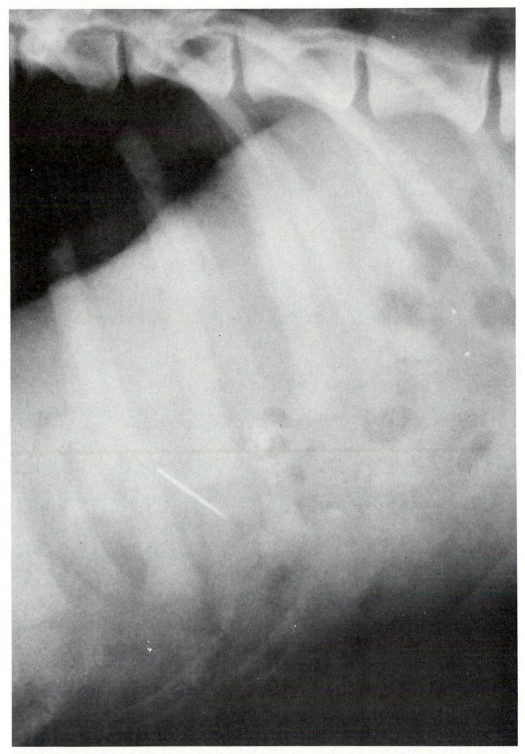

Figure 95–1 Detailed lateral view of canine cranioventral abdomen shows metallic foreign body (needle fragment) midway between stomach and sternum. The surrounding abdomen is indistinct. Diagnosis: pancreatic foreign body secondary to duodenal perforation with localized peritonitis.

III

The Skeleton

THE SKULL

96
DENTAL FRACTURE

General Considerations

Dental fractures are often associated with jaw injuries. Those occurring beyond the gum line are usually obvious when the mouth is examined; however, subgingival injuries, particularly fractures of the tooth roots, may escape visual detection. Hairline fractures of the dental crown or root are also difficult to appreciate grossly. Varying degrees of malocclusion may be seen with displaced dental fractures as well as with mandibular and maxillary injuries. Osteomyelitis secondary to an abscessed tooth root, especially the fourth upper premolar (carnassial tooth), may abruptly begin to drain through a skin sinus located cranial to the eye on the dorsal surface of the nasal bone. Occasionally teeth are chipped or split when dogs chew on hard objects; such injuries may be unnoticed until they become infected and affect the animal's eating. Rarely, a canine tooth may be traumatically repelled into the rostral part of the nasal cavity, with identification only possible on a radiograph. Alveolar fractures may occur without associated dental injury and may lead to dental disease through secondary devascularization or infection of the involved tooth.

Major Radiographic Observations

Dental fractures may be detected in a number of ways: a fracture line, deformity, defect, displacement or malocclusion (Figs. 96–1 to 96–3). When inferential evidence is used, the abnormality must be present in at least two views to reduce the likelihood of diagnostic error resulting from position-related anatomic distortion (see Fig. 96–1).

Diagnostic Strategy

All but the most clinically obvious dental injuries require multiple radiographic projections for proper assessment. Required views include dorsoventral or ventrodorsal (depending on the location and nature of the injury), lateral, and right and left lateral obliques; the oblique projections are made with the mouth open. Intraoral views, preferably using non-screen film, may be added as required. When diagnostic uncertainty exists, a comparable view of the opposite side should be made. This method of verifying a suspected lesion is superior to a textbook comparison because it eliminates the variables of age, breed, individual variation, and wear. Individual labeling of the right and left sides of the mandible reduces potential confusion. Anesthesia is required for optimal film quality.

Pitfalls

Anatomical distortion, common in oblique projections, may mimic fracture. Superimposition of one dental arcade over another, especially in the lateral view, may conceal a fracture. The middle mental foramen of the mandible, often seen in lateral projection as a poorly circumscribed radiolucency at the base of the canine tooth, may be mistaken for a fracture, infection, or tumor, depending on the clinical circumstances.

Alternative Diagnoses

Mandibular or maxillary fracture, dental infection, and immunomyositis.

Suggested Reading

Burk RL, Ackerman N. The skull. In: Burk RL, Ackerman N, ed. Small animal radiology. New York: Churchill Livingstone, 1986:339.

Owens JM. The teeth. In: Owens JM, ed. Radiographic interpretation for the small animal clinician. Saint Louis: Ralston Purina Co, 1982:65.

Zontine WJ. Dental radiographic technique and interpretation. Vet Clin North Am 1974; 4:760.

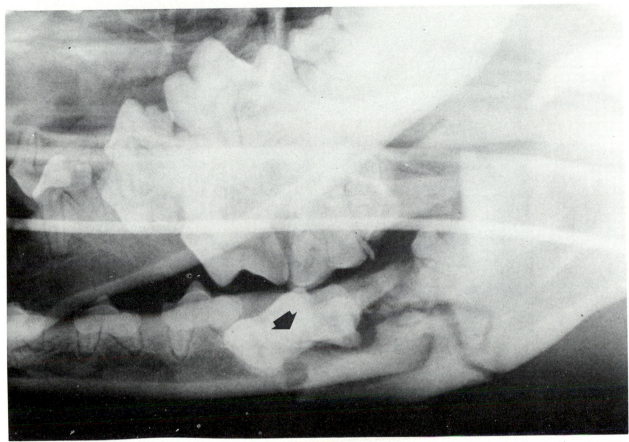

Figure 96–1 Lateral oblique view of canine mandibular dentition shows dislocation of the first molar (*arrow*) secondary to a comminuted mandibular fracture. Diagnosis: dental dislocation secondary to mandibular fracture.

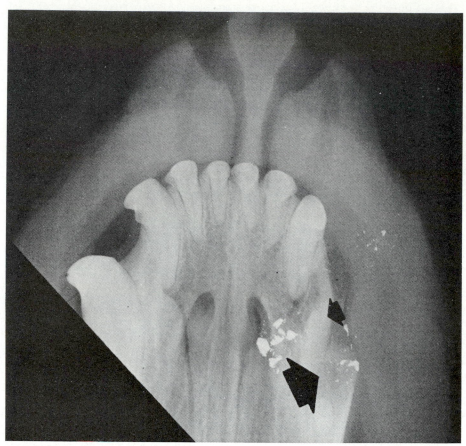

Figure 96–2 Intraoral, dorsal 20 degree rostral-ventrocaudal oblique view of canine maxillary incisor and canine teeth shows absence of left canine tooth (*large arrow*) and part of the adjacent maxilla (*small arrow*), and multiple lead fragments. Diagnosis: dental loss following gunshot injury.

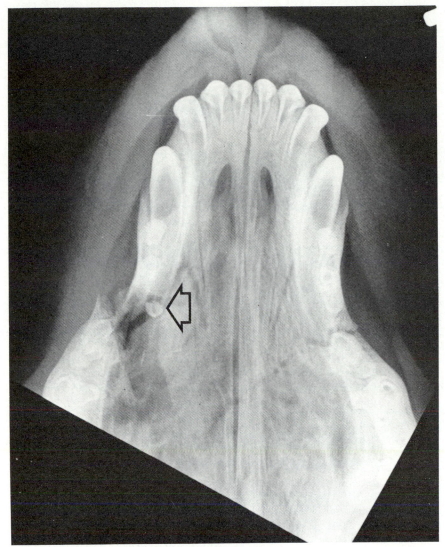

Figure 96–3 Open-mouth, ventral 20 degree rostral-dorsocaudal oblique view of canine maxillary dentition and nasal cavity shows comminuted nasomaxillary fractures and fracture-partial dislocation of the right second premolar tooth (*arrow*). Diagnosis: dental fracture-dislocation secondary to multiple facial fractures.

97

DENTAL INFECTION

General Considerations

Dental abscesses most often involve the tooth roots, resulting in localized or regional bone destruction and in the advanced stages, of the roots themselves. When bone loss occurs proximally, it is termed a *periapical abscess*. Occasionally, abscessed teeth result in an infraorbital draining sinus that may be mistaken for a bite wound. A subtotal dental extraction or fracture in which a root is inadvertently left behind or sequestered may evoke a foreign-body reaction, including sinus formation and associated drainage. Dental infections, although they usually develop gradually, may result in acute pain and in this regard may be viewed as emergencies. Affected animals may paw the face, eat abnormally, and resent oral examination. In animals with extensive periodontal disease and gingival hyperplasia, it may be very difficult, without the aid of radiology, to determine which tooth or teeth are responsible for the associated clinical signs.

Major Radiographic Observations

Bone loss is the hallmark of dental infection. It may be localized to the proximal part of the root as in periapical abscessation, or it may surround the entire tooth, as with sequestration (Figs. 97–1 and 97–2). With the accumulation and eventual drainage of associated pus, an opening often forms between the infected tooth and the bone surface. Typically this channel or cloaca is distinctly radiolucent, and it is frequently surrounded by denser than normal bone as a result of attempted osseous repair. There is usually additional periosteal new bone deposition on the related jaw surface, plus variable amounts of soft-tissue swelling.

Diagnostic Strategy

Make at least four views centering on the suspected tooth: ventrodorsal, lateral, and right and left lateral obliques. Make the oblique views to obtain the best profile of the lesion, being careful to make the contralateral comparison in a similar fashion. If there is drainage, place a small lead marker on the associated opening for the purpose of subsequent radiographic localization. The keys to the consistent and accurate diagnosis of both subtle and obvious dental infections are high-quality images and comparison films of the opposite, unaffected teeth. Diagnostic images must simultaneously isolate the affected tooth with a minimum of superimposition from surrounding teeth, provide a detailed image of related trabecular bone, and avoid unnecessary geometric distortion associated with excessive obliquity of the jaw (see Figs. 97–1 and 97–2). Comparable contralateral views are necessary to overcome the problems associated with nonstandard positioning, age-related dental and bone changes, and individual or breed differences. Individual labeling of the right and left sides of the mandible is best for oblique views. Anesthesia is required for optimal film quality.

Pitfalls

Dental distortion resulting from excessive obliquity, dental superimposition arising from insufficient obliquity, and the apparent loss of bone associated with the projection of a normal tooth upon an area of relatively lower density in the surrounding bone may all result in false-positive diagnoses.

Alternative Diagnoses

Dental fracture, aggravated gingival or periodontal disease; oral foreign body; acute tonsilitis or pharyngitis.

Suggested Reading

Burk RL, Ackerman N. The skull. In: Burk RL, Ackerman N, eds. Small animal radiology. New York: Churchill Livingstone, 1986:335.

Meyer W. The cranial vault and associated structures. In: Thrall DE, ed. Textbook of veterinary diagnostic radioiogy. Philadelphia: WB Saunders, 1986:29.

Owens JM. The teeth. In: Owens JM, ed. Radiographic interpretation for the small animal clinician. Saint Louis: Ralston Purina Co, 1982:65.

Watrous BJ. Dental disease: Apical abscess. In: Farrow CS, ed. Decision making in small animal radiology. Toronto: BC Decker, 1987:52.

Zontine WJ. Dental radiographic technique and interpretation. Vet Clin North Am [Small Anim Pract] 1974; 4:753.

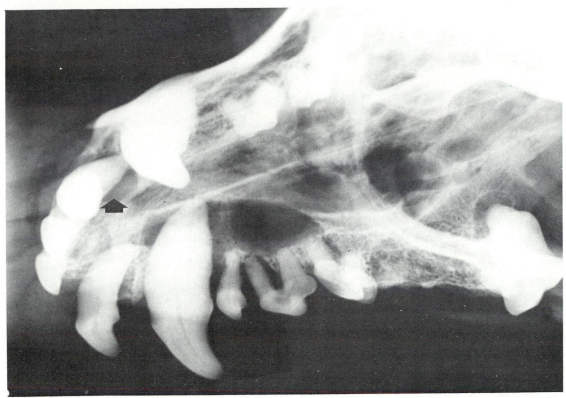

Figure 97–1   Lateral oblique view of canine maxillary dentition shows severe lysis around the uppermost third incisor (*arrow*). Diagnosis: dental infection.

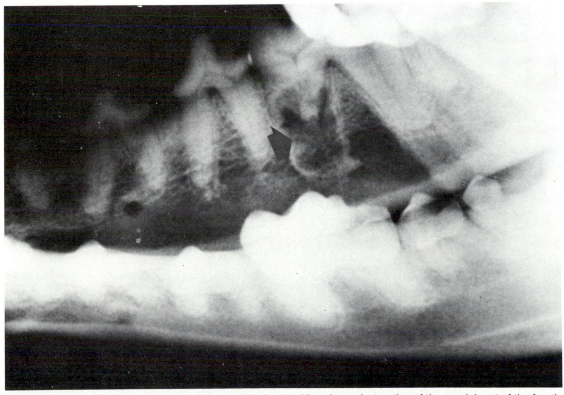

Figure 97–2   Lateral oblique view of canine mandibular dentition shows destruction of the cranial root of the fourth premolar (*arrow*). Diagnosis: dental infection.

98

MANDIBULAR FRACTURE

General Considerations

Mandibular fractures may involve the symphysis, vertical ramus, horizontal ramus, or temporomandibular joint, with one or both sides being affected. Fragment displacement is a function of both the severity and the location of the injury. For example, most fractures of the vertical ramus usually show only mild fragment separation because of the support of the surrounding musculature; conversely, fractures of the rostral mandible are often associated with severe malocclusion and jaw deformity. Temporomandibular injuries are particularly problematic because they often result in arthritis and associated jaw dysfunction. Not all mandibular fractures require surgical treatment. However, for those that do, sustained fragment reduction may be difficult to achieve, especially in smaller breeds. Delayed unions, nonunions, and secondary infections may develop as a result. Intraoral splints in dogs and extraoral splints in cats, secured to the adjacent teeth with wire, may provide an alternative to surgical implants in selected cases.

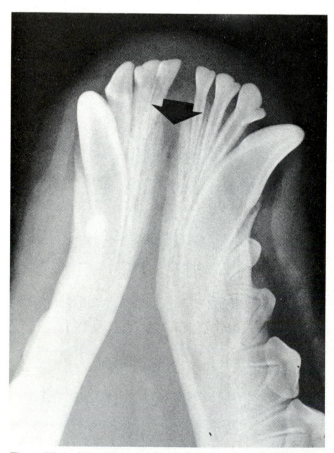

Figure 98–1 Intraoral, ventrodorsal view of canine mandible shows displaced symphyseal fracture (*arrow*). Diagnosis: symphyseal fracture.

Major Radiographic Observations

Bony discontinuity, when evident, is the most obvious sign of mandibular fracture (Figs. 98–1 to 98–4). Asymmetry between the right and left halves of the mandible (not resulting from nonstandard positioning) constitutes inferential evidence of fracture or symphyseal separation. Malocclusion may also be associated with such injuries, as well as with fractures of the temporomandibular joint. Nonfracture dislocations (second- and third-degree sprains) of the temporomandibular joint may also be associated with malocclusion.

Diagnostic Strategy

Four views should be made in cases of suspected mandibular fracture: dorsoventral (or ventrodorsal, depending on the nature of the injury), lateral, and right and left lateral obliques. The lateral oblique views should be double labeled (both sides of the mandible marked with the appropriate right or left lead markers) to avoid diagnostic confusion. An intraoral ventrodorsal view best shows symphyseal fractures, especially if they are only slightly displaced. Sedation or anesthesia is required. Anesthesia is required for optimal quality.

Pitfalls

The mandibular vascular canal may mimic a longitudinal fracture of the horizontal ramus. Following surgical stabilization, the vascular canal may resemble regional osteomyelitis.

Alternative Diagnoses

Contusion, cellulitis, retrobulbar abscess, immunomyositis, dental fracture, or infection.

Suggested Reading

Burk RL, Ackerman N. The skull. In: Burk RL, Ackerman N, eds. Small animal radiology. New York: Churchill Livingstone, 1986:332.

Kealy JK. The skull and vertebral column. In: Kealy JK, ed. Diagnostic radiology of the dog and cat. 2nd ed. Philadelphia: WB Saunders, 1987:446.

Leighton RL, Robinson GW. Orthopedic surgery. In: Holzworth J, ed. Diseases of the cat. Philadelphia: WB Saunders, 1987:134.

Meyer W. The cranial vault and associated structures. In: Thrall DE, ed. Textbook of veterinary diagnostic radiology. Philadelphia: WB Saunders, 1986:24.

Nunamaker DM. Fractures and dislocations of the mandible. In: Newton CD, Nunamaker DM, eds. Textbook of small animal orthopedics. Philadelphia: JB Lippincott, 1985:297.

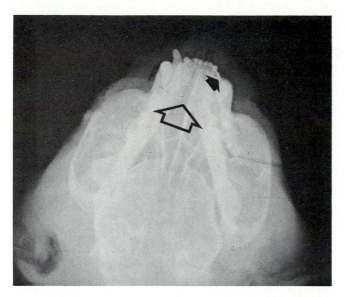

Figure 98–2 Ventrodorsal view of feline skull shows displaced symphyseal fracture (*large arrow*) and loss of left mandibular canine tooth (*small arrow*). Diagnosis: symphyseal fracture.

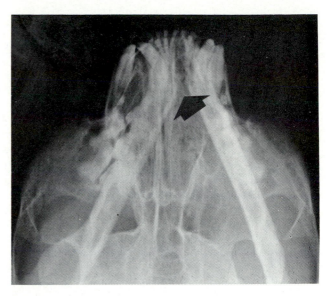

Figure 98–3 Ventrodorsal view of feline face and jaws shows displaced symphyseal fracture (*arrow*). Diagnosis: symphyseal fracture.

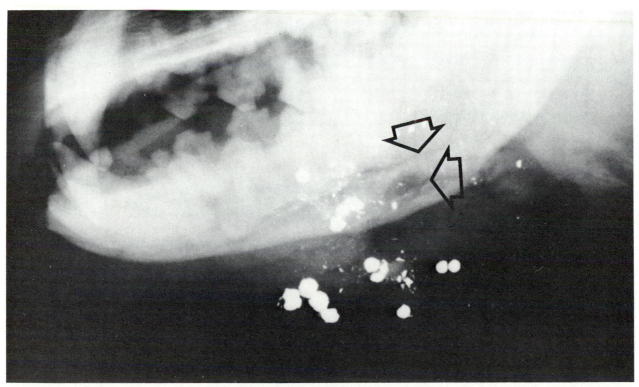

Figure 98–4 Lateral oblique view of canine mandible shows comminuted mandibular fracture (*arrows*), lead shot, gas pockets, and soft-tissue swelling. Diagnosis: compound, mandibular gunshot fracture.

99
TEMPOROMANDIBULAR JOINT FRACTURES AND DISLOCATIONS

General Considerations

Fractures and dislocations of the temporomandibular joint (TMJ) occur commonly in cats and occasionally in dogs. The lower incidence in dogs is probably due to relatively stronger bones and a larger surrounding muscle mass. Untreated or unsuccessfully treated TMJ injuries may result in nonunion, arthritis, reduced jaw motion, malocclusion, and regional muscular atrophy. Condylectomy is often the only alternative for chronic TMJ disorders. Sprain and meniscal injuries also affect the TMJ, although they are often missed for lack of diagnostic consideration.

Major Radiographic Observations

Subluxations of the TMJ are associated with an increased joint width (Fig. 99–1); complete dislocations may be associated with either increased joint width or loss of joint space caused by superimposition of the condyloid process on the glenoid cavity (Figs. 99–2 and 99–3). The assessment of the TMJ is often inconclusive because of its anatomical complexity and the difficulty in isolating it radiographically. Fractures, with or without dislocation, may be equally difficult to diagnose. Like other suspected fractures, a clear fracture line or fragment best confirms the diagnosis. Comparison with an unaffected opposite side should be made in questionable cases.

Diagnostic Strategy

The extended ventrodorsal and lateral oblique views best identify TMJ injury. The lateral radiograph usually contributes little because of the superimposition of one TMJ upon the other. A traction-stress, extended ventrodorsal view often reveals TMJ subluxation not seen in any other projection. A comparable view of the opposite side should be made routinely if one does not regularly read TMJ studies. Such comparison speeds diagnosis greatly by eliminating lengthy consideration of what is normal; it is superior to a radiographic atlas, which rarely contains a picture of the same breed

in the same position. Anesthesia is required for optimal quality.

Pitfalls

Because of its shape and position in the skull, the TMJ is difficult to project without some degree of distortion. Such distortion may resemble fracture or dislocation. When using the opposite TMJ for comparison, be sure it is clinically normal first; otherwise, you may be comparing one abnormal finding with another and falsely conclude that because both are similar, they are therefore normal.

Alternative Diagnoses

Mandibular or dental fracture; masseter-muscle contusion, abscess, or myositis; craniomandibular osteopathy (Fig. 99–4).

Suggested Reading

Burk RL, Ackerman N. The skull. In: Burk RL, Ackerman N, eds. Small animal radiology. New York: Churchill Livingstone, 1986:320.

Kealy JK. The skull and vertebral column. In: Kealy JK, ed. Diagnostic radiology of the dog and cat. 2nd ed. Philadelphia: WB Saunders, 1987:449.

Leighton RL, Robinson GW. Orthopedic surgery. In: Holzworth J, ed. Diseases of the cat. Philadelphia: WB Saunders, 1987:136.

Meyer W. The cranial vault and associated structures. In: Thrall DE, ed. Textbook of veterinary diagnostic radiology. Philadelphia: WB Saunders, 1986:30.

Nunamaker DM. Fractures and dislocations of the mandible. In: Newton CD, Nunamaker DM, eds. Textbook of small animal orthopedics. Philadelphia: JB Lippincott, 1985:302.

Owens JM. Temporomandibular luxations. In: Owens JM, ed. Radiographic interpretation for the small animal clinician. Saint Louis: Ralston Purina Co, 1982:59.

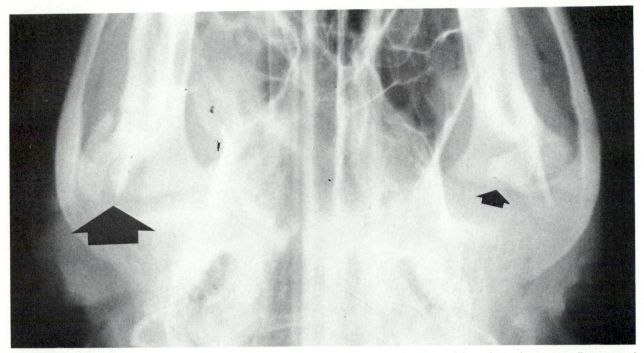

Figure 99–1 Ventrodorsal view of canine skull shows fractures of the right mandibular condyle and angular process (*large arrow*) and subluxation of the left temporomandibular joint (*small arrow*). Diagnosis: right temporomandibular fracture and left temporomandibular dislocation.

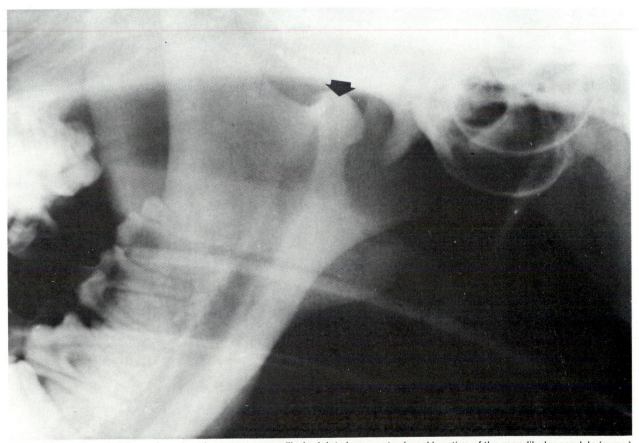

Figure 99–2 Lateral oblique view of canine temporomandibular joint shows rostrodorsal luxation of the mandibular condyle (*arrow*). Diagnosis: temporomandibular dislocation.

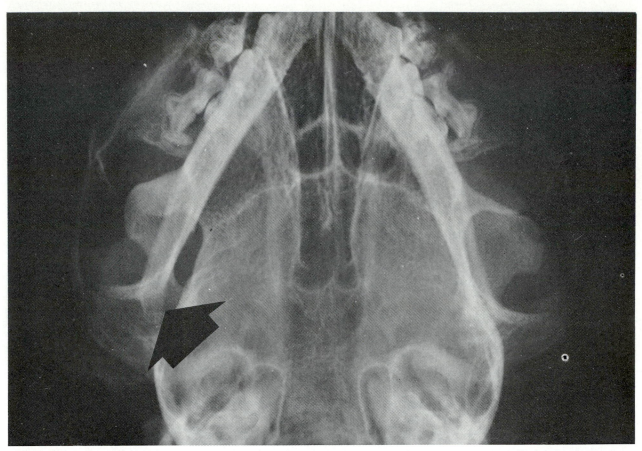

Figure 99–3   Ventrodorsal view of feline skull shows rostral luxation of right temporomandibular joint (*arrow*). Diagnosis: temporomandibular dislocation.

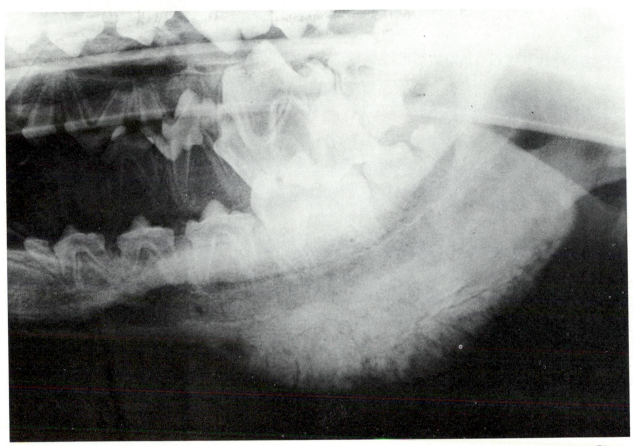

Figure 99–4 Lateral oblique view of canine caudoventral mandible shows large, apparently chronic new bone deposition. Diagnosis: craniomandibular osteopathy.

100

MAXILLARY FRACTURE

General Considerations

Fractures of the maxilla necessarily involve the rostral aspect of the nasal cavity and often its contained structures, including the teeth. Such fractures may be considered compound, because they are open to the atmosphere through the nasal cavity. Occasionally, depression fractures of the maxilla or nasal bones may result in the embedding of bone fragments or teeth in the nasal cavity, which in turn may lead to sequestration. Split mandibular symphysis is a common injury in cats following head trauma.

Major Radiographic Observations

Direct visualization of mandibular fractures may be difficult owing to the low background density of the nasal cavity upon which these injuries are superimposed; related nasal hemorrhage may create an equally confusing background. Often it is easier to locate the fracture by searching for a break in the maxillary margin at the point of greatest soft-tissue swelling (Figs. 100–1 to 100–3).

Diagnostic Strategy

Make four views centering on the suspected lesion site: dorsoventral, lateral, and right and left lateral oblique. A fifth projection, the ventrodorsal open-mouth view, eliminates mandibular superimposition in the dorsoventral plane. Be careful to make the oblique views similar, thereby providing an accurate comparison. Double labeling, right and left, reduces confusion, especially in nonstandard views. Anesthesia is required for optimal quality.

Pitfalls

Minimally displaced maxillary fractures may go unrecognized when there are more obvious surrounding injuries.

Alternative Diagnoses

Nasal foreign bodies, particularly plant awns; acute infectious sinusitis in cats; hemorrhaging nasal tumors or fungal disease.

Suggested Reading

Leighton RL, Robinson GW. Orthopedic surgery. In: Holzworth J, ed. Diseases of the cat. Philadelphia: WB Saunders, 1987:133.

Meyer W. The cranial vault and associated structures. In: Thrall DE, ed. Textbook of veterinary diagnostic radiology. Philadelphia: WB Saunders, 1986:24.

Newton CD. Fractures of the skull. In: Newton CD, Nunamaker DM, eds. Textbook of small animal orthopedics. Philadelphia: JB Lippincott, 1985:290.

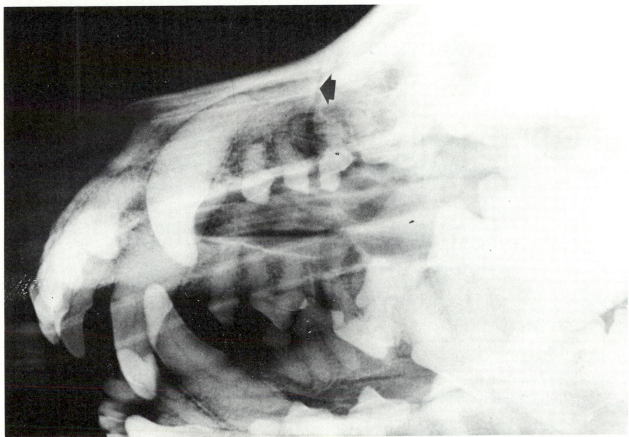

Figure 100-1 Lateral oblique view of canine maxilla shows vertically oriented fracture passing between third and fourth premolars (*arrow*). Diagnosis: maxillary fracture.

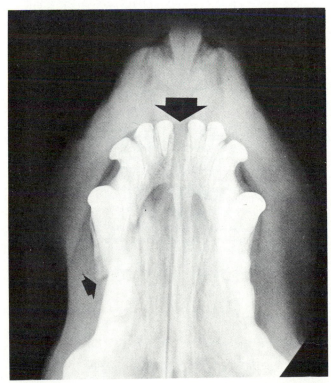

Figure 100-2 Open-mouth, ventral 20 degree rostral-dorsocaudal oblique view of canine maxillary dentition and nasal cavity shows displaced fracture of right maxilla immediately caudal to right canine tooth (*small arrow*). The maxillary symphysis is also fractured (*large arrow*). Diagnosis: maxillary fractures.

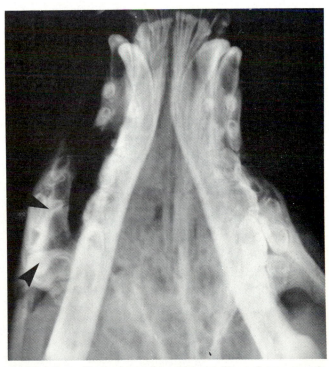

Figure 100-3 Ventrodorsal view of face and jaws shows severely displaced, piece fracture of the right lateroventral maxilla and associated dentition (*arrows*). Nasal cavity fractures and hemorrhage are also present, in addition to a mandibular symphyseal fracture. Diagnosis: multiple facial and jaw fractures.

101

NASAL CAVITY FRACTURE

General Considerations

The nasal cavity is divided into two halves by the nasal septum, with each half (or fossa) containing a pair of horizontally oriented conchae or turbinate bones. Above, below, and between the conchae are spaces called meattus nasi. The caudal part of the nasal cavity contains the numerous ethmoidal conchae. Disruption of the nasal cavity results from fracture of one or more of the surrounding bones, and it may be minimal or severe depending on the degree of fragment displacement. The more extensive the injury to the exterior of the nasal cavity, the more likely the possibility of internal injury. Fractured upper teeth may be driven through the hard palate into the nasal cavity and may act as foreign bodies. The turbinates or their intervening spaces (dorsal and ventral meattus) often trap inhaled foreign bodies such as plant awns, grass, or burrs. The result is usually acute sneezing, which often becomes bloody. Some tumors of the nasal cavity may also cause bleeding, which may be the first sign of illness. Occasionally the nasolacrimal canal and its contained duct may be fractured secondary to a depression fracture of the adjacent muzzle wall.

Major Radiographic Observations

Displaced fractures are more easily detected than those which are nondisplaced (Figs. 101–1 and 101–2). In either case, such fractures typically appear as breaks or discontinuity in the perimeter of the nasal cavity, often accompanied by a change in density and an elevation or depression of the adjacent bony contours. Obvious fracture lines are frequently absent unless there is facial deformity, and even then the extent of the injury often appears understated radiographically.

Diagnostic Strategy

Standard lateral and dorsoventral or ventrodorsal views should be made initially to determine the region(s) of injury. This also allows adjustment of radiographic technique in light of any density increase caused by contusion or intranasal hemorrhage. Oblique, dorsoventral views of the exterior of the nasal cavity are especially useful in detecting fractures. The dorsoventral position allows the radiographer to see the injury site better as the animal is positioned; in contrast, the ventrodorsal position may conceal the field of injury. The open-mouth ventrodorsal view best images the nasal cavity, especially when a high-detail, film-and-screen combination is used. Alternatively, nonscreen film may be used with equally good results. If regular film-and-screen combinations are employed, the radiographic technique must be reduced to compensate for the comparatively transparent nature of the nasal cavity. Nonmetallic nasal foreign bodies do not show up radiographically, although they sometimes may be inferred by the presence of localized or regional intranasal density, probably representing inflammation and accumulated fluid. Anesthesia is required for optimal quality.

Pitfalls

The use of skull technique when attempting to image the nasal cavity typically results in radiographic overexposure and an underestimation of any injuries.

Alternative Diagnoses

Sources of acute nasal hemorrhage, including contusion, foreign body, and occasionally infection or tumor.

Suggested Reading

Burk RL, Ackerman N. The skull. In: Burk RL, Ackerman N, eds. Small animal radiology. New York: Churchill Livingstone, 1986:321.

Kealy JK. The skull and vertebral column. In: Kealy JK, ed. Diagnostic radiology of the dog and cat. 2nd ed. Philadelphia: WB Saunders, 1987:457.

Meyer W. The nasal cavity and paranasal sinuses. In: Thrall DE, ed. Textbook of veterinary diagnostic radiology. Philadelphia: WB Saunders, 1986:34.

Owens JM. The nasal cavity and paranasal sinuses. In: Owens JM, ed. Radiographic interpretation for the small animal clinician. Saint Louis: Ralston Purina Co, 1982:61.

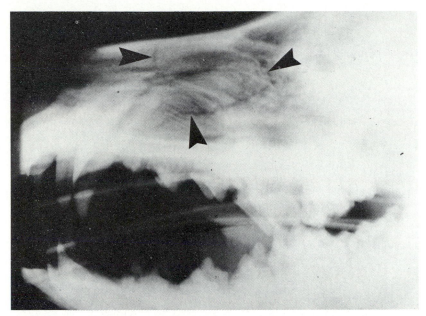

Figure 101–1 Lateral view of canine nasal cavity shows nondisplaced lateral wall fractures (*arrows*) and increased intranasal density. Diagnosis: fractured nasal cavity with hemorrhage.

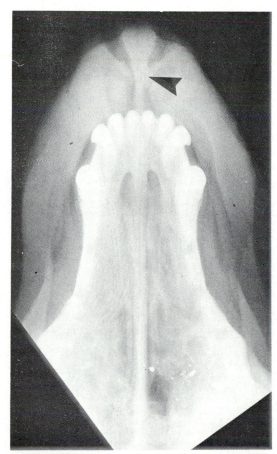

Figure 101–2 Open-mouth, ventral 20 degree rostral-dorsocaudal oblique view of canine nasal cavity shows lead fragments in the left ethmoturbinate bone, increased intranasal density, and decreased structural detail indicative of hemorrhage. The left nare is partially occluded with clot (*arrow*). Diagnosis: nasal cavity gunshot injury.

102

FRONTAL SINUS FRACTURE

General Considerations

The frontal sinuses, located caudodorsally to the ethmoid turbinates, are often fractured from blows to the rostrocranial part of the head, and they may be associated with related injuries to the nasal cavity and cranium. Typically, fractures of the frontal sinuses result in fragment depression and hemorrhage; however, few become infected even though such fractures may be compound in nature. Affected animals often bleed from the nose. Occasionally, orbital emphysema occurs as a result of frontal sinus fracture.

Major Radiographic Observations

Loss of symmetry, marginal disruption, and abnormal luminal density (usually the result of hemorrhage) are the signs of an abnormal frontal sinus. Involvement may be unilateral or bilateral (Figs. 102–1 to 102–4).

Diagnostic Strategy

Examination should begin with standard lateral, dorsoventral or ventrodorsal, and frontal (rostrocaudal, skyline) views. This last projection, if well positioned, is the most informative. Be careful not to overexpose the sinuses, which are air filled and therefore nearly transparent. Frontal sinuses that do not project well away from the head do not radiography well, often appearing to be abnormally dense and misshapen. Anesthesia is required for optimal quality.

Pitfalls

Normal frontal sinuses projected in a nonstandard manner appear abnormal.

Alternative Diagnoses

Subcutaneous hematoma.

Suggested Reading

Owens JM. The nasal cavity and paranasal sinuses. In: Owens JM, ed. Radiographic interpretation for the small animal clinician. Saint Louis: Ralston Purina Co, 1982:61.

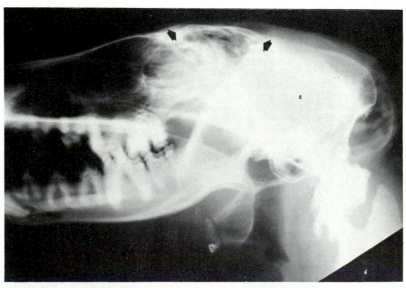

Figure 102–1 Lateral view of canine skull shows increased density and marginal disruption of the frontal sinus field (*arrows*). It is impossible to tell whether the injury is unilateral or bilateral.

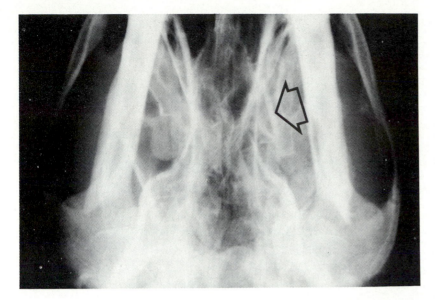

Figure 102–2 Ventrodorsal view of frontal sinuses of dog shown in Figure 102–1 shows fracture fragment (*arrow*) and increased density in the left frontal sinus. Diagnosis: unilateral depression fracture of left frontal sinus with associated hemorrhage.

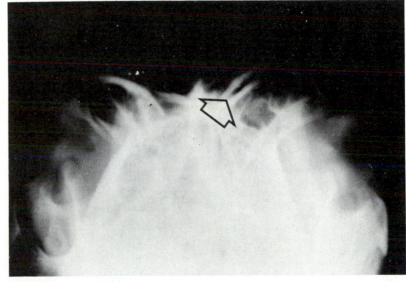

Figure 102–3 Frontal view of frontal sinuses of dog shown in Figures 102–1 and 102–2 shows comminuted depression fracture of left sinus compartment (*arrow*). Diagnosis: frontal sinus depression fracture.

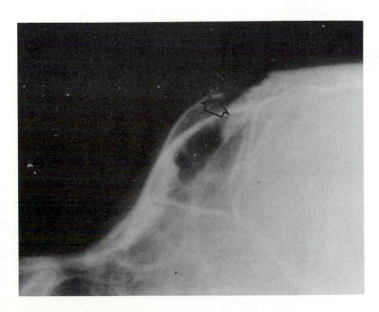

Figure 102–4 Lateral oblique view of canine right frontal sinus shows incomplete dorsal margin, and expressed bone fragments (*arrow*). Diagnosis: expression fracture of right frontal sinus.

103

ZYGOMATIC ARCH FRACTURE

General Considerations

The zygomatic arch or zygoma, formed by the zygomatic and temporal bones, is vulnerable to blows to the side of the head. Resulting fractures are often displaced medially and may occasionally result in secondary injury to the eye, or inhibition of jaw motion.

Major Radiographic Observations

In cases in which there is no obvious disruption, asymmetry of the zygomatic arches, as seen in either the standard or special views, is the most reliable evidence of fracture. (Figs. 103–1 to 103–3). The various frontal plane views—rostrocaudal, rostrocaudal oblique, with or without open mouth—have specific advantages over standard views; however, they are more difficult to position and are associated with considerable magnification of the rostral part of the arch as well as with varying degrees of distortion, depending on the amount of obliquity. For these reasons, I prefer the ventrodorsal and ventrodorsal oblique views (see Fig. 103–1).

Diagnostic Strategy

Make ventrodorsal and right and left ventrodorsal oblique views of the zygomatic arches centered over the cranium midway between the zygomatic arches. Take care to position the head symmetrically with the muzzle parallel to the table surface. Once a fracture is located, the image may be improved by reducing the field size and centering the beam laterally over the affected arch. When making standard survey views, use skull technique; however, when the zygomatic arches are examined individually, reduce the kVp to compensate for the thinner part. Anesthesia is required for optimal quality.

Pitfalls

The normal linear separation (suture) between the zygomatic and temporal bones may be mistaken for a nondisplaced fracture.

Alternative Diagnoses

Subcutaneous hematoma, abscess (especially in cats).

Suggested Reading

Kealy JK. The skull and vertebral column. In: Kealy JK, ed. Diagnostic radiology of the dog and cat. 2nd ed. Philadelphia: WB Saunders, 1987:448.

Meyer W. The cranial vault and associated structures. In: Thrall DE, ed. Textbook of veterinary diagnostic radiology. Philadelphia: WB Saunders, 1986:25.

Newton CD. Fractures of the skull. In: Newton CD, Nunamaker DM, eds. Textbook of small animal orthopedics. Philadelphia: JB Lippincott, 1985:292.

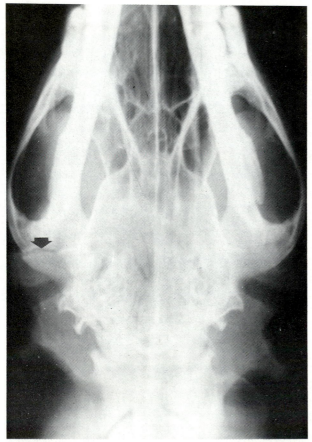

Figure 103–1 Ventrodorsal view of canine skull shows transverse fracture of caudal aspect of right zygomatic arch (*arrow*). Diagnosis: fractured zygoma.

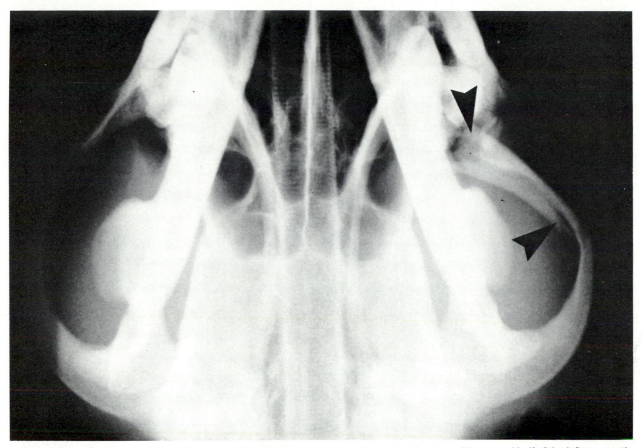

Figure 103–2 Ventrodorsal view of canine proximal facial region shows depressed fracture of the rostral half of the left zygomatic arch (*arrows*). Diagnosis: depression fracture of left zygoma.

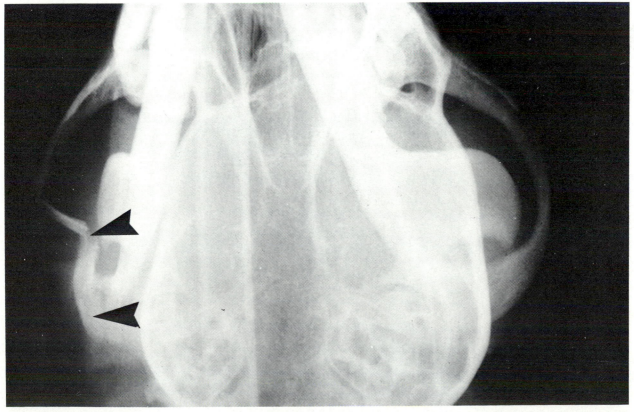

Figure 103–3 Ventrodorsal oblique view of canine proximal facial region shows a two piece, depressed fracture of the caudal half of the right zygomatic arch (*arrows*). Diagnosis: depressed fracture of right zygoma.

104

ORBITAL FRACTURE

General Considerations

Orbital fractures, particularly those of a depressed nature, are of greatest concern, because they may relate to secondary eye injuries. Potential facial disfigurement or ocular malalignment must also be considered, especially in show animals. Although composed of many comparatively small, thin, fragile bones, the orbit is surprisingly strong because of its nearly circular configuration. Realignment and postoperative stabilization following fracture are facilitated by an absence of muscle pull, unlike long-bone fractures, which are often subjected to considerable distractive muscular forces. Fractures involving the dorsal part of the orbit may also involve either the frontal sinuses or the cranium. Accordingly, these areas must also be routinely evaluated for fracture, even if there are no related clinical signs. In the case of paranasal sinus injury, orbital emphysema may develop secondarily. Direct trauma to the eye may produce a bursting type fracture in which pressure is transmitted through the globe, shattering and often displacing the bone of the caudal orbit. Occasionally animals are shot in or around the eye, in which case the bullet or pellet must be localized radiographically, relative to its effect on the eye or optic nerve.

Major Radiographic Observations

Minimally displaced orbital fractures are difficult to diagnose. Most such injuries show as thin radiolucent lines radiating diagonally outward from the orbit. The appearance of depression fractures varies widely depending on the size, number, and location of the fragments. Deeply depressed, relatively small bone fragments may be impossible to profile; consequently, the only radiographic evidence of such fractures may be a localized increase in bone density resulting from fragment superimposition. Distracted bone fragments are not usually difficult to identify.

Diagnostic Strategy

Begin with the two standard views: lateral and ventrodorsal, centered over the orbits. If the soft-tissue swelling is eccentric, center over the affected side in the ventrodorsal projection. If no abnormalities are found, yet a fracture is still suspected, make a penetrated rostrocaudal view (increase kVp by 10 percent or until the bones of the orbit are visible). Radiographic localization of the orbit can be further enhanced by placing a loop of wire suture secured with tape around the perimeter of the orbit (Fig. 104–1). This is very useful in determining whether or not a bullet lies within the eye. When doubtful about the validity of a particular radiographic finding, be certain to compare with the opposite side. Anesthesia is required for optimal quality.

Pitfalls

The relatively sunken position of the orbit makes radiographic isolation difficult.

Alternative Diagnoses

Subcutaneous or retrobulbar hematoma, periorbital abscess.

Suggested Reading

Converse JM, Baker DC. Maxillofacial fractures. In: Heppenstall RB, ed. Fracture treatment and healing. Philadelphia: WB Saunders, 1980:273.

Juhl JH. The teeth, jaws, and facial bones. In: Juhl JH, ed. Essentials of roentgen interpretation. 4th ed. Philadelphia: Harper & Row, 1981:1173.

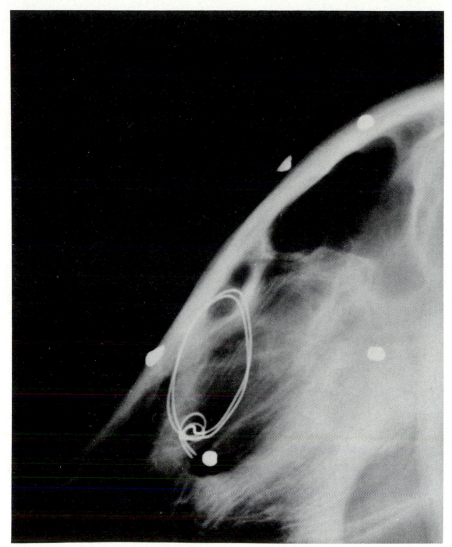

Figure 104–1 Close-up lateral view of canine proximal facial region shows wire loops temporarily placed over the right eye and underlying orbit; marking these structures radiographically to determine if either contains lead shot following a shotgun wound to the face. Diagnosis: negative study.

105
CRANIAL FRACTURE

General Considerations

Skull fractures are usually associated with varying degrees of subdural hemorrhage as well as with concussion. Depression fractures may lacerate the meninges and brain, producing extravasation of the cerebrospinal fluid and parenchymal bleeding. Cranial-nerve dysfunction is usually due to damage to the nerve at the site of exit from the skull, although midbrain contusion may produce ocular or pupillary deficits.

Major Radiographic Observations

Skull injuries are variable in appearance, ranging from nondisplaced fractures showing hairline cracks to large, comminuted depression fractures (Figs. 105–1 to 105–5). When cranial defects are present, search carefully for associated fragments that may be embedded in the brain.

Diagnostic Strategy

Begin examination with a lateral view of the skull centered on the cranium, specifically on any area of soft-tissue swelling; most medium- and large-sized fractures are detectable in this view (see Figs. 105–1 to 105–4). For questionable areas, add lateral oblique views, either right or left depending on earlier findings. Generally, the ventrodorsal and frontal views are less informative than the lateral projection. Use careful judgment in the choice and amount of chemical or gas restraint, if any.

Pitfalls

Interosseous skull sutures in immature animals, as well as vascular furrows on the inner surface of the cranium in animals of any age, may mimic hairline fractures.

Alternative Diagnoses

Subcutaneous hematoma, concussion, and isolated subdural hemorrhage.

Suggested Reading

Burk RL, Ackerman N. The skull. In: Burk RL, Ackerman N, eds. Small animal radiology. New York: Churchill Livingstone, 1986:324.

Kealy JK. The skull and vertebral column. In: Kealy JK, ed. Diagnostic radiology of the dog and cat. 2nd ed. Philadelphia: WB Saunders, 1987:446.

Meyer W. The cranial vault and associated structures. In: Thrall DE, ed. Textbook of veterinary diagnostic radiology. Philadelphia: WB Saunders, 1986:24.

Newton CD. Fractures of the skull. In: Newton CD, Nunamaker DM, eds. Textbook of small animal orthopedics. Philadelphia: JB Lippincott, 1985:287.

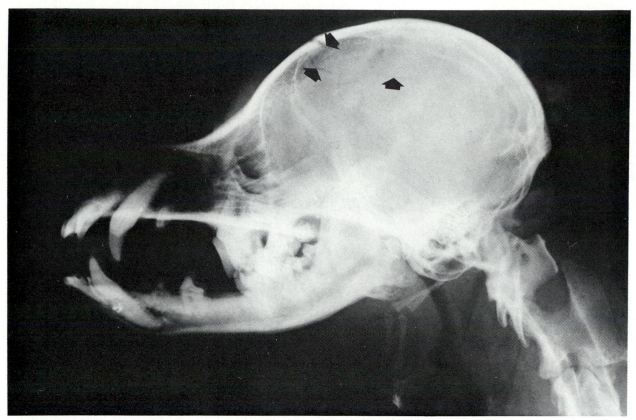

Figure 105–1 Lateral view of canine skull shows fracture lines (*arrows*) in the rostral cranium associated with mild fragment elevation. Diagnosis: cranial elevation fracture.

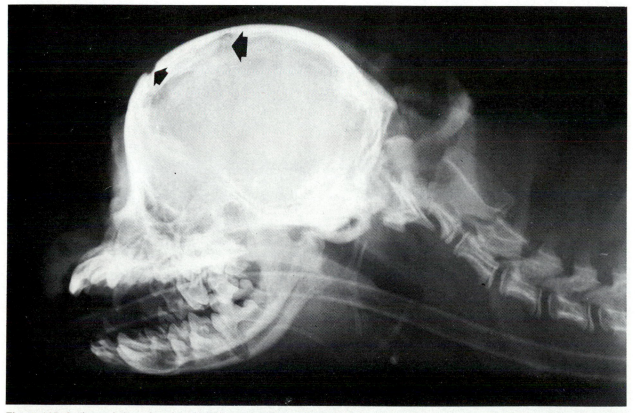

Figure 105–2 Lateral view of canine skull shows marginal defect (*small arrow*) and fracture lines (large arrow) in the rostral cranium associated with mild fragment depression. Diagnosis: cranial depression fracture.

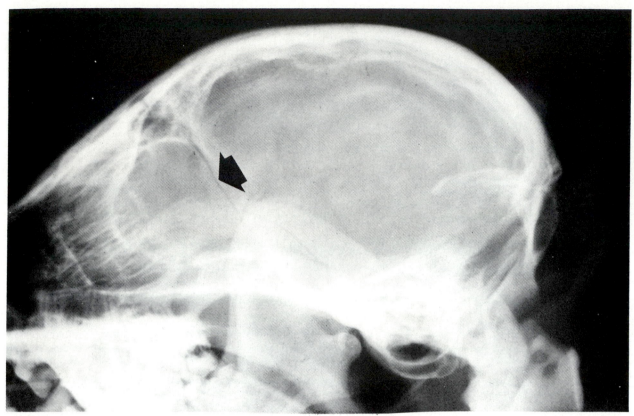

Figure 105–3 Lateral view of canine skull shows a long rostrolateral fracture line (*arrow*). Diagnosis: cranial fracture.

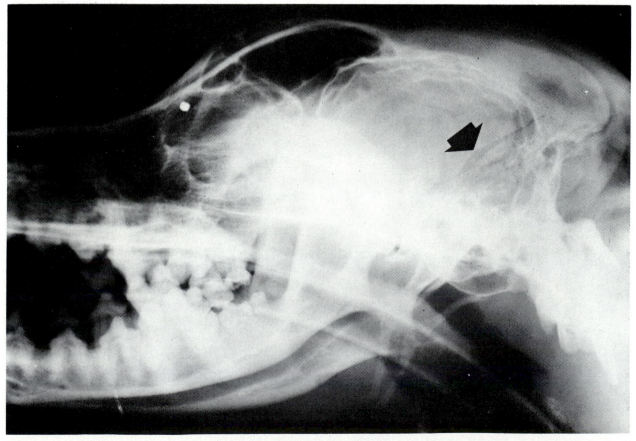

Figure 105–4 Lateral view of canine skull shows multiple caudolateral fracture lines (*arrow*). Diagnosis: cranial fracture.

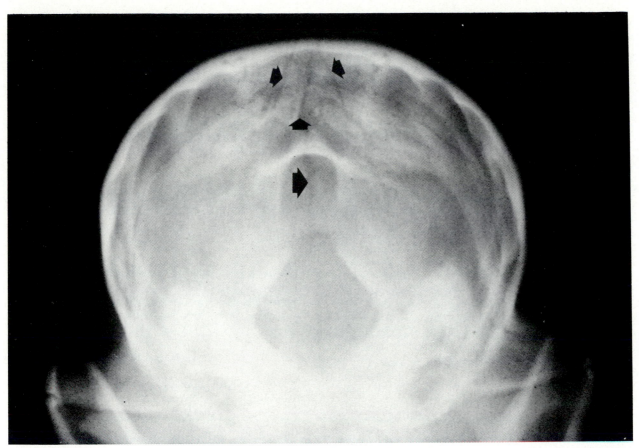

Figure 105–5 Frontal view of canine skull shows multiple, sagitally oriented fracture lines (*small arrows*) that were not seen in lateral projections. Observe the difference between the fracture lines and a normal suture line ((*large arrow*). Diagnosis: cranial fracture.

106

TYMPANIC BULLA INFECTION

General Considerations

Fractures of the bullae are rare because of the bulla's relatively protected location at the base of the skull. Bullae infections (otitis media, tympanitis) are believed to occur in three ways: secondary to outer ear infections (otitis externa), as a result of ascending infection from the pharynx through the eustachian tube, or secondary to bacteremia; all of these ways are capable of producing an acute head tilt. Structural alterations to the bullae are largely limited to thinning or thickening of the outer margins subsequent to bone loss or deposition. Increased or decreased bulla density results accordingly. Such changes require a great deal of time to develop: months or even years. Associated fluid does not appear to influence the appearance of the radiographic image. Foreign bodies such as plant awns may produce a head tilt and vigorous head shaking and usually can be seen otoscopically. Abscessation or osteomyelitis may develop if the awn is not removed promptly.

Major Radiographic Observations

Acute middle ear infections are typically associated with a normal radiograph. Infections of intermediate duration may or may not produce changes in the bullae. When present, these alterations most commonly take the form of marginal thickening, as seen in the lateral oblique or open-mouth view, and a small increase in overall density, seen in the ventrodorsal projection (Figs. 106–1 to 106–3). Luminal fluid cannot be identified directly. Chronic infections are most likely to produce detectable changes similar to, or more severe than, those described in infections of intermediate duration. Occasionally, osteomyelitis may penetrate the bulla margin.

Diagnostic Strategy

The extended ventrodorsal view, centered on the bullae and using a high-detail imaging system, is best for evaluating bulla density. An exactly positioned open-mouth view of the bullae is best for assessing the bulla margins. Avoid superimposing the endotracheal tube or tongue over either bulla. The lateral oblique projection of the bulla is subject to distortion and is difficult to reproduce consistently in different breeds; accordingly it must be evaluated with caution. The lateral view superimposes one bulla over another, often obscuring unilateral pathology, and is generally of minimal use. Anesthesia is required for optimal quality.

Pitfalls

Superimposition of the tongue over a bulla in the open-mouth view causes an increase in density that may be mistaken for disease. Superimposition of an endotracheal tube may obscure all or part of a bulla.

Alternative Diagnoses

Other causes of head tilt, including severe otitis externa and foreign body in the ear canal.

Suggested Reading

Barber DL, Oliver JE, Mayhew IG. Neuroradiography In: Oliver JE, Hoerlein BF, Mayhew IG, eds. Veterinary neurology. Philadelphia: WB Saunders, 1987:91.

Braund KG. Diseases of the peripheral nerves, cranial nerves, and muscle. In: Oliver JE, Hoerlein BF, Mayhew IG, eds. Veterinary neurology. Philadelphia: WB Saunders, 1987:361.

Burk RL, Ackerman N. The Skull. In: Burk RL, Ackerman N, eds. Small animal radiology. New York: Churchill Livingstone, 1986:328.

Meyer W. The cranial vault and associated structures. In: Thrall DE, ed. Textbook of veterinary diagnostic radiology. Philadelphia: WB Saunders, 1986:28.

Owens JM The cranial vault. In: Owens JM, ed. Radiographic interpretation for the small animal clinician. Saint Louis: Ralston Purina Co, 1982:60.

Watrous BJ. Otitis media-interna. In: Farrow CS, ed. Decision making in small animal radiology. Toronto: BC Decker, 1987:58.

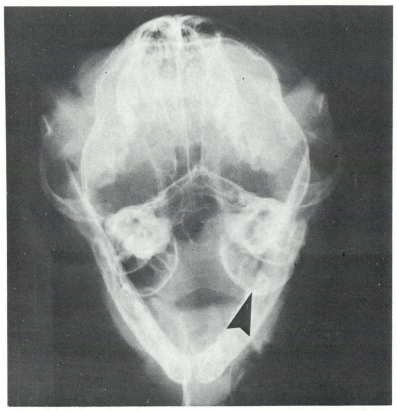

Figure 106–1 Open-mouth, rostral 30 degree ventral-caudodorsal view of feline tympanic bullae shows increased density and marginal thickness on the left (*arrow*). Diagnosis: infected left tympanic bulla.

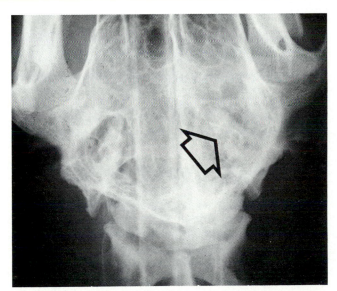

Figure 106–2 Ventrodorsal view of canine cranium centered on the tympanic bullae shows increased density and reduced definition of the left bulla (*arrow*). Diagnosis: infected left tympanic bulla.

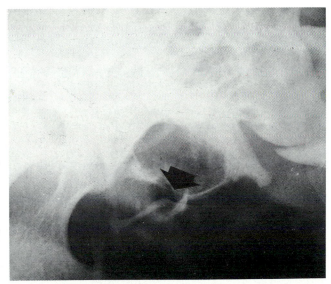

Figure 106–3 Lateral oblique view of canine right bulla shows increased luminal density and marginal destruction (*arrow*). Diagnosis: infected right tympanic bulla.

THE SPINE

Most emergencies involving the spine are the result of trauma or disk herniation. Occasionally, congenital disease such as absence of the dens and its associated ligaments may predispose to atlantoaxial luxation. Typically, instability disorders (cervical vertebral instability, cervical spondylopathy, wobblers) are associated with a gradual onset of clinical signs, but they may occasionally present acutely. Likewise, most infections and tumors of this region result in gradually developing illness, although they may sometimes result in an acute onset of clinical signs.

Concept of the Spinal Unit

The following sections dealing with the spine frequently mention the *spinal unit*. This is a conceptual term used to describe any two adjacent vertebrae and their associated soft tissues, and it emphasizes their important functional relationship. This concept is especially useful when considering fractures of the facetal joints and disk disease, conditions affecting structures shared by an adjacent pair of vertebrae.

Facetal Joints

The term *facetal joints*, describing the vertebral joints formed by the articular processes and their associated facets, is used in this text to replace the rather awkward expression "diarthrodial joint spaces."

107
SPINAL FRACTURE

Spinal fractures may occur at one or more locations in an individual vertebra: the body, arch, articular processes or facets, and transverse or dorsal spinous processes. They may also involve structures common to a spinal unit, such as the facetal joints or intervertebral disk. Prior to reaching skeletal maturity, vertebrae contain secondary growth centers that are prone to fracture or dislocation. This is especially true of the vertebral end-plates and less commonly of the cranial growth centers of the second cervical vertebra. Mature vertebrae often fracture centrally with little or no resulting malalignment; they are termed *nondisplaced compression fractures*. Thus, the only radiographic abnormality may be a relatively shortened vertebra compared to those on either side. Fractures of the facetal joints are nearly always bilateral and are typically indicated by a widening of the facetal joint spaces. Fractures of the dorsal and transverse spinal processes may be isolated injuries or may be associated with other spinal fractures. They often appear detached or malaligned but may also be nondisplaced. The caudal fragment of sacral-body fractures is often distracted caudally, remaining attached to the coccygeal spine. Fractures of the sacral wing are commonly associated with iliac separation and are seen most often in the ventrodorsal view.

General Considerations

Cervical Region

Cervical fractures and dislocations are less common than similar injuries elsewhere in the spine. Most occur cranially. The anatomic complexity and dissimilarity existing among the first three cervical vertebrae make consistent radiographic projections difficult) especially of the first cervical vertebra—C1 or atlas), and make relative comparison impossible. The large, ventrally protruding transverse processes of the sixth cervical vertebra (C6) may resemble fracture fragments when projected obliquely, and the relatively short, blocky appearance of the seventh cervical vertebra (C7) may mimic a compression fracture.

Thoracolumbar Region

Thoracic spinal fractures are not as common as lumbar injuries, largely because of the relative support provided by the rib cage and its associated axial musculature. Thoracic fractures tend to be relatively less displaced for the same reason. Still, although deeply embedded in muscle and linked to one another by an elaborate ligamentous network, the dorsal spinous processes of thoracic vertebrae may be fractured, often without any additional vertebral injury. The frequency of proximal lumbar fractures reflects the high degree of mobility of this region, as well as its comparatively superficial location and relative lack of surrounding soft-tissue support.

Sacrococcygeal Region

Sacral fractures may occur as isolated injuries, as avulsion fractures associated with the tail, and as injuries in conjunction with pelvic fractures, particularly sacroiliac separations. They may be associated with neurologic deficits to the bladder, bowel, or tail.

Major Radiographic Observations

Cervical Region

Atlanto-occipital fracture or dislocation may often be identified indirectly on the basis of a reduced distance or overlap between C1 and the occipital condyles (Figs. 107–1 and 107–2). Fracture of the odontoid process (dens) usually results in rostral fragment displacement and dorsal subluxation of the second cervical vertebra (C2 or axis), typically producing an increased distance between the dorsal arch of C1 and the dorsal spinous process of C2 (Fig. 107–3). In immature animals the dens may be fractured through its growth plate with the same results. Identification of such fractures is often difficult or impossible in standard projections, so special views are required. The lateral projections (wings) of C1 may be fractured, sometimes in combination with dislocation of the atlanto-occipital joint. Occasionally, the atlantoaxial ligaments are sprained severely resulting in an abnormally large gap between the dorsal aspects of C1 and C2. Mid and caudal cervical injuries are comparatively less common (Fig. 107–4).

Thoracolumbar Region

Fractures of the thoracic region are often compressive with minimal fragment displacement. Reduced length in comparison to adjacent vertebrae is often the only radiographic sign (Figs. 107–5 and 107–6). Lumbar fractures are variable, ranging from subtle compression fractures to comminuted dislocations (Figs. 107–7 to 107–13). Severe comminution is not unusual.

Sacrococcygeal Region

Fractures of the sacral body are often obvious based on a large interfragment gap or caudal displacement (Figs. 107–14 to 107–16). Conversely, fractures of the sacral wings with or without lumbosacral separation are often overlooked.

Diagnostic Strategy

Cervical Region

Begin by making a lateral view centered over the suspected lesion. If the animal can stand, this view may be made with a horizontal beam, which often provides an image superior to that obtained from a recumbent projection. Make an opposite projection if it can be done safely; this may be done in the standing position with a vertical x-ray beam. A regional spinal survey in the lateral position should rule out any additional cervical injury. Fractures of the dens are best seen with the open-mouth view; however, great care must be taken not to injure the cord further during the radiographic examination. Alternatively, one may use a lateral oblique projection centered on the junction of C1 and C2, although this view may be compromised by superimposition of associated bony parts. Dislocations may be difficult to demonstrate using standard views and therefore often require stress radiography to confirm suspected lesions. Such views must be taken carefully and only under general anesthesia. The assessment of caudal cervical fractures requires an increase in kVp to compensate for the increased thickness of the neck in this region. Anesthesia is advisable.

Thoracolumbar Region

When spinal injury has been established prior to radiographic examination, the animal should first be secured to a radiographically transparent body splint. If this is not available, place a large, closed-cell foam pad between the animal and the table surface. A lateral radiograph centered on the suspected fracture should then be made, followed as needed by a ventrodorsal view in which the animal's position remains unchanged, while the x-ray beam and receiver are redirected horizontally (cross-table projection). If the tube head cannot be moved into the horizontal position, then a ventrodorsal or dorsoventral view must be considered. Great caution should be exercised when assessing a spinal fracture on the basis of a lateral view only! Anesthesia or sedation is required.

Sacrococcygeal Region

Make two views: lateral and ventrodorsal, centered over the sacrum. Be certain to penetrate the sacrum fully in the ventrodorsal projection. The ventrodorsal view is less painful if made with the hindlimbs in the frog position, with the animal lying on a closed-cell foam pad.

Pitfalls

Cervical Region

The wings of the atlas are often seen obliquely in the lateral view, resembling fracture; in the ventrodorsal projection, C1 often appears asymmetrical, mimicking fracture or dislocation.

Thoracolumbar Region

Fracture pain, along with related muscle spasm, may produce functional scoliosis, which in turn can result in spinal obliquity and poor image quality.

Sacrococcygeal Region

Congenital segmentation and lumbarization of the sacrum may mimic fracture. The normal variation in sacral length, density, and curvature may also resemble fracture, especially when the sacrum lies at the lateral film margin or if it is obliquely seen.

Alternative Diagnoses

Cervical Region

Sprain, strain, or contusion of the neck, typically associated with muscle spasm.

Thoracolumbar Region

Cord contusion, extradural hematoma, traumatic disk rupture, and degenerative disk herniation.

Sacrococcygeal Region

Lower lumbar or pelvic fractures.

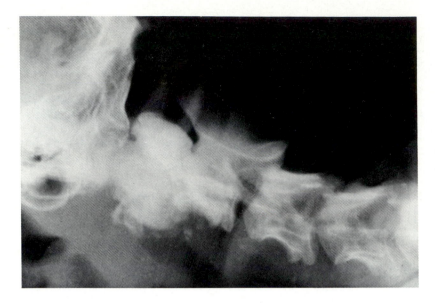

Figure 107–1   Lateral view of canine cervical spine shows reduced distance between the first and second cervical vertebrae, dorsal displacement of the dorsal spinous process of C2, and increased density, loss of detail, and ventral fractures of C1. Diagnosis: sprain-fracture-luxation of the C1–2 spinal unit.

Figure 107–2   Lateral cervical myelogram (lumbar injection site) of patient described in Figure 107–1 shows abrupt termination of contrast medium at the caudal aspect of C1 (*arrows*). Diagnosis: spinal cord stenosis secondary to trauma.

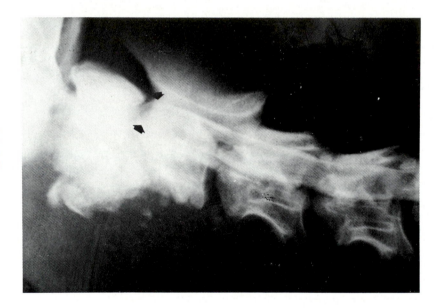

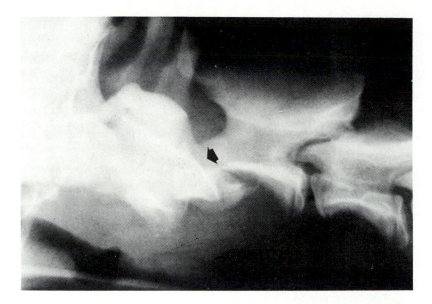

Figure 107–3 Lateral view of canine proximal cervical spine shows dorsal displacement of C2 and a complete fracture of the dens (*arrow*). Diagnosis: fracture-dislocation of the C1–2 spinal unit.

Figure 107–4 Lateral view of canine midcervical spine shows a comminuted fracture of the cranial end-plate of C4 (*arrows*) with a loss of disk space and numerous surrounding lead fragments. Diagnosis: C4–C5 gunshot fracture.

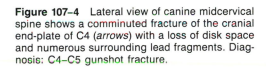

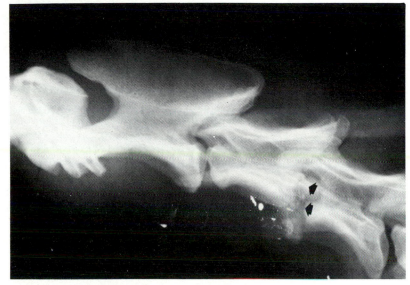

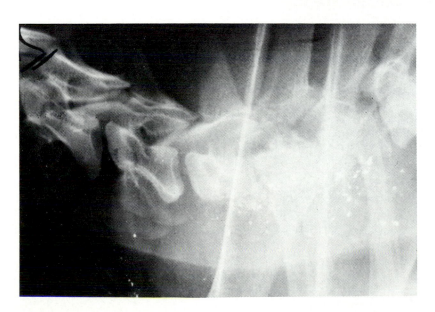

Figure 107–5 Lateral view of canine proximal thoracic spine shows lead fragments superimposed on the scapulae, last cervical, and first and second thoracic vertebrae, and the proximal aspect of the related ribs.

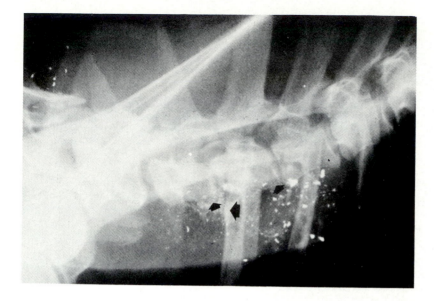

Figure 107–6 Lateral view of the animal shown in Figure 107–5, but with the scapulae drawn forward, shows most of the lead lying against the vertebrae and ribs. There are fractures of the caudoventral aspects of the seventh cervical and first thoracic vertebral bodies (*small arrows*), and the left rib (*large arrow*). Diagnosis: multiple vertebral gunshot fractures with associated rib fracture.

Figure 107–7 Lateral view of canine thoracolumbar spine shows luxation of T12–13 (*arrow*) with detachment of the last rib pair. Diagnosis: dislocated T12–13 spinal units.

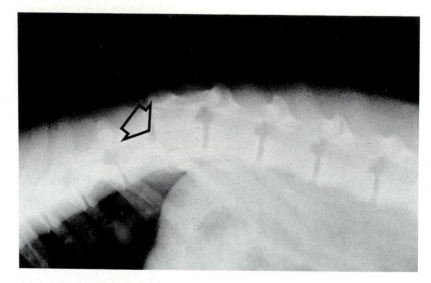

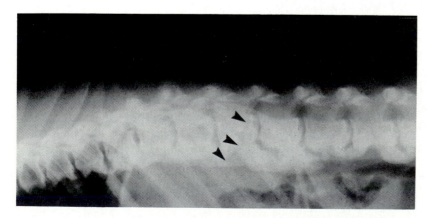

Figure 107–8 Lateral view of canine thoracolumbar spine shows nondisplaced fracture of L1 and its associated spondylotic bridge (*arrows*). Diagnosis: fractured first lumbar vertebra.

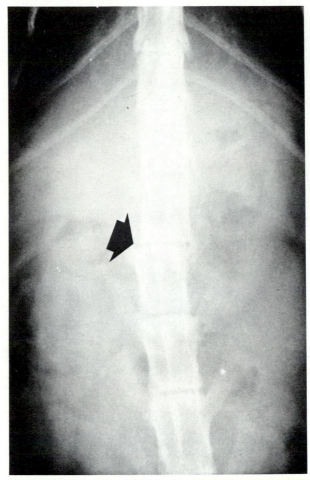

Figure 107–9 Ventrodorsal view of feline lumbar spine shows subluxation of L2–3 (*arrow*) with associated facetal joint fractures. Diagnosis: subluxated L2–3 spinal unit.

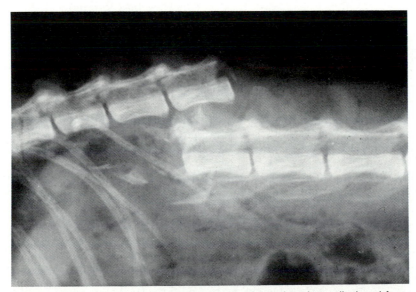

Figure 107–10 Lateral view of feline thoracolumbar spine shows displaced fractures of the facetal joints of the L2–3 spinal unit and transverse processes of L3 with resulting dislocation. Diagnosis: sprain-fracture-luxation of the L2–3 spinal unit.

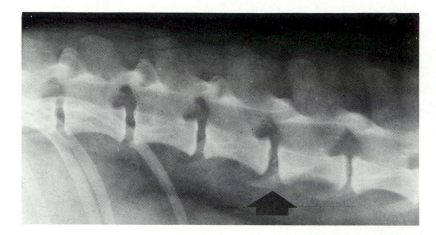

Figure 107–11 Lateral view of canine midlumbar spine shows subluxation of the L3–4 vertebrae as evidenced by widening of the associated facetal joints, distortion of the intervertebral foramen, stepping of the vertebral canal, and avulsion fragments within the disk space (*arrow*). Diagnosis: sprain-fracture-luxation of the L3–4 spinal unit.

Figure 107–12 Lateral view of canine lumbar spine shows narrowing of the L3–4 disk space, reduction of the associated intervertebral foramen, and dorsal narrowing of the related facetal joints (*arrow*). Diagnosis: sprain-fracture-luxation of the L3–4 spinal unit.

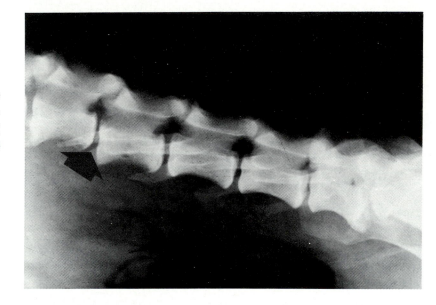

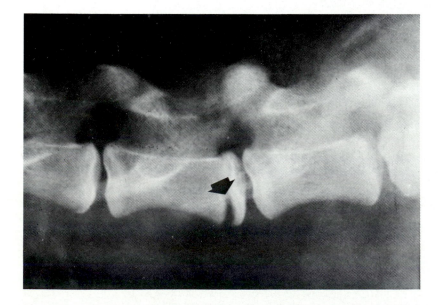

Figure 107–13 Lateral view of canine caudal lumbar spine shows abnormal separation between the body and caudal end-plate of L5 (*arrow*) Diagnosis: end-plate fracture of L5.

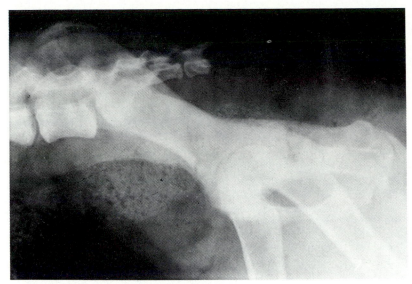

Figure 107–14 Lateral view of canine sacrococcygeal spine shows absence of all but first coccygeal vertebra. Diagnosis: avulsion fracture of tail.

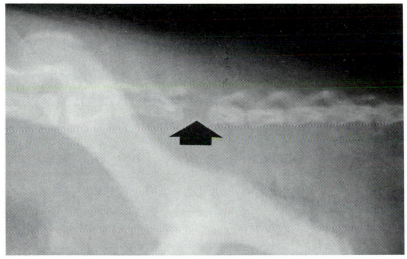

Figure 107–15 Lateral view of feline sacrococcygeal spine shows a large gap (*arrow*) between the sacrum and the first coccygeal vertebra. Diagnosis: sacrococcygeal avulsion.

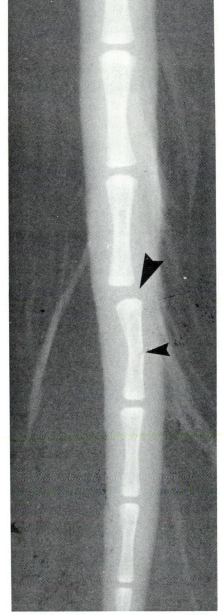

Figure 107–16 Ventrodorsal view of feline midcoccygeal spine shows subluxation (*large arrow*) and greenstick fracture (*small arrow*). Diagnosis: coccygeal fracture, dislocation.

Suggested Reading

Bailey CS, Morgan JP. Diseases of the spinal cord. In Ettinger SJ, ed. Textbook of Veterinary internal medicine. Philadelphia: WB Saunders, 1983:585.

Barber DL, Oliver JE, Mayhew IG. Neuroradiography. In: Oliver JE, Hoerlein BF, Mayhew IG, eds. Veterinary neurology. Philadelphia: WB Saunders, 1987:74.

Burk RL, Ackerman N. The spine. In: Burk RL, Ackerman N, eds. Small animal radiology. New York: Churchill Livingstone, 1986:367.

Kealy JK. The skull and vertebral column. In: Kealy JK, ed. Diagnostic radiology of the dog and cat. 2nd ed. Philadelphia: WB Saunders, 1987:519.

Leighton RL, Robinson GW. Orthopedic surgery. In: Holzworth J, ed. Diseases of the cat. Philadelphia: WB Saunders, 1987:135.

McNeel SV. Radiology of the skull and cervical spine. Vet Clin North Am [Small Anim Pract] 1982; 12:285.

Owens JM. Atlanto-axial subluxation. In: Owens JM, ed. Radiographic interpretation for the small animal clinician. Saint Louis: Ralston Purina Co, 1982:78, 80.

Smith GK, Walter MC. Fractures and luxations of the spine. In: Newton CD, Nunamaker DM, eds. Textbook of small animal orthopedics. Philadelphia: JB Lippincott, 1985:317.

Watrous BJ. Atlantoaxial instability. In: Farrow CS, ed. Decision making in small animal radiology. Toronto: BC Decker, 1987:66.

Watrous BJ. Vertebral compression fracture. In: Farrow CS, ed. Decision making in small animal radiology. Toronto: BC Decker, 1987:88.

108
DISK HERNIATION

General Considerations

The true incidence of traumatic disk herniation in dogs is not known; however, it does occur with sufficient frequency to require consideration in cases of spinal injury. Particularly in Dachshunds and similarly shaped chondodystrophoid breeds, nontraumatic disk herniation is common. Herniation also occurs in other breeds, although not as often. Accordingly, disk herniation should not be ruled out on the basis of breed alone. Loss of disk material ranges from partial to complete, so the associated radiographic signs may vary. For example; a partial disk herniation is associated with less intervertebral narrowing than a complete rupture. Likewise, a calcified disk is potentially more obvious than a noncalcified disk, other factors being equal. However, not all calcified herniated disks are detectable, largely because of the amount, location, and distribution of the disk material, as well as its orientation relative to the x-ray beam. Occasionally, a presumptive diagnosis may be made on the basis of a single, marginally narrowed disk space, flanked by multiple calcified disks. Disk herniations are commonly described as Hansen type I or II: the former typically occurs in Dachsund-type breeds secondary to anular rupture and nuclear extrusion into the spinal canal; the latter occurs in nonchondrodystrophoid breeds following partial tearing of the anulus with resulting dorsal bulging of the disk. The incidence of disk herniation is greatest in Dachshunds, most often involving the thoracolumbar region, with the T12–13 spinal unit being affected most commonly, followed by T13–L1, L1–2, and T11–12. Cervical lesions are most common proximally, beginning with C2–3, and becoming progressively less frequent caudally.

Major Radiographic Observations

The majority of acute disk herniations are detected indirectly by one of three associated abnormalities involving a particular spinal unit: narrowing of the intervertebral disk space (Fig. 108–1), narrowing of the intervertebral foramen, and narrowing of the facetal joints. Occasionally, a herniated disk may be seen directly as a mineralized mass within the spinal canal (Figs. 108–2 to 108–4 and Figs. 108–9 and 108–10). Nonmineralized disks are radiographically invisible. Partial, small-volume disk herniations may be associated with a normal-appearing radiograph because they alter the affected spinal unit imperceptibly (Figs. 108–5 to 108–8).

Diagnostic Strategy

Use general anesthesia or heavy sedation, if at all possible. Begin with lateral views and take great care in positioning the animal parallel to the table top in order to pre- vent oblique, nonstandard projection of the spine. If anesthesia or sedation is not possible, make a limited-field radiograph directly over the suspected lesion site. Lesions that cannot be readily localized require spinal survey, which may be limited to the lateral view initially. This should be done segmentally with the animal in lateral position, approximately 3 inches at a time in small dogs and cats, 6 inches in medium-sized dogs, and 10 inches in large dogs. These limited fields keep anatomic distortion to a minimum. Once a lesion is located, a ventrodorsal view may be made in an attempt to establish if a mineralized disk is located eccentrically, which may in turn determine the hemilaminectomy site.

Pitfalls

The disk space of the C2–3 spinal unit is relatively narrow compared to those located caudally, although it may be increased by as much as 50 percent using traction-stress radiography. There is no disk space between C1 and C2.

Alternative Diagnoses

Progressive hemorrhage myelomalacia, ischemic myelopathy secondary to fibrocartilagenous emboli, epidural hemorrhage or abscess, and spinal meningitis.

Suggested Reading

Adams WM. Myelography. Vet Clin North Am [Small Anim Pract] 1982; 12:295.

Bailey CS, Morgan JP. Diseases of the spinal cord. In Ettinger SJ, ed. Textbook of veterinary internal medicine. Philadelphia: WB Saunders, 1983; 584.

Bartels JE. Intervertebral disk disease. In: Thrall DE, ed. Textbook of veterinary diagnostic radiology. Philadelphia: WB Saunders, 1986:51.

Burk RL, Ackerman N. The spine. In: Burk RL, Ackerman N, eds. Small animal radiology. New York: Churchill Livingstone, 1986:356.

Kealy JK. The skull and vertebral column. In: Kealy JK, ed. Diagnostic radiology of the dog and cat. 2nd ed. Philadelphia: WB Saunders, 1987:503.

Shores A. Intervertebral disk disease. In: Newton CD, Nunamaker DM, eds. Textbook of small animal orthopedics. Philadelphia: JB Lippincott, 1985:739.

Owens JM. Intervertebral disk disease. In: Owens JM, ed. Radiographic interpretation for the small animal clinician. Saint Louis: Ralston Purina Co, 1982:81.

Watrous BJ. Intervertebral disc disease. In: Farrow CS, ed. Decision making in small animal radiology. Toronto: BC Decker 1987:84.

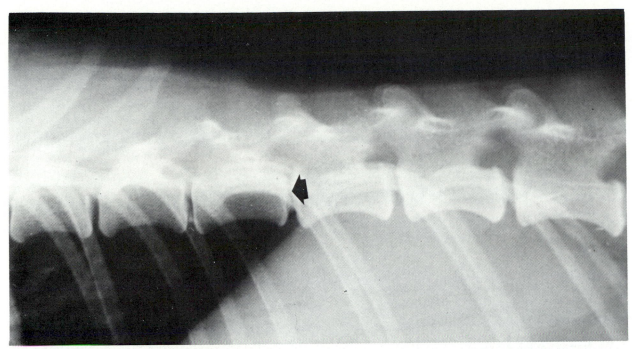

Figure 108–1 Lateral view of canine thoracolumbar spine shows narrowing of the T11–12 disk space (*arrow*). Diagnosis: herniated T11–12 disk.

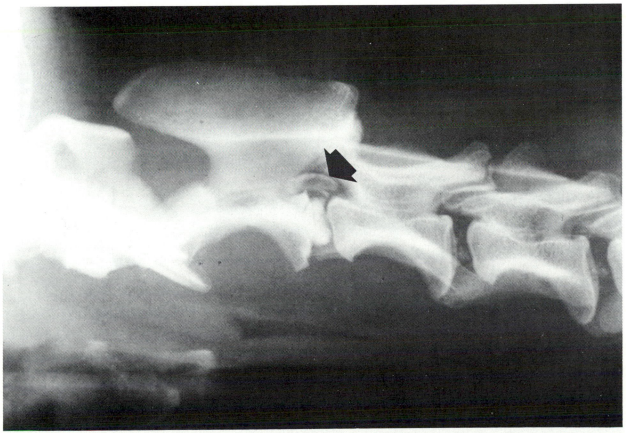

Figure 108–2 Lateral view of canine proximal cervical spine shows large mineralized mass superimposed on the intervertebral foramen of the C2–3 spinal unit (*arrow*), in addition to calcification of the associated intervertebral disk. Diagnosis: C2–3 partial disk herniation.

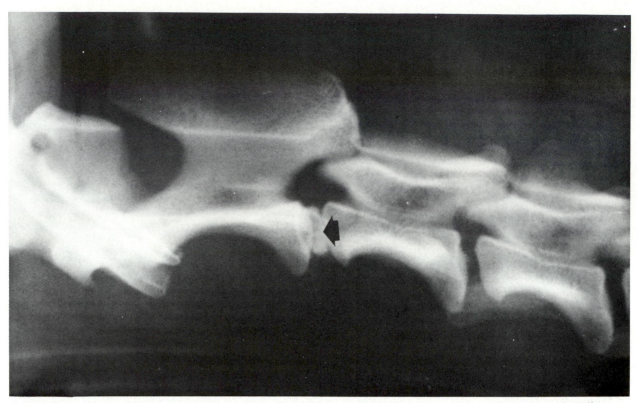

Figure 108–3 Lateral view of canine proximal cervical spine shows large mineralized disk at C2–3 (*arrow*) without visible calcific density in the overlying spinal canal. Myelography was negative. Diagnosis: calcified C2–3 intervertebral disk without evidence of herniation.

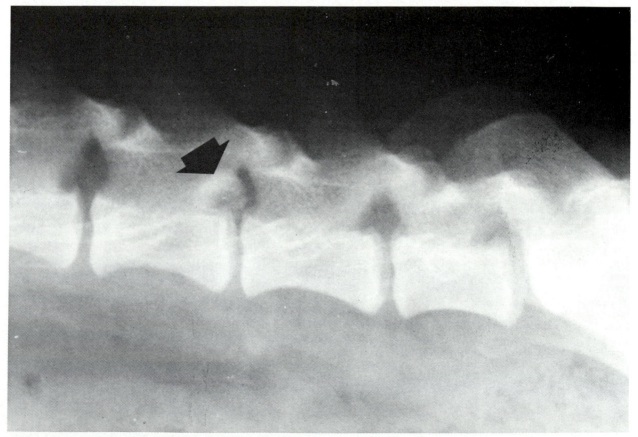

Figure 108–4 Lateral view of canine caudal lumbar spine shows large mineralized density in the caudal aspect of the vertebral canal of L5 (*arrow*). Diagnosis: L5–6 disk herniation.

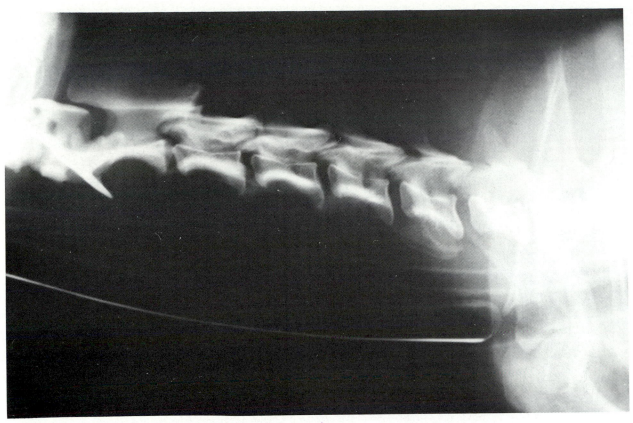

Figure 108–5 Lateral view of canine cervical spine appears normal.

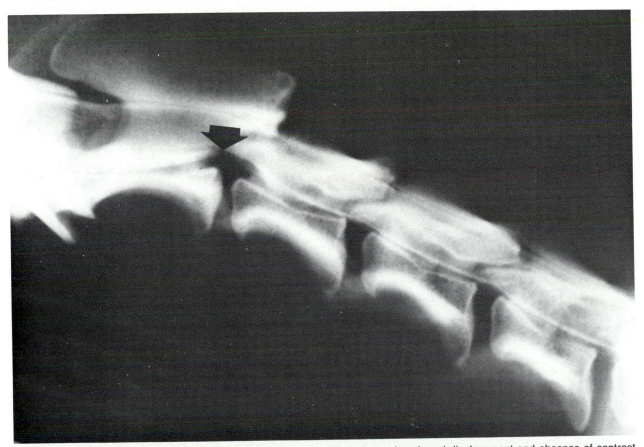

Figure 108–6 Lateral cervical myelogram of patient in Figure 108–5 shows dorsal cord displacement and absence of contrast medium in the ventral aspect of the dural sac over the C2–3 disk space. Diagnosis: extradural mass, C2–3 (a partial disk herniation was identified surgically).

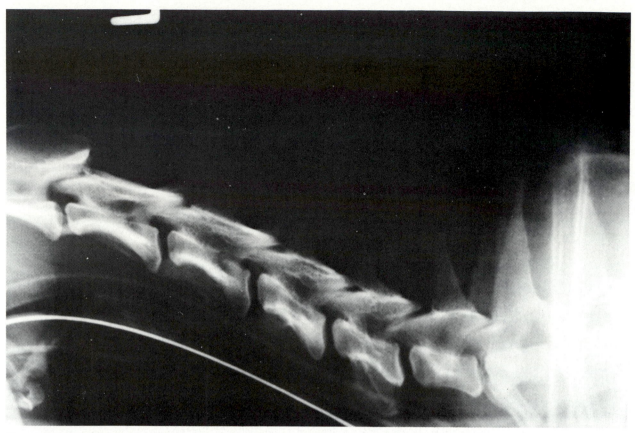

Figure 108–7   Lateral view of canine cervical spine appears normal.

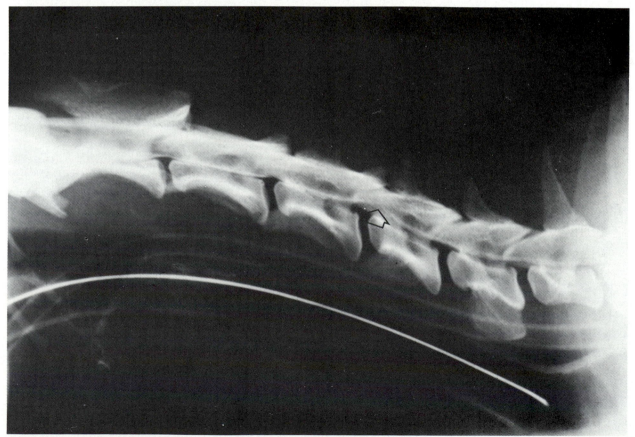

Figure 108–8   Lateral cervical myelogram of patient in Figure 108–7 shows dorsal cord displacement over the C4–5 disk space (*arrow*). Diagnosis: partial disk herniation.

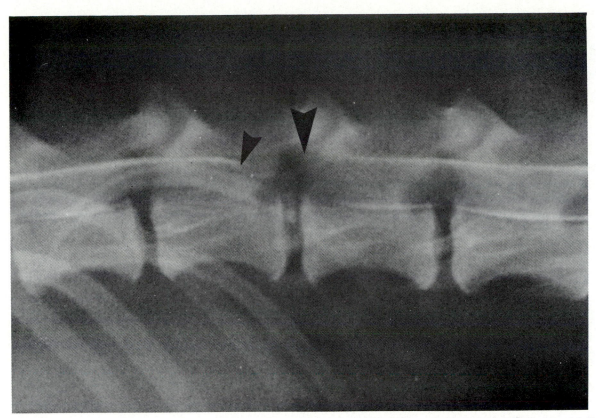

Figure 108–9   Lateral thoracolumbar myelogram of dog shown in Figure 108–8 shows absence of dural filling above L1–2 (*large arrow*) with dural displacement cranially (*small arrow*). Diagnosis: herniated intervertebral disk, L1–2 with cord compression.

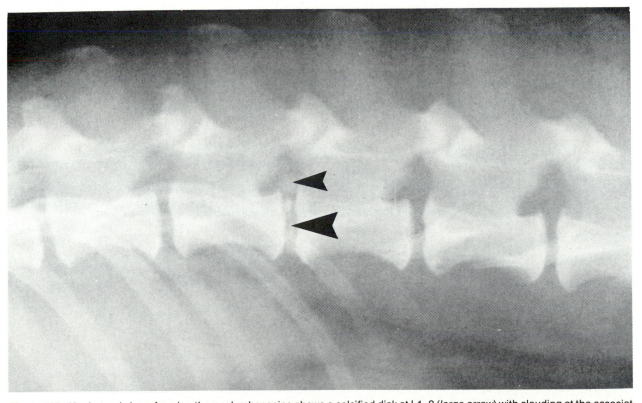

Figure 108–10   Lateral view of canine thoracolumbar spine shows a calcified disk at L1–2 (*large arrow*) with clouding of the associated intervertebral foramen (*small arrow*).

109

SUBACUTE AND CHRONIC SPINAL DISORDERS THAT MAY MIMIC ACUTE CONDITIONS

General Considerations

Fibrocartilaginous emboli, infections, spinal and extraspinal tumors, cervical spondylopathy (cervical vertebral instability, wobbler disease), and congenital spinal anomalies may occasionally cause acute clinical signs or at least alter an animal's behavior or appearance so that it becomes noticeable to the owner. This seemingly abrupt onset of signs is probably the result of a breakdown of compensatory mechanisms, which are no longer able to sustain a relatively normal-appearing animal. The clinical signs in this disease group are highly variable as are the associated neurologic abnormalities. Localizing signs are often absent or, when present, may be vague, contradictory, or misleading.

Major Radiographic Observations

Cervical spondylopathy is usually characterized by one or more of the following abnormalities: subluxation of a spinal unit; vertebral deformity, particularly narrowing of the vertebral foramen; facetal joint asymmetry or deformity; and vertebral remodeling (Figs. 109–2 and 109–3). Stress or postural radiography is often required to demonstrate spatial derangement among the elements of a spinal unit. Advanced spinal tumors may cause either bone deposition or destruction (Figs. 109–4 and 109–5); early tumors may be radiographically invisible, requiring nuclear medicine techniques for detection. The same is true of extraspinal tumors. Congenital abscence of the dens predisposes the C1–2 spinal unit to traumatic subluxation (Fig. 109–1). Fibrocartilaginous emboli are not identifiable with conventional methods.

Diagnostic Strategy

When localizing signs are present, make paired right-angle projections centered over the suspected lesion site. A compression ventrodorsal view greatly enhances the structural detail of cervical and lumbar lesions. If the animal is capable of standing, consider making a postural radiograph (animal in the standing position with the x-ray beam directed horizontally at the suspected lesion site). In the absence of a known lesion location, make multiple lateral views of the entire spine. Supplement with ventrodorsal views as re-quired. If cervical spondylopathy is suspected and cannot be verified on conventional views, make at least two stress films (lateral ventroflexion with fulcrum positioned at a point approximately midway between the head and thoracic inlet, and lateral ventroflexion with the fulcrum positioned at the thoracic inlet).

Pitfalls

Fibrocartilaginous emboli produce no radiographic abnormalities.

Alternative Diagnoses

Subacute fracture, disk disease.

Suggested Reading

Bailey CS, Morgan JP. Diseases of the spinal cord. In: Ettinger SJ, ed. Textbook of veterinary internal medicine. Philadelphia: WB Saunders, 1983:532.

Burk RL, Ackerman N. The spine. In: Burk RL, Ackerman N, eds. Small animal radiology. New York: Churchill Livingstone, 1986:341.

Kealy JK. The skull and vertebral column. In: Kealy JK, ed. Diagnostic radiology of the dog and cat. 2nd ed. Philadelphia: WB Saunders, 1987:511, 516.

Trotter EJ. Canine wobbler syndrome. In: Newton CD, Nunamaker DM, eds. Textbook of small animal orthopedics. Philadelphia: JB Lippincott, 1985:317.

Watrous BJ. Cervical vertebral malformation: malarticulation. In: Farrow CS, ed. Decision making in small animal radiology. Toronto: BC Decker, 1987:70.

Watrous BJ. Spondylitis. In: Farrow CS, ed. Decision making in small animal radiology. Toronto: BC Decker, 1987:80.

Watrous BJ. Discospondylitis. In: Farrow CS, ed. Decision making in small animal radiology. Toronto: BC Decker, 1987:82.

Watrous BJ. Intraspinal soft tissue neoplasia. In: Farrow CS, ed. Decision making in small animal radiology. Toronto: BC Decker, 1987:100.

Watrous BJ. Paravertebral soft tissue neoplasia. In: Farrow CS, ed. Decision making in small animal radiology. Toronto: BC Decker, 1987:102.

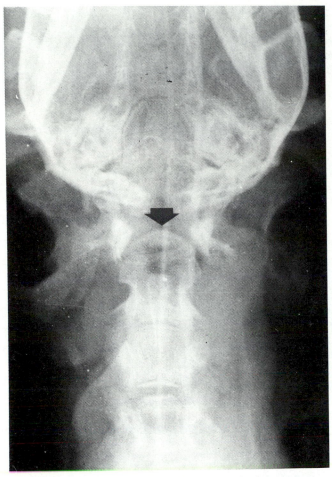

Figure 109–1 Ventrodorsal view of canine proximal cervical spine shows absence of dens (*arrow*). Diagnosis: aplasia of odontoid process.

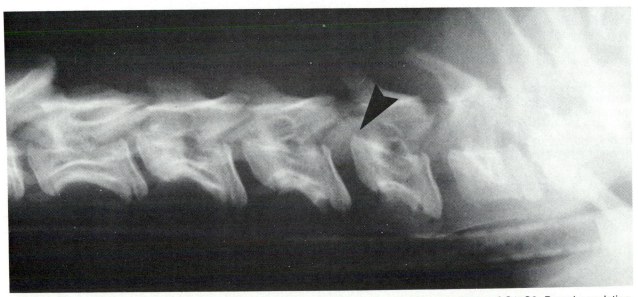

Figure 109–2 Lateral view of immature canine cervical spine shows abnormal vertebral obliquity of C4–C6. Dorsal angulation is greatest at C6 (*arrow*).

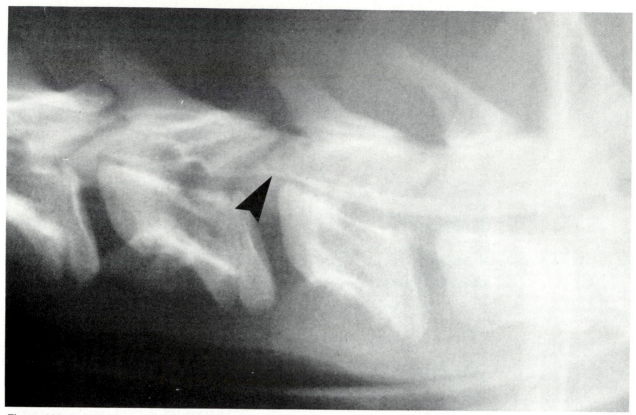

Figure 109–3 Lateral cervical myelogram (traction stress maneuver) of dog shown in Figure 109–2 shows maximum cord displacement over C6 (*arrow*). Diagnosis: cervical spondylopathy (cervical vertebral instability, wobbler syndrome).

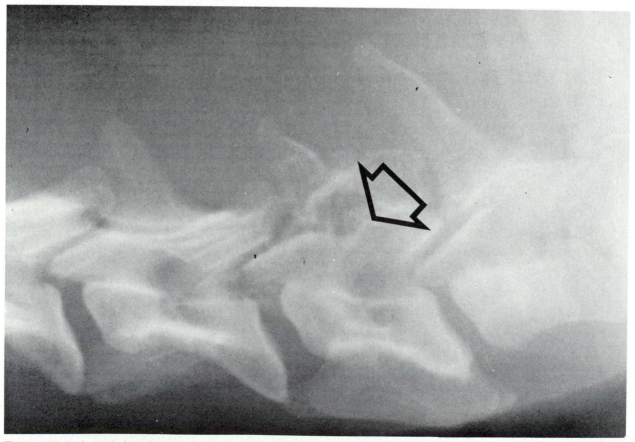

Figure 109–4 Lateral view of canine caudal cervical spine shows lysis of much of C6 (*arrow*).

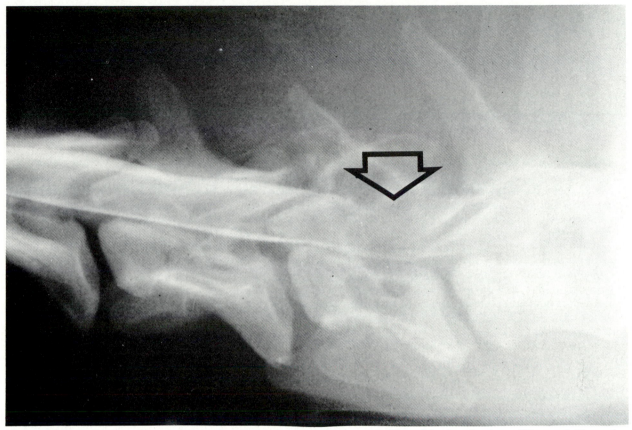

Figure 109–5 Lateral cervical myelogram shows ventral cord displacement and loss of dural contrast over C6 (*arrow*). Diagnosis: cervical cord compression secondary to spinal tumor.

PELVIS AND HIP
110

PELVIC FRACTURE

General Considerations

Pelvic fractures commonly occur in groups, for example, combined fractures of the pubis, pubic symphysis, and ischium, and they often result in considerable short-term pelvic deformity. The entire pelvis may become partially or completely dislocated as a result of injury to the sacroiliac joints. Occasionally, the lower urinary tract is punctured or lacerated secondary to medial fracture fragment displacement. The greater the degree of pelvic disruption or dislocation, the more difficult it is for the animal to stand. The early post-injury period is often very difficult because of the pain associated with getting up, moving about, and defecating. This last factor often results in constipation. With time, most pelvic fractures heal without clinical complication; the exceptions are the nontreated acetabular fracture that becomes arthritic and the permanently narrowed pelvic canal that may cause dystocia in breeding females. Permanent neuromuscular or vascular damage is unusual.

Major Radiographic Observations

Simple sacroiliac separations are best seen in the ventrodorsal view, usually as a widened sacroiliac joint or discontinuity of the caudal iliosacral margin. They are typically associated with two or more additional fractures, most often the pubis and ischium (Figs. 110–1 to 110–4). Displaced ilial fractures are usually evident as a large gap in the central third of the ilium in either standard projection. Nondisplaced ilial fractures are variable in appearance depending on the plane of the fracture and the position of the animal (Figs. 110–5 and 110–6). Pubic fractures may be difficult to see because of superimposition of colonic stool and the tail. When there is comminution, pubic fractures are often best appreciated in the lateral view in which portions of the pubis may be displaced ventrally. Ischial neck fractures are often associated with large gaps best visualized in the ventrodorsal view. Avulsive ischial injuries involving the tuberosities may be seen equally well in both lateral and ventrodorsal projections. Multiple pelvic fractures often result in gross deformity or asymmetry (Figs. 110–7 and 110–8). The latter may be attributed to fracture (as opposed to pelvic obliquity) if the dorsal spinous processes of the caudal lumbar vertebrae appear centered on their respective vertebral bodies in the ventrodorsal view.

Diagnostic Strategy

Make lateral and ventrodorsal views of the pelvis centered over the hips, with the animal's legs in a relaxed, flexed outward position; the flexing greatly reduces patient discomfort associated with the examination. If pelvic deformity or asymmetry is present, yet no fractures are identified, make 30-degree right and left ventrodorsal oblique views centered over the area of suspected injury. If stool obscures the field of interest, gently remove it and remake the appropriate film.

Pitfalls

Oblique ventrodorsal views of the pelvis make the sacroiliac joint closest to the table surface appear wider than normal, thereby mimicking sacroiliac separation. Colonic gas, especially when in relatively linear configurations and superimposed on the pelvis, often resembles a fracture. Fractures involving the ventral aspect of the pelvic canal are often concealed by the colonic contents and tail in the ventrodorsal view. Bilateral sacroiliac separation is often missed because the viewer falsely concludes that since the sacroiliac joints are similar in appearance, they must be normal.

Alternative Diagnoses

Caudal lumbar, sacral, coccygeal, coxofemoral, or proximal femoral fracture.

Suggested Reading

Betts CW. Pelvic fractures. In: Slatter DH, ed. Textbook of small animal surgery. Philadelphia: WB Saunders, 1985:2138.

Kealy JK. Bones and joints. In: Kealy JK, ed. Diagnostic radiology of the dog and cat. 2nd ed. Philadelphia: WB Saunders, 1987:333.

Leighton RL, Robinson GW. Orthopedic surgery. In: Holzworth J, ed. Diseases of the cat. Philadelphia: WB Saunders, 1987:127.

Newton CD. Fractures of the pelvis. In: Newton CD, Nunamaker DM, ed. Textbook of small animal orthopedics. Philadelphia: JB Lippincott, 1985:393.

Owens JM. The pelvis and hips. In: Owens JM, ed. Radiographic interpretations for the small animal clinician. Saint Louis: Ralston Purina Co, 1982:42.

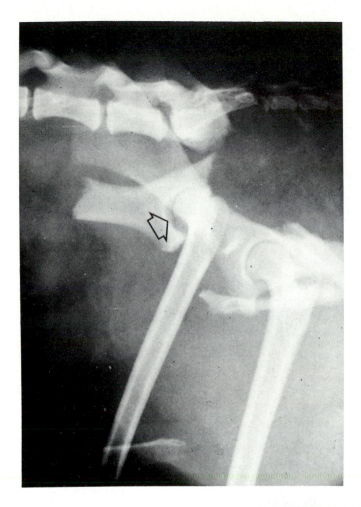

Figure 110–1 Lateral view of feline pelvis shows fractures of the right ileum, acetabulum, and ischium; left sacroiliac joint; and pubic and ischial symphyses. There is also subluxation of the right hip as evidenced by a widened cartilage space (*arrow*). Diagnosis: multiple pelvic fractures.

Figure 110–2 Lateral view of canine pelvis shows fractures of the left acetabulum, pubis, and ischium; and right ileum, pubis, and ischium. The left hip is dislocated and the left distal femur, fractured. Gas in the surrounding soft tissues is from regional lacerations. Diagnosis: multiple pelvic fractures, left femoral fracture, dislocated left hip and lacerations.

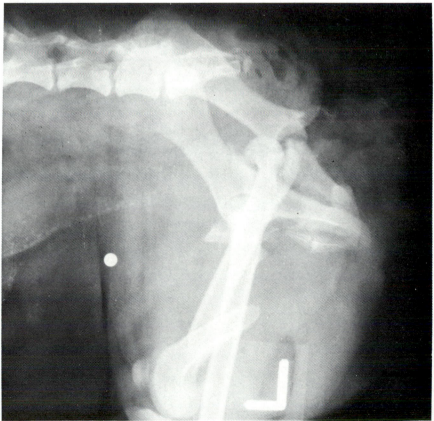

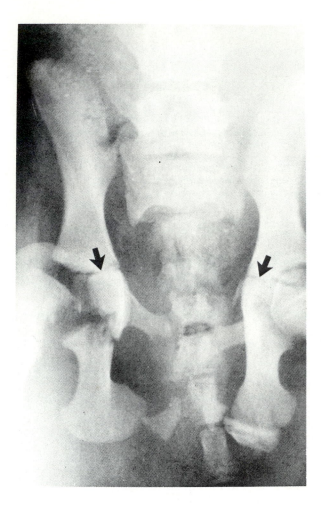

Figure 110–3 Ventrodorsal view of immature canine pelvis shows subluxation of the sacroiliac joints, fractures of the right caudal acetabulum, and multiple fractures of the pubis and ischium bilaterally. A right capital physeal fracture with dislocation of the femoral head is also present. Arrows indicate normal acetabular growth plates. Diagnosis: multiple pelvic fractures, fracture-dislocation of the right hip.

Figure 110–4 Ventrodorsal view of immature feline pelvis shows subluxation of the right sacroiliac joint, bilateral pubic and ischial fractures, and a right capital physeal fracture. Diagnosis: multiple pelvic fractures, fractured right hip.

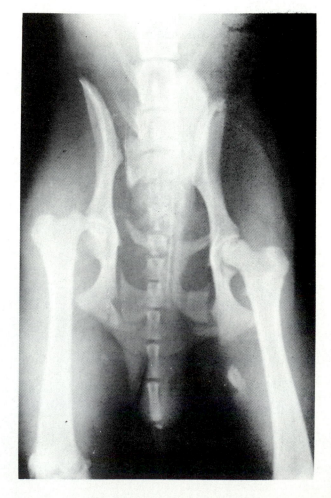

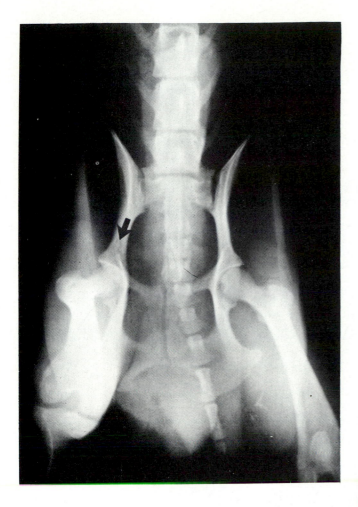

Figure 110–5 Ventrodorsal view of canine pelvis shows bilateral sacroiliac, pubic, and ischial separations and a nondisplaced fracture of the right ilium (*arrow*). The right femur appears deformed because of geometric distortion resulting from limb flexion. Diagnosis: multiple pelvic fractures.

Figure 110–6 Ventrodorsal view of canine pelvis shows nondisplaced, left ilial fracture (*arrow*). Diagnosis: left ilial fracture.

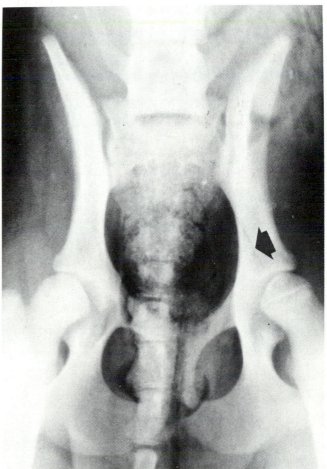

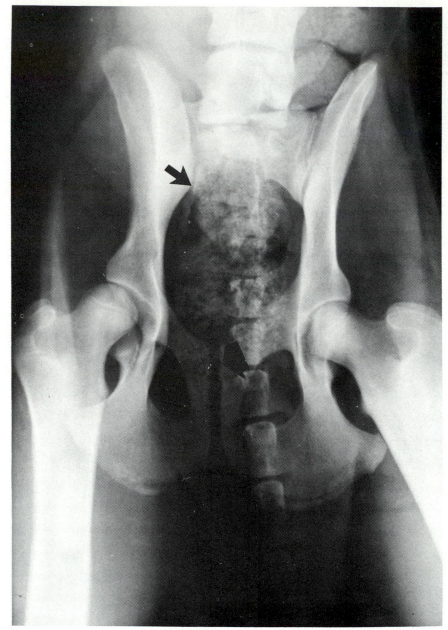

Figure 110–7 Ventrodorsal view of canine pelvis shows slight separation of the right sacroiliac joint (*small arrow*) and moderate displacement of the puboischial symphysis (*large arrow*). Diagnosis: multiple pelvic fractures.

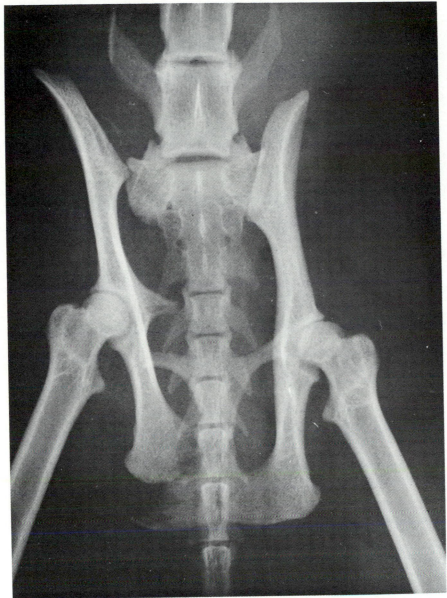

Figure 110–8   Ventrodorsal view of feline pelvis shows fractures of the right ischium, pubis, and sacroiliac joint. Diagnosis: multiple pelvic fractures.

111

HIP FRACTURES AND DISLOCATIONS

General Considerations

Acetabular fractures, as any joint injury, may lead to arthritis if untreated, or unsuccessfully treated. Generally, the greater the resulting incongruency, the more severe the arthritis. For this reason, it is extremely important that acetabular fractures be identified early. Most dislocated hips occur craniodorsally. Alternatively, but much less frequently, luxated hips may be displaced in a cranioventral, ventral or caudal direction. Displacement of the femoral head through a medial acetabular fracture is termed a central dislocation. Dislocated hips are often associated with pelvic or proximal femoral fractures. A dysplastic hip is predisposed to traumatic dislocation.

Major Radiographic Observations

Most acetabular fractures may be detected in one or both standard views as a thick radiolucent band crossing the acetabulum (Figs. 111–1 and 111–2). Peripheral acetabular fractures usually occur in the cranial or caudal margins as variable-sized chips or fragments. Central dislocations show the affected proximal femur within the pelvic canal (Fig. 111–3).

Diagnostic Strategy

A craniodorsally dislocated hip often projects as a distinctive hump in the central or proximal one third of the dorsal iliac margin (Figs. 111–4 and 111–5). In the ventrodorsal view, the femoral head is usually displaced in a craniolateral direction, and is occasionally associated with a small avulsion fracture originating from the central margin of the femoral head at the insertion of the round ligament (Figs. 111–6 and 111–7).

Begin with a ventrodorsal view centered on the hips, with the animal's legs in a flexed (frogleg) position; this is much less painful for the animal than the more frequently employed extended position. A plastic-covered foam pad beneath the animal further reduces patient discomfort. Examine both coxofemoral joints for fracture and dislocation, and examine the surrounding pelvis for additional injuries. If hip luxation is suspected but not confirmed in the ventrodorsal view, make a lateral projection centered on the hips and check for two lucent crescents, which represent the cartilage spaces of the coxofemoral joints. If these are absent, dislocation is confirmed. When there is uncertainty about acetabular fracture, oblique lateral and ventrodorsal views centered over the hip in question are usually diagnostic. If there is still doubt, make comparable views of the uninvolved hip for comparison.

Pitfalls

Dorsally luxated hips may appear normal in an extended ventrodorsal radiograph, depending on the amount of hindlimb traction applied by the radiographer. A fracture bed in the midproximal border of the femoral head may be mimicked by the normal insertion site of the round ligament.

Alternative Diagnoses

Pelvic or proximal femoral fractures.

Suggested Reading

Hauptman J. The hip joint. In: Slatter DH, ed. Textbook of small animal surgery. Philadelphia: WB Saunders, 1985:2153.

Kealy JK. Bones and joints. In: Kealy JK, ed. Diagnostic radiology of the dog and cat. 2nd ed. Philadelphia: WB Saunders, 1987:335.

Leighton RL, Robinson GW. Orthopedic surgery. In: Holzworth J, ed. Diseases of the cat. Philadelphia: WB Saunders, 1987: 127, 147.

Nunamaker DM. Fractures and dislocations of the hip joint. In: Newton CD, Nunamaker DM, eds. Textbook of small animal orthopedics. Philadelphia: JB Lippincott, 1985:403.

Owens JM. The pelvis and hips. In: Owens JM, ed. Radiographic interpretations for the small animal clinician. Saint Louis: Ralston Purina Co, 1982:42.

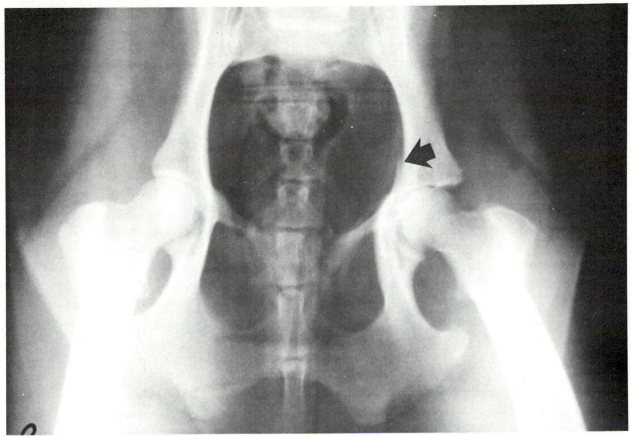

Figure 111–1 Ventrodorsal view of hips shows a minimally displaced fracture of the left acetabulum (*arrow*) and pubis. Diagnosis: left acetabular fracture.

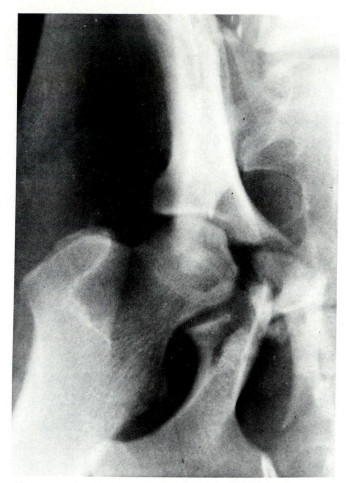

Figure 111–2 Ventrodorsal view of canine right acetabulum shows impaction-type fracture. Diagnosis: right acetabular fracture.

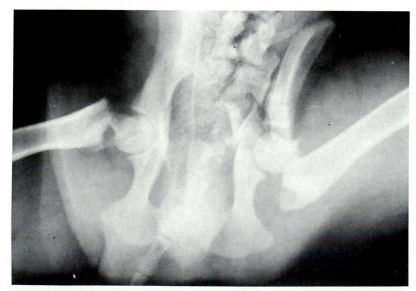

Figure 111–3 Ventrodorsal view of canine pelvis shows comminuted fracture of the left acetabulum and bilateral femoral neck fractures. Additional pelvic fractures are obscured by patient positioning and colonic stool. Diagnosis: multiple pelvic fractures with bilateral femoral neck fractures.

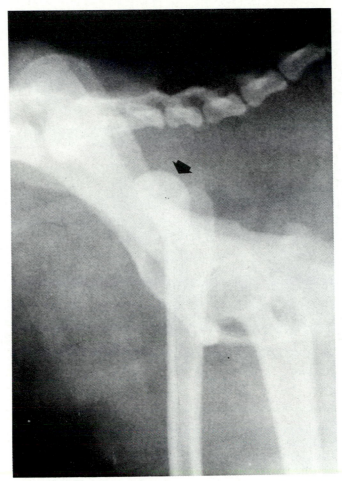

Figure 111–4 Lateral view of feline pelvis shows unilateral luxation of the right hip (*arrow*). Diagnosis: dislocated right hip.

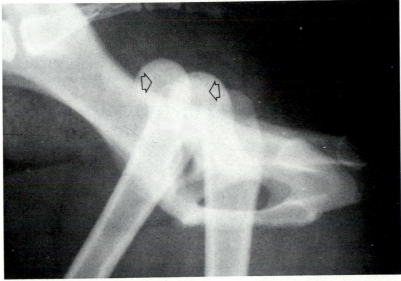

Figure 111–5 Lateral view of canine pelvis shows bilateral hip luxation (*arrows*). Diagnosis: bilateral hip dislocation.

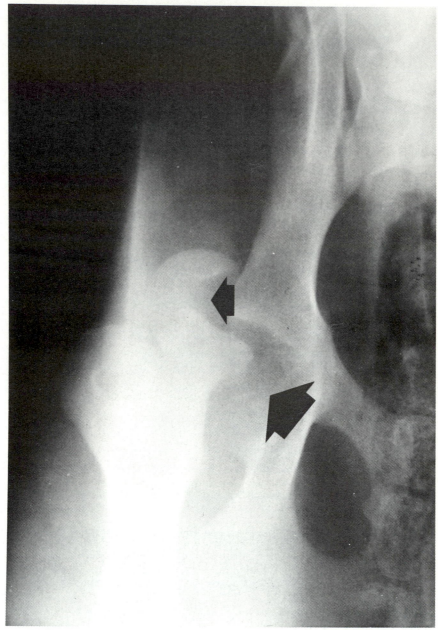

Figure 111–6 Ventrodorsal view of canine hip shows femoral head luxation (*large arrow*) and complete fracture of the associated capital physis (*small arrow*). Diagnosis: right femoral fracture-dislocation.

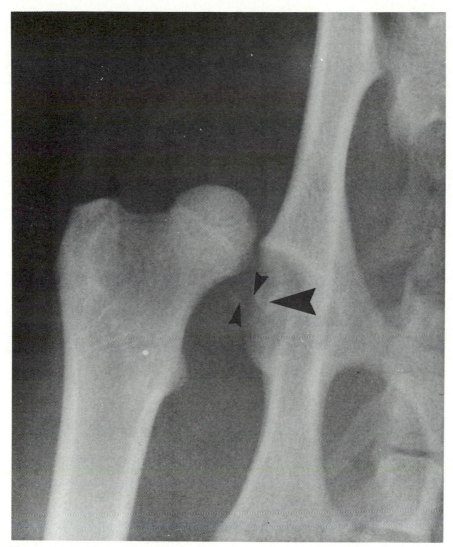

Figure 111–7 Ventrodorsal view of canine right hip shows luxation of the femur with multiple acetabular bone fragments (*arrows*). Diagnosis: dislocated hip with associated avulsion fractures of the femoral head.

THE HINDLIMB

Special Problems Related to Fractures in Immature Animals.

These special features include the following:
1. The presence of growth plates, which in young animals are a frequent site of injury, sometimes leading to growth disturbance and angular limb deformities.
2. The presence of multiple, variably shaped growth plates, dense and irregular metaphyses (cut-back zones), secondary centers of ossification, and large outstanding nutrient foramina, which may be mistaken for fracture lines.
3. The occurrence of incomplete or greenstick fractures, which commonly occur in immature bones due to their increased resiliency or elasticity.
4. The ability to heal and remodel rapidly following fracture injury.

Because of the difficulties inherent in the assessment of fractures of the extremities in young animals, I *strongly recommend* that radiographs of the opposite limb be obtained for comparison.

Growth Plate Injuries

Fractures of the *pressure* epiphyses and associated growth plates (for example, the distal radius and ulna) are customarily classified according to a system developed by Drs. Salter and Harris, in which the injury is graded I to VI, depending on the fracture plane and involvement of the associated metaphysis. This classification serves both to describe the fracture briefly and to provide a general prognosis. Alternatively, growth plate injuries may be described simply by indicating the location of the separation; the direction of epiphyseal displacement; the presence, direction, and location of any associated fractures; and the angulation occurring secondary to the injury. Fractures of the *traction* epiphyses and related growth plates (for example, the greater or lesser trochanters) are usually less complicated, being of the avulsion type; in this respect they may be described simply as avulsion fractures.

112
FEMORAL FRACTURE

General Considerations

A wide variety of femoral injuries may occur, probably more often than to any other single bone in the body. This is particularly true of immature dogs and cats, which can sustain various types of growth plate injuries and greenstick fractures in addition to the more conventional shaft and metaphyseal breaks. Such injuries may be accompanied by dislocations of the hip, second- or third-degree stifle sprains, and pelvic fractures. The relative anatomic complexity of both the proximal and distal aspects of the femur, especially in young animals, often warrants making a radiograph of the opposite femur for comparison.

Major Radiographic Observations

Proximal femoral growth plate fractures may involve the femoral head or greater trochanter; occasionally, the lesser trochanter is avulsed (Figs. 112–1 to 112–9). Fractures to the distal femoral growth plates may affect the femoral trochlea or condyles. When displaced, these fractures are not hard to identify; however, when there is little or no fragment displacement, the injury may be indistinguishable from the normal growth plate, even when compared to the opposite limb. Greenstick diaphyseal fractures may require an optimal projection angle, in addition to a high-quality image, to be detected. Proximal femoral fractures in the adult usually involve the neck as opposed to the femoral head, with trochan-

teric injuries being much less common. Distal femoral fractures in the adult are less difficult to identify than those in immature animals, but the detection of articular fractures remains problematic, often requiring special views (Figs. 112–10 to 112–12).

Diagnostic Strategy

Suspected femoral-head fractures not seen in lateral and conventional extended ventrodorsal views may often be verified in the flexed (frogleg) ventrodorsal view. The same is often true of femoral-neck fractures. Questionable trochanter injuries are often clarified with ventrodorsal oblique projections. Suspected greenstick breaks that are not apparent on initial radiographs are often identified a few days later following resorption of dead bone along the fracture margins with resulting fracture visibility. Alternatively, a suspected but unverified fracture may be seen on later films as a callus, suggesting an earlier healing fracture.

Pitfalls

Partially flexed ventrodorsal views of the femur often result in marked geometric distortion and magnification, which may result in both false-positive and false-negative findings. Consequently, caution should be exercised in analyzing and interpreting such projections.

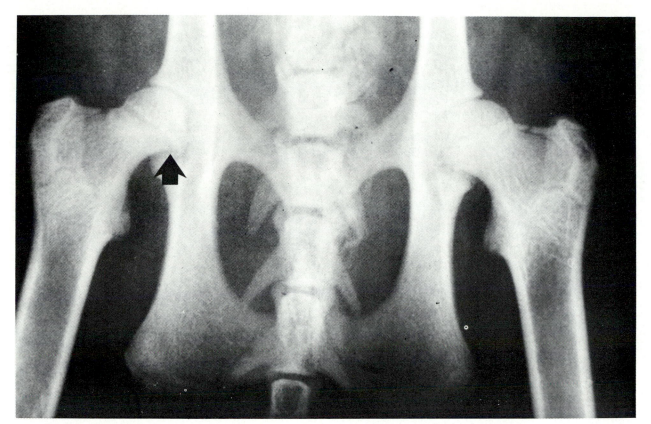

Figure 112–1 Ventrodorsal view of immature feline hips shows minimally displaced fracture of right capital physis (*arrow*). Diagnosis: right capital physeal fracture.

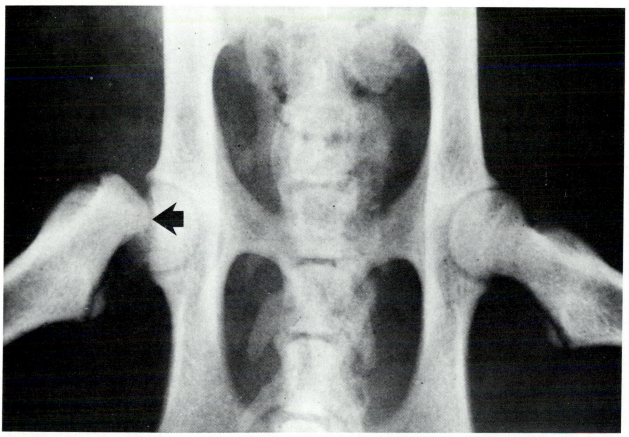

Figure 112–2 Ventrodorsal view of immature feline hips shows severely displaced fracture of right capital physis (*arrow*). Diagnosis: right capital physeal fracture.

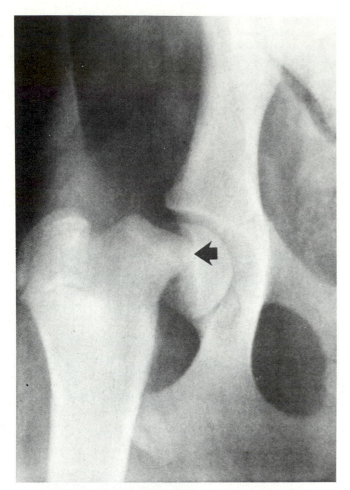

Figure 112-3   Ventrodorsal view of immature canine hip shows severely displaced fracture of right capital physis (*arrow*). Diagnosis: right capital physeal fracture.

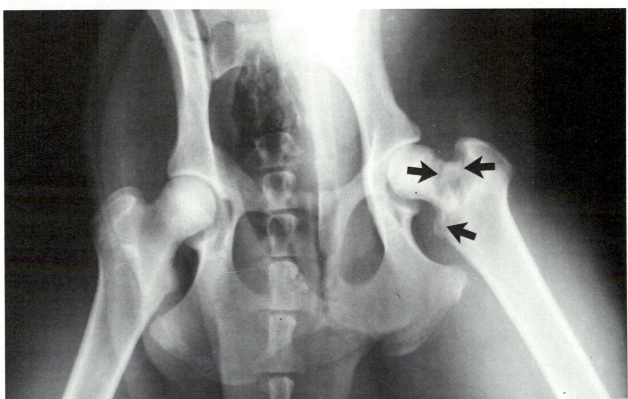

Figure 112-4   Ventrodorsal view of immature canine hips in mildly flexed position shows nondisplaced fracture of left femoral neck including the lesser trochanter (arrows).

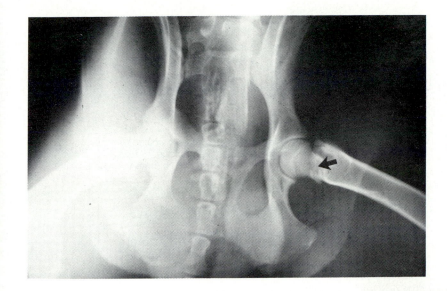

Figure 112-5 Ventrodorsal view of the patient shown in Figure 112-4, with hips in moderately flexed position, shows minimally displaced fracture of left femoral neck including the lesser trochanter (*arrow*). Diagnosis: left femoral neck fracture including lesser trochanter.

Figure 112-6 Ventrodorsal view of feline pelvis shows fractures of the right femoral head (*large arrow*) and greater trochanter (*small arrow*). Diagnosis: proximal right femoral fractures.

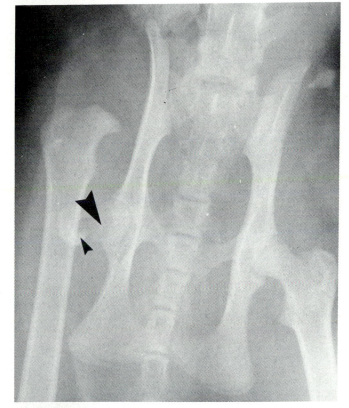

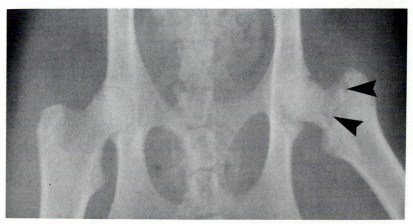

Figure 112-7 Ventrodorsal view of feline hips shows minimally displaced fracture of the left femoral neck (*arrows*). Pelvic asymmetry is due to multiple pelvic fractures. Diagnosis: left femoral neck fracture.

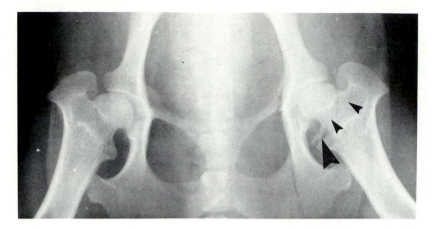

Figure 112-8 Ventrodorsal view of canine hips shows hairline fractures of the left femoral neck (*small arrows* and a displaced fracture of the associated lesser trochanter (*large arrow*). Fractures of the left pubis and ischium are also present. Diagnosis: multiple pelvic and left femoral fractures.

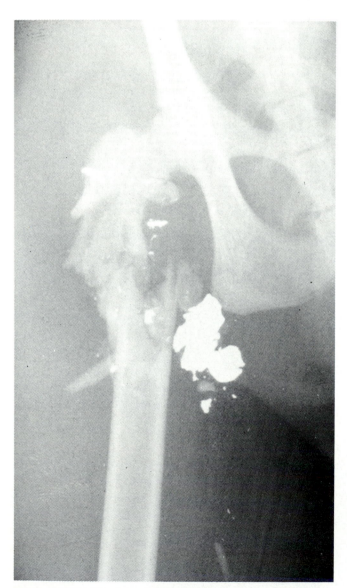

Figure 112-9 Craniocaudal view of feline right proximal femur shows severely comminuted fracture with lead fragments. Diagnosis: severe right femoral gunshot fracture.

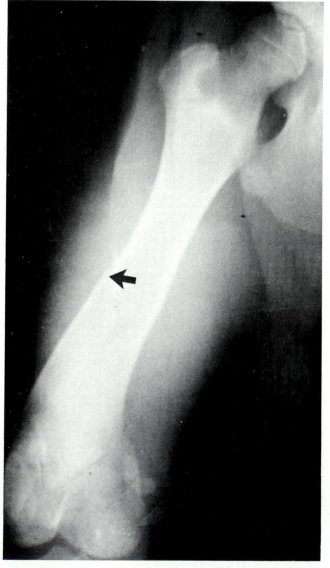

Figure 112-10 Craniocaudal oblique view of immature canine right femur shows minimally displaced fracture (*arrow*). Diagnosis: right femoral shaft fracture.

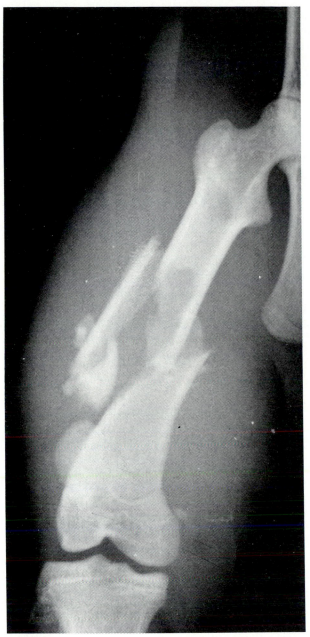

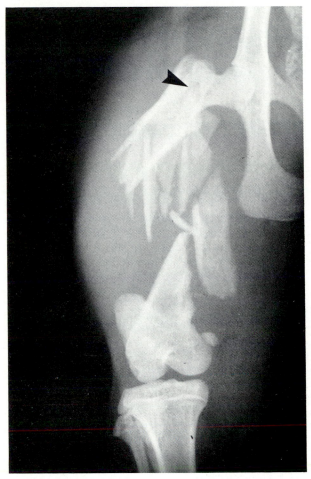

Figure 112–12 Craniocaudal view of feline femur shows severely comminuted fracture with a fissure line extending into the greater trochanter (*arrow*). Regional soft-tissue swelling (hemorrhage) is marked. Diagnosis: severely comminuted right femoral shaft fracture.

Figure 112–11 Craniocaudal view of feline femur shows comminuted mid-diaphyseal fracture with a large butterfly fragment and much regional soft-tissue swelling (hemorrhage). Diagnosis: comminuted right femoral shaft fracture.

Alternative Diagnoses

Pelvic and hip fractures, stifle injuries, and severe contusion of the thigh region, including hematoma.

Suggested Reading

Leighton RL, Robinson GW. Orthopedic surgery. In: Holzworth J, ed. Diseases of the cat. Philadelphia: WB Saunders, 1987:111.

Kealy JK. The skull and vertebral column. In: Kealy JK, ed. Diagnostic radiology of the dog and cat. 2nd ed. Philadelphia: WB Saunders, 1987:397, 404, 409.

Milton JL, Newman ME. Fractures of the femur. In: Slatter DH, ed. Textbook of small animal surgery. Philadelphia: WB Saunders, 1985:2180.

Newton CD. Fracture of the femur. In: Newton CD, Nunamaker DM, eds. Textbook of small animal orthopedics. Philadelphia: JB Lippincott, 1985:415.

Owens JM. The pelvis and hips. In: Owens JM, ed. Radiographic interpretation for the small animal clinician. Saint Louis: Ralston Purina Co, 1982:43, 48.

113

PATELLAR FRACTURE

General Considerations

Fractures of the patella are relatively uncommon injuries; they are typically transverse through the center of the patella and often result in considerable distraction of the proximal fragment. Less commonly, a small chip or flake of bone is detached from one of the poles with only minimal distraction. This type of fracture indicates a partial tearing of the patellar ligament at its point of attachment and is most accurately termed a *sprain-avulsion injury*. Longitudinal or comminuted fractures of the patella are rare. Typically, affected animals are unable to extend their stifles fully.

Major Radiographic Observations

There is often a large gap in the center of the patella. The uppermost fragment is usually displaced proximally (Figs. 113–1 and 113–2). Polar avulsions are more difficult to detect because of their smaller size and close proximity to the parent bone, but they usually are seen as small bone-dense flakes just beyond the proximal border of the patella in the lateral view.

Diagnostic Strategy

Make a single lateral view of the patella using a 10-percent reduction in kVp relative to standard stifle technique. The decrease in technique improves the chances of identifying small avulsion fractures that might otherwise be lost to overpenetration.

Pitfalls

The lateral extended view of the stifle results in a more proximal position of the patella and therefore mimics traumatic displacement. This does not occur when the leg is in a neutral or flexed position.

Alternative Diagnoses

Avulsion of the tibial tuberosity, ruptured patellar ligament (third-degree sprain).

Suggested Reading

Hulse DA, Shires PK. The stifle joint. In: Slatter DH, ed. Textbook of small animal surgery. Philadelphia: WB Saunders, 1985:2193.

Kealy JK. Bones and joints. In: Kealy JK, ed. Diagnostic radiology of the dog and cat. 2nd ed. Philadelphia: WB Saunders, 1987:398.

Leighton RL, Robinson GW. Orthopedic surgery. In: Holzworth J, ed. Diseases of the cat. Philadelphia: WB Saunders, 1987:120.

Newton CD. Fractures of small bones. In: Newton CD, Nunamaker DM, eds. Textbook of small animal orthopedics. Philadelphia: JB Lippincott, 1985:453.

Owens JM. The stifle. In: Owens JM, ed. Radiographic interpretation for the small animal clinician. Saint Louis: Ralston Purina Co, 1982:48.

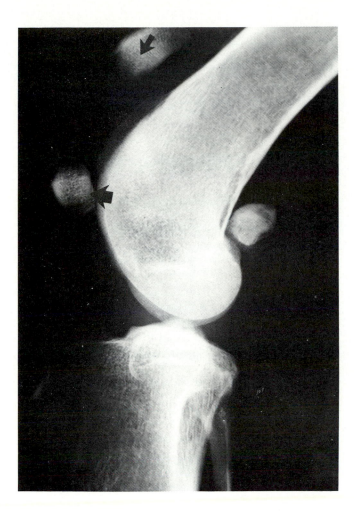

Figure 113-1 Lateral view of canine stifle shows a complete fracture of the distal third of the patella with associated fragment displacement (*arrows*). Diagnosis: displaced central patella fracture.

Figure 113-2 Lateral view of canine stifle shows absence of the distal third of the patella (*arrow*) and lead fragments. The remaining patella is displaced in a cranioproximal direction. Diagnosis: gunshot fracture to the patella and patella ligament.

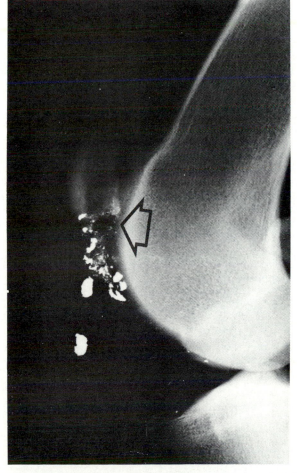

114

STIFLE JOINT FRACTURES AND DISLOCATIONS

General Considerations

Articular fractures involving the stifle joint are uncommon. They may involve either of the two major bony components—the femoral condyle and tibial plateau—or the various sesamoids including the patella. Of these, oblique fractures of the femoral condyle are most common. A vertical intercondylar fracture may be combined with a transverse supracondylar fracture, resulting in a T-type or three-piece intercondylar fracture of the distal femur; alternatively, a V-shaped supracondylar separation may be combined with a vertical intercondylar break to produce a Y fracture. Avulsion of the long digital extensor tendon from its femoral attachment site typically results in a small bone fragment being torn from the cranial aspect of the lateral femoral condyle. Articular fractures of the proximal tibia are also uncommon, with lateral or medial oblique fractures of the tibial plateau being the most usual. Third-degree sprains of the femerotibial collateral ligaments and of the cranial cruciate ligament may result in small avulsion fractures if the involved ligaments tear at their points of attachment, as opposed to separating centrally. Such injuries may occur in combination or separately; in most cases they produce subluxation or dislocation. Second-degree sprains of the cruciate or collateral ligaments usually produce some subluxation and instability, although this may not be demonstrable until related swelling and muscle spasm have subsided. Such injuries potentiate future rupture or arthritis if the stifle is not immobilized, supported, or at least rested for an appropriate period of time. Meniscal tears are rarely seen in pet animals as isolated injuries but many occur in conjunction with other injuries such as cruciate or collateral sprains.

Major Radiographic Observations

Articular fractures of the distal femur and proximal tibia show best in the caudocranial view, usually as a widened condyle, and occasionally as a distinct fracture line entering the stifle joint (Figs. 114–4 and 114–5). Sprain-avulsions of the various femerotibial ligaments are usually seen as small bone fragments near their points of origin, with or without comparable defects in the adjacent parent bone (Fig. 114–3). Severe sprains without fractures may or may not show spatial derangement of the stifle joint. (Figs. 114–1 and 114–2).

Diagnostic Strategy

Make two views of the stifle—lateral and caudocranial—being certain to penetrate the distal femur sufficiently to al-low identification of articular fracture lines. If an articular fracture is suspected but cannot be verified, make well-penetrated, limited-field, right and left caudocranial oblique views; in most cases they resolve the question. The oblique projections are also useful in detecting small sprain-avulsion fractures. Suspected joint instability that is not appreciable in standard and oblique views is often shown using stress radiography. Because stress maneuvers are painful, they should only be done under sedation or, preferably, general anesthesia. Suspected cruciate injuries are best verified by surgical inspection, although an experienced arthrographer may be able to identify such injuries.

Pitfalls

The stifle joint shows an extremely wide range of widths in the caudocranial view, depending on the manner in which the animal is positioned and restrained, as well as the angle and center point of the x-ray beam. Accordingly, neither a widened nor a narrowed stifle joint should be presumed to indicate injury without collaborating clinical data. The popliteal sesamoid, normally found immediately proximal to the tibia in the lateral view, may be mistaken for a fracture fragment.

Alternative Diagnoses

Distal femoral or proximal tibial fractures.

Suggested Reading

Farrow CS, Newton CD. Ligamentous injury(sprain). In: Newton CD, Nunamaker DM, eds. Textbook of small animal orthopedics, Philadelphia: JB Lippincott, 1985:843.

Hulse DA, Shires PK. The stifle joint. In: Slatter DH, ed. Textbook of small animal surgery. Philadelphia: WB Saunders, 1985:2193.

Leighton RL, Robinson GW. Orthopedic surgery. In: Holzworth J, ed. Diseases of the cat. Philadelphia: WB Saunders, 1987:143.

Kealy JK. Bones and joints. In: Kealy JK, ed. Diagnostic radiology of the dog and cat. 2nd ed. Philadelphia: WB Saunders, 1987:341.

Nunamaker DM. Fractures and dislocations of the stifle. In: Newton CD, Nunamaker DM, eds. Textbook of small animal orthopedics. Philadelphia: JB Lippincott, 1985:433.

Owens JM. The stifle. In: Owens JM, ed. Radiographic interpretation for the small animal clinician. Saint Louis: Ralston Purina Co, 1982:44.

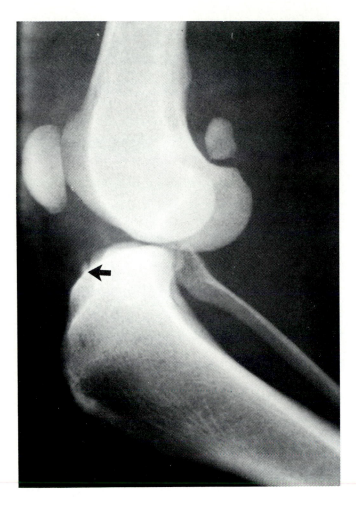

Figure 114–1 Lateral view of canine stifle shows cranial dislocation of the tibia associated with a small avulsion fracture (*arrow*).

Figure 114–2 Craniocaudal view of Figure 114–1 shows medial dislocation of the tibia. Diagnosis: sprain-fracture-luxation of the stifle.

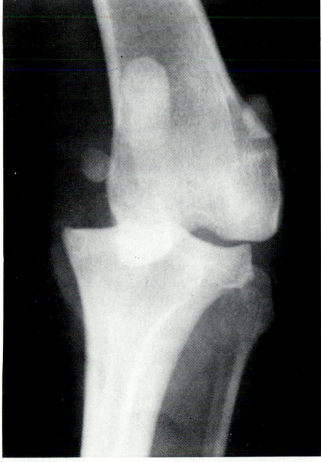

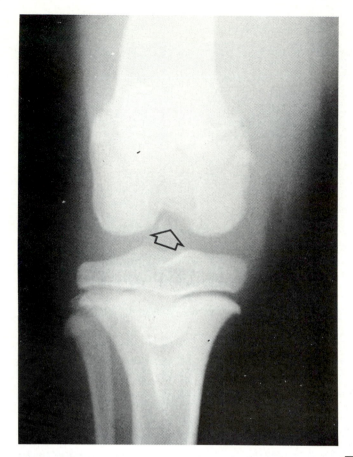

Figure 114–3   Craniocaudal view of immature canine stifle shows bone fragment in central part of joint (*arrow*). Diagnosis: avulsion fracture of medial tibial tubercle.

Figure 114–4   Craniocaudal view of canine stifle shows an oblique, distal femoral articular fracture extending from the medial metaphysis through the central aspect of condyle (*arrow*). Diagnosis: displaced intracondylar fracture.

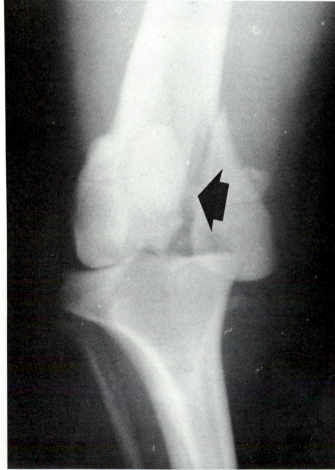

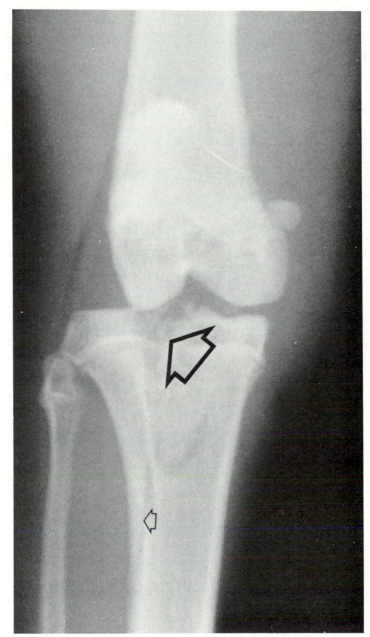

Figure 114–5 Craniocaudal view of immature feline stifle shows a minimally displaced, centrally depressed, split fracture of the proximal tibia with lateral dislocation (*arrows*). Diagnosis: proximal tibial articular fracture.

115

TIBIAL AND FIBULAR FRACTURES

General Considerations

Proximal tibial avulsion fractures occur regularly in immature dogs and may involve the tibial tuberosity alone or the tibial tuberosity and the proximal tibial epiphysis (tibial plateau). Tibial shaft fractures range from greenstick breaks in the young to severely comminuted, segmental injuries in adults, with most occurring in the central third and being steeply oblique or spiral in nature. The associated part of the fibula is usually fractured, although this is not always detectable until after a callus begins to form; isolated tibial fractures are unusual. Distal tibiofibular fractures usually involve the growth plates in young animals; the malleoli are frequently fractured in mature individuals, usually in conjunction with collateral ligament sprain. The destabilizing nature of sprain-fracture injury to one or both malleoli often results in subluxation or dislocation.

Major Radiographic Observations

Isolated tibial tuberosity fractures are of the avulsion type and are typically displaced proximally by the pull of the quadriceps. Fractures of both the tibial tuberosity and proximal tibial epiphysis are usually distracted in a proximocaudal direction, assuming hingelike configuration in lateral view (Figs. 115–1 to 115–3). The proximal tibial growth plate may be sheared laterally with resulting epiphyseal displacement (Fig. 115–4). If displacement is minimal, comparison with the contralateral limb or stress radiographs may be required for confirmation (Fig. 115–5). The same is true of fractures of the distal tibial epiphysis or the lateral or medial maleolus. Because of the avulsive nature of most malleolar fractures and the resulting instability, the tibiotarsal joint space is usually widened (Figs. 115–9 and 115–10). Diaphyseal fractures vary with the plane of breakage and degree of fragment displacement (Figs. 115–6 to 115–8).

Diagnostic Strategy

Make two limited-field views centered over the tibia at the point of suspected injury, which can usually be isolated to the proximal, middle, or distal third; reduce the radiographic technique as the field is moved distally. Make comparison views of the opposite limb, and use stress radiography as required. Oblique projections are often necessary to assess malleolar injuries accurately and completely.

Pitfalls

It is often very difficult to differentiate a distal tibial growth plate fracture with epiphyseal separation from a tibiotarsal subluxation or dislocation secondary to a malleolar fracture.

Alternative Diagnoses

Stifle and tarsal injuries.

Suggested Reading

Burk RL, Ackerman N. The appendicular skeleton. In: Burk RL, Ackerman N, eds. Small animal radiology. New York: Churchill Livingstone, 1986:337.

Gofton N. Fractures of the tibia and fibula. In: Slatter DH, ed. Textbook of small animal surgery. Philadelphia: WB Saunders, 1985:2235.

Kealy JK. Bones and joints. In: Kealy JK, ed. Diagnostic radiology of the dog and cat. 2nd ed. Philadelphia: WB Saunders, 1987:344, 398, 399.

Leighton RL, Robinson GW. Orthopedic surgery. In: Holzworth J, ed. Diseases of the cat. Philadelphia: WB Saunders, 1987:120.

Nunamaker DM. Fractures of the tibia and fibula. In: Newton CD, Nunamaker DM, eds. Textbook of small animal orthopedics. Philadelphia: JB Lippincott, 1985:439.

Owens JM. The stifle. In: Owens JM, ed. Radiographic interpretation for the small animal clinician. Saint Louis: Ralston Purina Co, 1982:44.

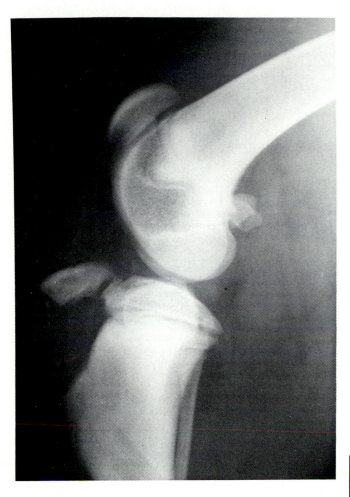

Figure 115–1 Lateral view of immature canine stifle shows cranioproximal displacement of the tibial tuberosity with proximal displacement of the patella (see Fig. 115–2 for normal left stifle). Diagnosis: avulsion fracture of the tibial tuberosity.

Figure 115–2 Lateral view of normal opposite stifle for comparison with Figure 115–1.

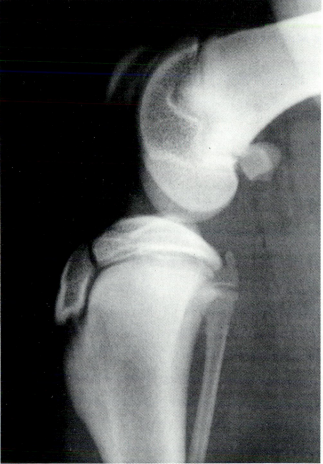

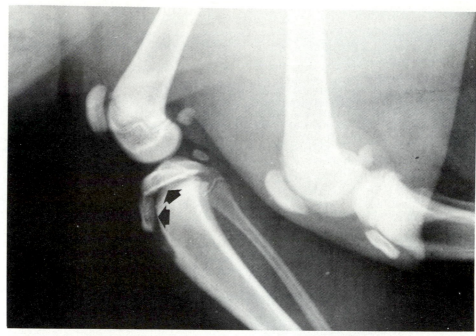

Figure 115–3   Lateral view of immature feline stifles shows growth plate fractures of the proximal tibial epiphysis and tuberosity (*arrows*). Diagnosis: proximal physeal fractures of the tibia.

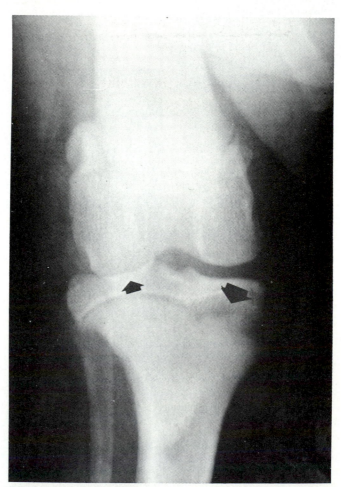

Figure 115–4   Craniocaudal view of immature canine stifle shows widening of the medial aspect of the proximal tibial growth plate (*large arrow*) with overlap of the lateral aspect of the stifle joint (*small arrow*). Diagnosis: probable proximal tibial growth plate fracture.

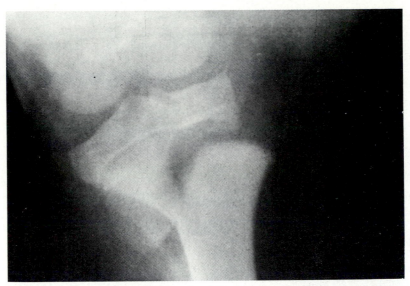

Figure 115–5   Craniocaudal stress view (lateral wedge maneuver) of stifle shown in Figure 115–4. Diagnosis: confirmation of suspected proximal tibial growth plate fracture.

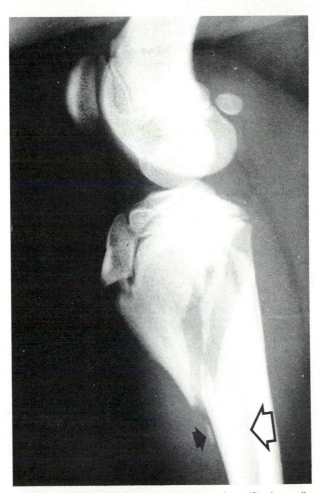

Figure 115–6   Lateral view of immature canine stifle shows displaced, comminuted fracture of the tibia extending from the metaphyseal side of the proximal tibial growth plate to the cranial aspect of the proximal diaphysis. There is a small cortical fragment distally (*small arrow*) and a long fissure in the center of the tibial shaft (*large arrow*). Diagnosis: displaced, proximal tibial metaphyseal fracture.

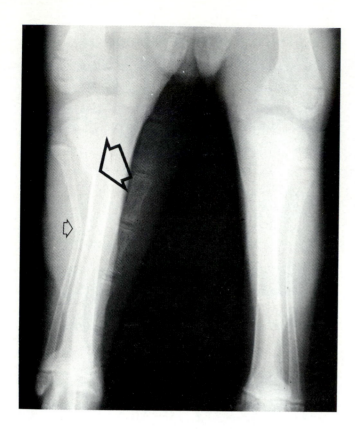

Figure 115–7 Craniocaudal view of immature canine tibias and fibulas shows folding fractures of right proximal tibia (*large arrow*) and central fibula (*small arrow*). There is an overall reduction in bone density and thinning of the cortices. Diagnosis: pathological fractures due to nutritional secondary hyperparathyroidism.

Figure 115–8 Lateral view of canine tibia and fibula shows displaced central diaphyseal fractures (*arrows*). Diagnosis: tibial and fibular shaft fractures.

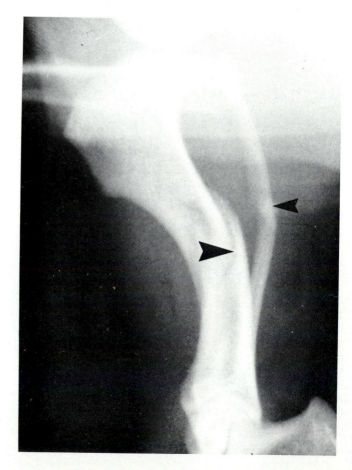

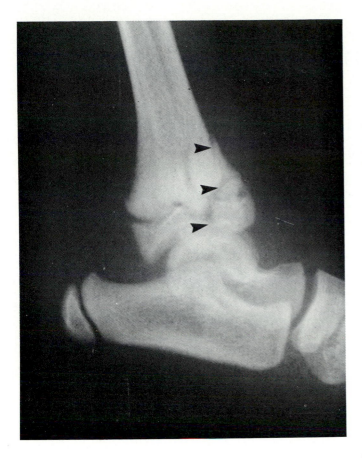

Figure 115–9 Lateral view of immature canine left tarsus shows fracture extending through the distal tibial metaphysis, growth plate, and epiphysis (*arrows*). Diagnosis: Salter-Harris fracture, type IV.

Figure 115–10 Lateral view of canine right tarsus shows widened distal tibial growth plate (*arrow*). Diagnosis: minimally displaced distal tibial growth plate fracture.

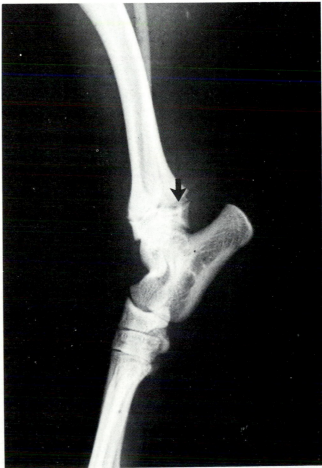

116

TARSAL FRACTURES AND DISLOCATIONS

General Considerations

As with any anatomically complex joint, the tarsus or hock may be fractured in a wide variety of ways. These injuries have been elaborately categorized according to severity and pattern, for example, calcaneal and central tarsal bone fractures in racing greyhounds. Articular fractures of the distal tibia are rare, except for the medial malleolus. Collateral sprain avulsions may involve the lateral or medial malleoli as well as the outer margins of the talus or calcaneus and the plantar surface of the hock. Subluxation may occur at any of fours levels in the tarsus: the tibiotarsal joint, the proximal intertarsal joint, the distal intertarsal joint, or the tarsometatarsal joint. Abrasion injuries from being dragged over pavement may remove substantial amounts of bone from the lateral or medial aspects of the carpus in addition to the more obvious soft-tissue loss.

Major Radiographic Observations

Malleolar fractures are often first noted indirectly, on the basis of regional soft-tissue swelling or a subluxated or dislocated tibiotarsal joint (Figs. 116–1 to 116–5). Closer inspection, especially if aided by oblique views, usually shows a malleolar fracture line or detachment. Calcaneal fractures are most often avulsive and therefore distractive, with the os calcaneus being pulled proximally; some however are only minimally displaced (Figs. 116–7 and 116–8). Occasionally, the base of the calcaneus is fractured transversely where it enters the talocalcaneal joint; or, the sustentaculum is fractured vertically, thus becoming separated from the remaining calcaneus. Rarely, the anconeal process of the calcaneus is fractured. Talar fractures, often best seen in oblique projection, may involve either trochlear ridge or may break longitudinally into both the tibiotarsal and proximal intertarsal joints (slab fracture). Avulsion fractures may occur from the lateral margin of the talus (see Fig. 116–1). The remaining tarsal bones may be chipped, "slabbed", or comminuted, with or without derangement of the associated joints (Fig. 116–6). Abrasion injuries may show tissue defects, soft-tissue swelling, gas, road debris, and bone loss.

Diagnostic Strategy

Make four views: lateral, dorsoplantar, and right and left lateral obliques centered directly over the tarsus and excluding most of the tibia, fibula, and metatarsus. If a lower hindlimb survey is required, make a lateral projection centered over the middle third of the tibia, extending proximally to the stifle and distally to the digits, using a compromise technique kVp sufficient to penetrate the stifle, but not to overexpose the metatarsus.

Pitfalls

Lateral and dorsoplantar views alone often fail to reveal the full extent of complex tarsal injuries. Make paired oblique projections when diagnostic uncertainty exists. Some tarsal sprain injuries may only be detected with stress radiography.

Alternative Diagnoses

Bite wounds (especially in cats), Achilles tendon injury, distal tibial and proximal metatarsal injuries.

Suggested Reading

Ellison GW. Conditions of the tarsus and metatarsus. In: Slatter DH, ed. Textbook of small animal surgery. Philadelphia: WB Saunders, 1985:2247.

Farrow CS, Newton CD. Ligamentous injury(sprain) In: Newton CD, Nunamaker DM, eds. Textbook of small animal orthopedics. Philadelphia: JB Lippincott, 1985:843.

Leighton RL, Robinson GW. Orthopedic surgery. In: Holzworth J, ed. Diseases of the cat. Philadelphia: WB Saunders, 1987:127, 141.

Kealy JK. Bones and joints. In: Kealy JK, ed. Diagnostic radiology of the dog and cat. 2nd ed. Philadelphia: WB Saunders, 1987:344, 401.

Newton CD. Fracture and luxation of the tarsus and metatarsus. In: Newton CD, Nunamaker DM, eds. Textbook of small animal orthopedics. Philadelphia: JB Lippincott, 1985:447.

Owens JM. The tarsus. In: Owens JM, ed. Radiographic interpretation for the small animal clinician. Saint Louis: Ralston Purina Co, 1982:49.

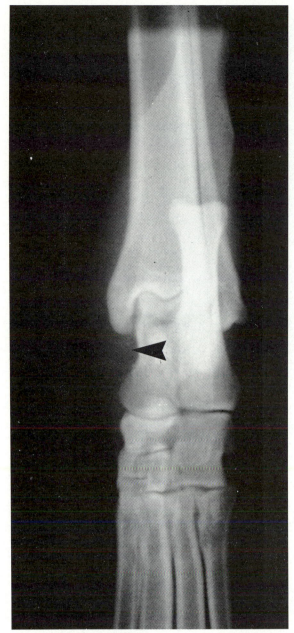

Figure 116–1 Dorsoplantar view of canine left tarsus shows regional soft-tissue swelling centered at the medial aspect of the tibiotarsal joint (*arrow*).

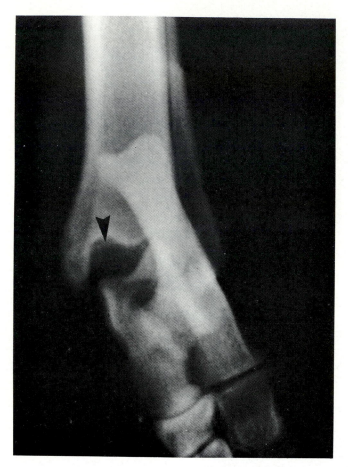

Figure 116–2 Dorsoplantar stress view (lateral wedge maneuver) of tarsus shown in Figure 116–2 shows medial subluxation and a small bone fragment (*arrow*). Diagnosis: sprain-fracture-subluxation of tibiotarsal joint.

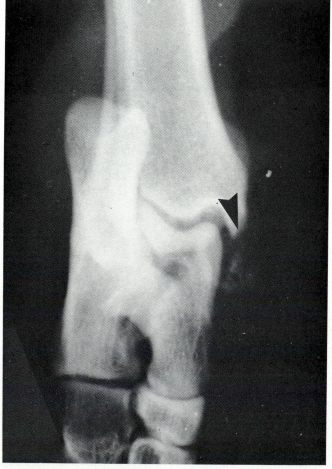

Figure 116–3 Dorsoplantar view of canine tarsus shows displaced, comminuted fracture of the distal aspect of the medial malleolus (*arrow*) and minimal widening of the tibiotarsal joint medially. Diagnosis: sprain-fracture-subluxation of tibiotarsal joint.

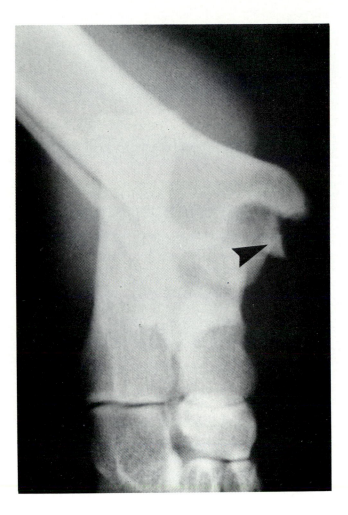

Figure 116–4 Dorsoplantar view of canine tarsus shows luxated tibiotarsal joint, and a displaced fracture of the tip of the medial malleolus (*arrow*). Diagnosis: sprain-fracture-luxation of tibiotarsal joint.

Figure 116–5 Dorsoplantar view of feline tarsus shows bilateral malleolar fractures, a distal fibular shaft fracture, and an overriding luxation of the tibiotarsal joint. Diagnosis: sprain-fracture-luxation of the tibiotarsal joint.

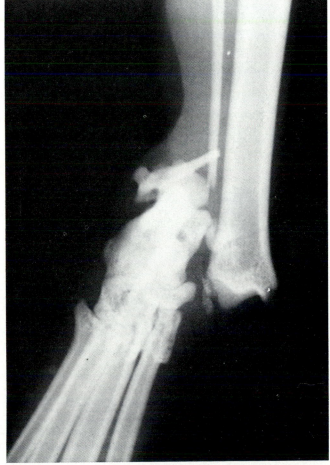

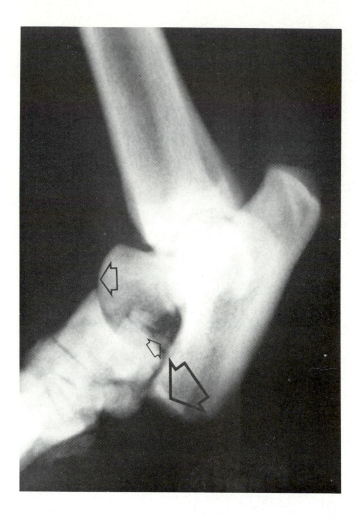

Figure 116–6   Lateral view of canine tarsus shows luxation of the distal aspect of the calcaneus (*large arrow*), subluxation of the distal talus (medium arrow), separation of the talocalcaneal joint (*small arrow*), and numerous small fragments at the level of the proximal intertarsal joint. Diagnosis: sprain-fracture-luxation of the talocalcaneal and proximal intertarsal joints.

Figure 116–7   Lateral view of canine right tarsus shows nondisplaced, comminuted fracture of proximal calcaneus (*arrows*), and multiple lead fragments. Diagnosis: calcaneal gunshot fracture.

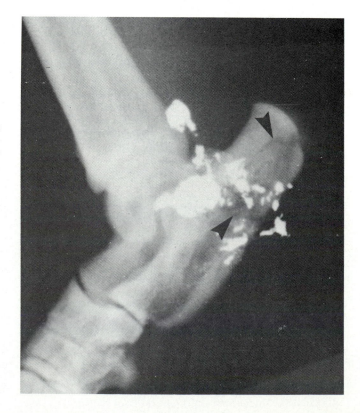

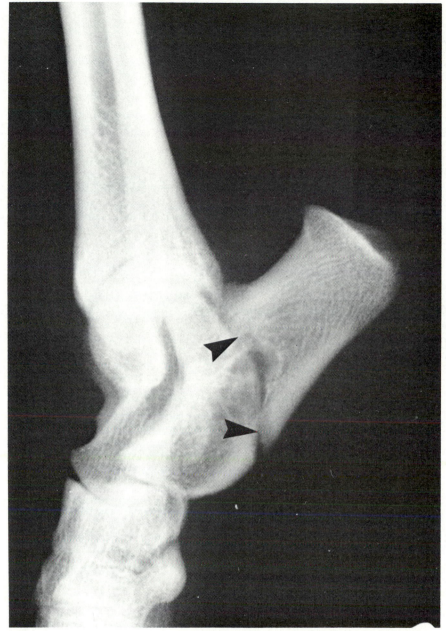

Figure 116–8 Lateral view of canine right tarsus shows mildly displaced fracture of central calcaneus (*arrows*). Diagnosis: calcaneal fracture.

117

METATARSAL FRACTURE

General Considerations

The proximal metatarsal articulation may be injured in conjunction with the distal tarsus, because of fracture, sprain, or both. The plantar protuberances of the fourth and fifth metatarsi may be avulsed, as may the distal dorsal or plantar sesamoids. Young animals often fracture their distal metatarsal growth plates, resulting in epiphyseal displacement. Articular fractures are uncommon and are encountered more often distally. Shaft fractures most often occur in groups, either from crushing of the paw or catching it in a door.

Major Radiographic Observations

Tarsometatarsal subluxations often require stress radiography to demonstrate (Figs. 117–1 and 117–2). Avulsions are most common over the proximolateral aspect of the metatarsus, usually appearing as small to medium-sized chips or fragments (Figs. 117–3 and 117–4). Shaft fractures are usually grouped and are transverse or short oblique in direction (Fig. 117–5). Growth plate fractures may occur distally in immature animals, displaying the entire range of such injuries. Sesamoidian fractures usually occur centrally, separating the bone into halves, but with much distraction.

Diagnostic Strategy

Make two views, lateral and dorsoplantar, centered on the midmetatarsus. Make right and left lateral oblique views to overcome lateral superimposition. Comparable views of the opposite metatarsus are useful in both immature and adult animals.

Pitfalls

Shaft fractures are usually obvious, although one or two in a group may be missed because they are higher or lower than more outstanding injuries. Similarly, small proximal avulsions may go undetected in the context of larger and more striking fractures. Much individual variation exists in normal sesamoid bones. Normal sesamoids may be composed of two or three equal or unequal parts; these are termed *bipartite* and *tripartite*, respectively.

Alternative Diagnoses

Bite wounds (especially cats), tarsal and digital injuries.

Suggested Reading

Ellison GW. Conditions of the tarsus and metatarsus. In: Slatter DH, ed. Textbook of small animal surgery. Philadelphia: WB Saunders, 1985:2247.

Farrow CS, Newton CD. Ligamentous injury(sprain). In: Newton CD, Nunamaker DM, eds. Textbook of small animal orthopedics. Philadelphia: JB Lippincott, 1985:843.

Leighton RL, Robinson GW. Orthopedic surgery. In: Holzworth J, ed. Diseases of the cat. Philadelphia: WB Saunders, 1987:127.

Newton CD. Fracture and luxation of the tarsus and metatarsus. In: Newton CD, Nunamaker DM, eds. Textbook of small animal orthopedics. Philadelphia: JB Lippincott, 1985:450.

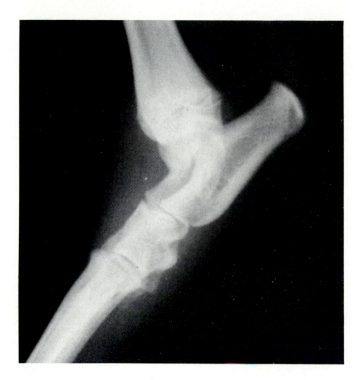

Figure 117–1 Lateral view of canine left tarsus shows regional soft-tissue swelling only.

Figure 117–2 Lateral stress view (fulcrum assisted hyperextension) of tarsus shown in Figure 117–1 shows subluxation of tarsometatarsal joints (*arrow*). Diagnosis: tarsometatarsal sprain-luxation.

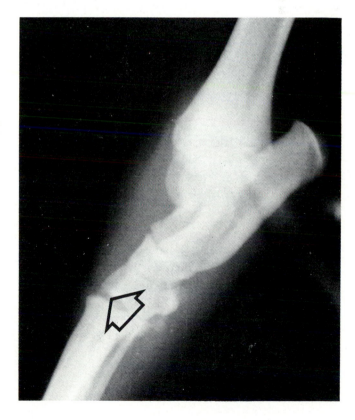

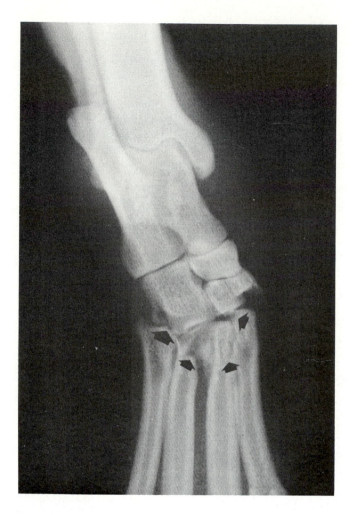

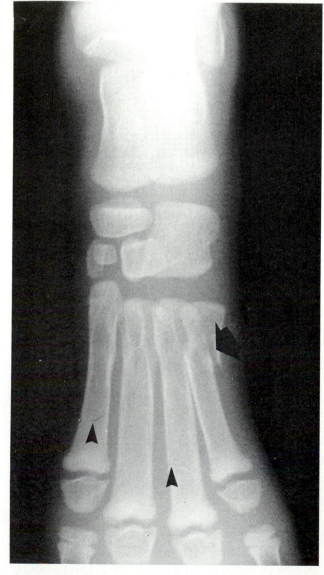

Figure 117–3 Dorsoplantar view of canine left tarsus and proximal metatarsus shows lateral displacement of the metatarsal bones with associated fractures (*arrows*). Diagnosis: sprain-fracture-luxation of the tarsometatarsal joints.

Figure 117–4 Dorsoplantar view of immature canine left tarsus and metatarsus shows displaced fracture of the fifth metatarsal bone proximally (*large arrow*), and hairline fractures in the distal aspects of the second and fourth metatarsals distally (*small arrows*). Diagnosis: multiple metatarsal fractures.

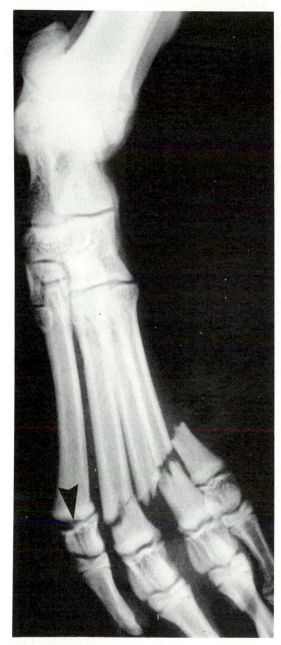

Figure 117–5 Dorsoplantar oblique view of immature canine right metatarsus shows displaced fractures of distal metatarsals 3 to 5, and a type II, growth plate fracture of the second metatarsal bone (*arrow*). Multiple metatarsal fractures. Diagnosis: multiple metatarsal fractures.

118

METATARSOPHALANGEAL JOINT FRACTURES AND DISLOCATIONS

General Considerations

Articular fractures of the distal metacarpal bones and proximal phalanges occur occasionally. Such injuries are often associated with subluxation of the associated metatarsophalangeal joint, although this varies. Sesamoidian injuries are uncommon, and because of their infrequency they are often missed during the initial radiographic examination. A later, closer inspection of the original films often reveals the injury.

Major Radiographic Observations

Condylar metatarsal fractures are most often steeply oblique, with or without obvious widening. Proximal phalangeal fractures frequently break through and detach the caudoproximal protuberance. Related growth plate injuries are common (Fig. 118–1).

Diagnostic Strategy

Make lateral and dorsoplantar views, with supplementary lateral obliques as required. The oblique views are mandatory for complete assessment of the sesamoids. Stress films, standing dorsoplantar and lateral oblique, may reveal fragment distraction not demonstrable in nonstress views.

Pitfalls

Because of the considerable anatomic variability among sesamoids, and because of developmental anomalies such as bipartite and tripartite sesamoids, it is highly advisable first to radiograph the opposite side before establishing a diagnosis of fracture.

Alternative Diagnoses

Bite wounds (especially cats), tarsal, metatarsal, and digital injuries.

Suggested Reading

Farrow CS, Newton CD. Ligamentous injury(sprain). In: Newton CD, Nunamaker DM, eds. Textbook of small animal orthopedics. Philadelphia: JB Lippincott, 1985:843.

Newton CD. Fractures of small bones. In: Newton CD, Nunamaker DM, eds. Textbook of small animal orthopedics. Philadelphia: JB Lippincott, 1985:455.

Owens JM. The digits. In: Owens JM, ed. Radiographic interpretation for the small animal clinician. Saint Louis: Ralston Purina Co, 1982:39.

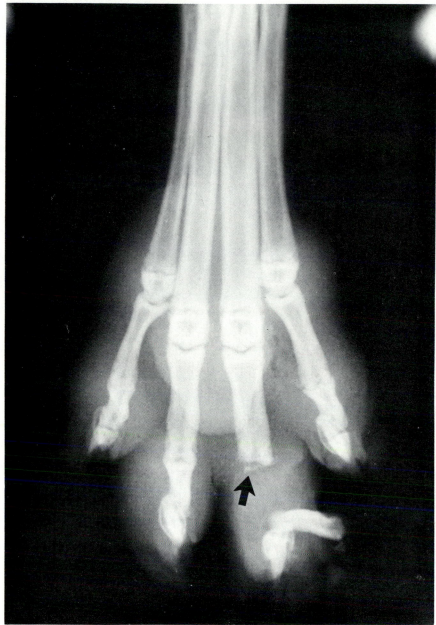

Figure 118–1 Dorsoplantar view of immature feline digits shows a compound fracture-dislocation of the proximal interphalangeal joint of the third digit. A small epiphyseal fragment remains attached to the injured joint (*arrow*). Diagnosis: digital sprain-fracture-luxation.

119

DIGITAL FRACTURE

General Considerations

The digit is composed of three small bones called phalanges, with two intervening articulations: the proximal and distal interphalangeal joints. The third or distal phalanx contains the nail, or more appropriately, the claw. The first (proximal) phalanx is most frequently fractured, followed by the second and third phalanges. The claw is frequently broken or torn from its attachment on the distal part of the third phalanx. Articular fractures occur most commonly on the proximal aspect of the first phalanx, often in the frontal plane, resulting in the detachment of the caudal protuberance.

Major Radiographic Observations

Young animals often sustain incomplete (or incomplete-appearing) diaphyseal fractures, as well as displaced and non-displaced epiphyseal fractures (Fig. 119–2). A normal comparison radiograph is often necessary to differentiate such injuries from normal developmental variation. Digital fractures in mature dogs are less difficult to diagnose, resembling for the most part other long-bone injuries (Fig. 119–1). As with younger animals, comparison films are useful in questionable cases.

Diagnostic Strategy

Begin with a standard examination with a lateral and dorsoplantar view. If the injuries are unusual or complex, include right and left dorsoplantar obliques. When superimposition is a problem in the lateral view, isolate the affected digit from the remaining digits with a gauze loop using gentle traction. Cotton balls are useful in separating the digits in the dorsoplantar projection. Stress radiography may be required to establish sprain injury involving the interphalangeal joints.

Pitfalls

Dorsoplantar views of the digits are difficult to assess accurately owing to the considerable natural angulation in both the proximal and distal intertarsal joints, which produces both distortion and magnification of many of the component parts. The lateral view is flawed by extensive digital superimposition, which may conceal surprisingly large injuries.

Alternative Diagnoses

Bite wounds (especially cats), broken or avulsed claw, tarsal injuries.

Suggested Reading

Farrow CS, Newton CD. Ligamentous injury(sprain). In: Newton CD, Nunamaker DM, eds. Textbook of small animal orthopedics. Philadelphia: JB Lippincott, 1985:843.

Leighton RL, Robinson GW. Orthopedic surgery. In: Holzworth J, ed. Diseases of the cat. Philadelphia: WB Saunders, 1987:110.

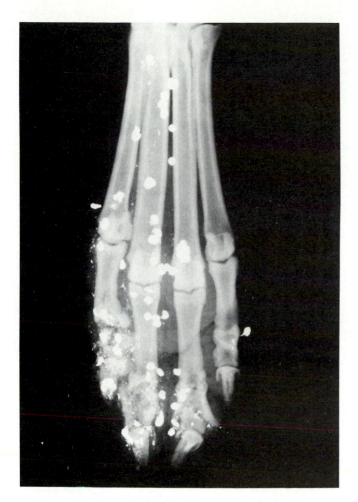

Figure 119–1 Dorsoplantar view of canine metatarsus and digits shows shotgun pellets, nondisplaced fractures of the proximal phalanges of the second and fourth digits and comminuted articular fractures of the middle phalanges of digits 2, 3, and 4. Diagnosis: multiple phalangeal gunshot fractures.

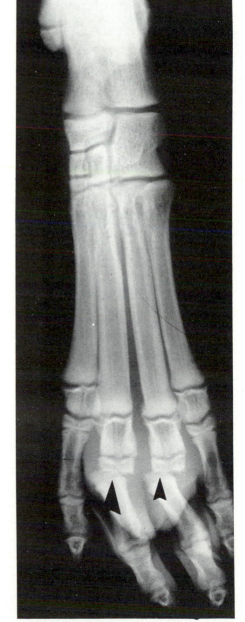

Figure 119–2 Dorsoplantar view of immature canine right metatarsus and phalanges shows displaced growth plate fractures of the third and fourth phalanges (*arrows*). Diagnosis: multiple phalangeal fractures.

THE FORELIMB

120

SCAPULAR FRACTURE

General Considerations

Scapular fractures are more varied than many clinicians realize, potentially involving the scapular body, spine, neck, or articular surface, as well as one or more of the distal muscle attachment sites. These sites include the acromion, located distally on the scapular spine; the coracoid process, found on the craniomedial aspect of the neck; and the scapular tuberosity, which forms the cranial part of the glenoid. Although the scapula may be severely comminuted with wide fragment separation, it may also be subtly fractured. This is especially true of the body and spine of the scapula; because they normally are irregularly curved and show considerable anatomic variability, it is often difficult to separate suspected fracture from normal variation. The often relatively small diagnostic yield from the mediolateral projection and the difficulty in obtaining a high-quality caudocranial view of the scapula may further limit diagnosis. Dislocations may occur with or without associated fracture and may not be consistently demonstrable depending on severity, related injuries, and radiographic positioning.

Major Radiographic Observations

The severe fractures are almost always obvious in one or both standard views. Mildly displaced, vertically oriented fractures of the body, spine, or acromion are often detectable only when projected at right angles; horizontally oriented fractures are usually seen better with a parallel beam (Figs. 120–1 to 120–5). Minimally displaced neck fractures are often only appreciated in the caudocranial view, and tuberosity injury is more apt to be seen with a lateral image (Figs. 120–6 and 120–7). Coracoid avulsion, frequently concealed in the standard projections, may require oblique views for complete evaluation. Glenoid fractures usually show in one or both standard positions.

Diagnostic Strategy

The caudocranial view is best for demonstrating most scapular-body, spine, and neck fractures; the mediolateral view projection is usually better in showing distal injuries. Accordingly, both views should be made if possible. When there is doubt about normal anatomy, the opposite side should be radiographed for comparison.

Pitfalls

The body of the scapula is often overpenetrated in the mediolateral view, potentially obscuring injury. Also in the mediolateral projection, the distal scapula may be wholly or partially superimposed on the caudal part of the cervical spine, mimicking a fracture.

Alternative Diagnoses

Shoulder fracture or dislocation.

Suggested Reading

Kealy JK. Bones and joints. In: Kealy JK, ed. Diagnostic radiology of the dog and cat. 2nd ed. Philadelphia: WB Saunders, 1987:393.

Leighton RL, Robinson GW. Orthopedic surgery. In: Holzworth J, ed. Diseases of the cat. Philadelphia: WB Saunders, 1987:102.

Newton CD. Fractures of the scapula. In: Newton CD, Nunamaker DM, eds. Textbook of small animal orthopedics. Philadelphia: JB Lippincott, 1985:333.

Owens JM. The shoulder. In: Owens JM, ed. Radiographic interpretation for the small animal clinician. Saint Louis: Ralston Purina Co, 1982:31.

Parker RB. Scapula. In: Slatter DH, ed. Textbook of small animal surgery. Philadelphia: WB Saunders, 1985:2049.

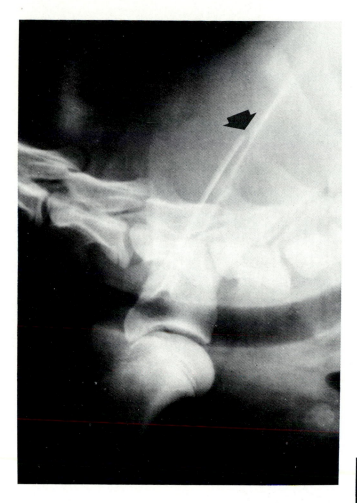

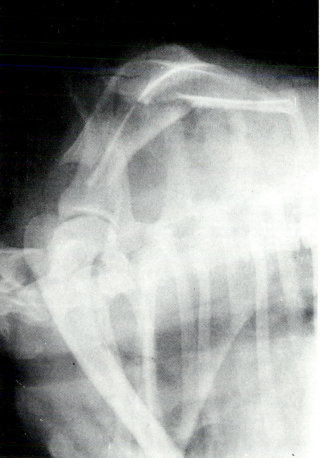

Figure 120–1 Lateral view of immature canine scapula shows mildly displaced fracture of scapular spine (*arrow*). Diagnosis: fracture of scapular spine.

Figure 120–2 Lateral view of canine scapula shows a displaced transverse fracture of the scapular body. Diagnosis: fracture of scapular body.

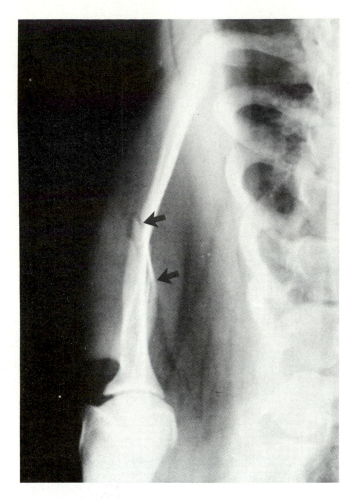

Figure 120–3 Caudocranial view of canine scapula shows mild to moderately displaced oblique fracture of the scapular body (*arrows*). Diagnosis: fracture of scapular body.

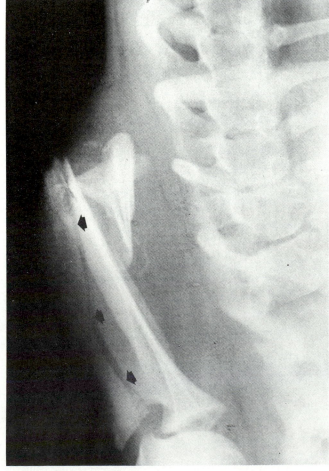

Figure 120–4 Caudocranial view of canine scapula shows severely comminuted fracture of the proximal scapular body with a complete fracture of the scapular spine (*arrows*). Diagnosis: multiple scapular fractures.

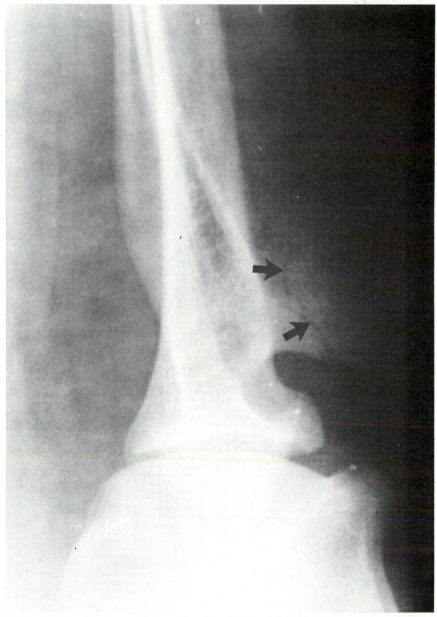

Figure 120–5 Caudocranial view of canine shoulder joint shows incomplete fracture of scapular spine (*arrows*). Diagnosis: fracture of scapular spine.

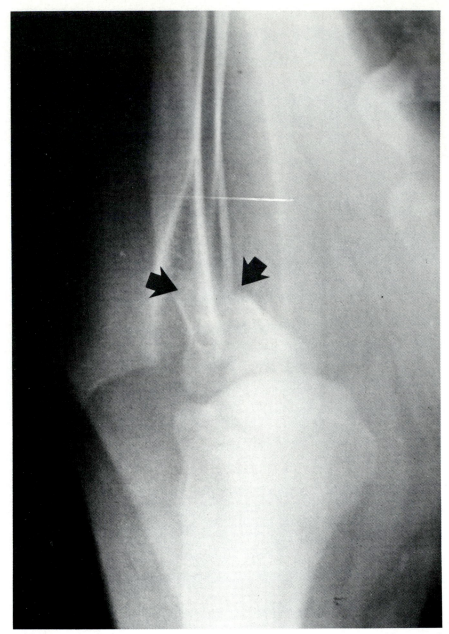

Figure 120–6 Caudocranial view of canine shoulder joint shows comminuted fracture of scapular neck (*arrows*). Diagnosis: fracture of scapular neck.

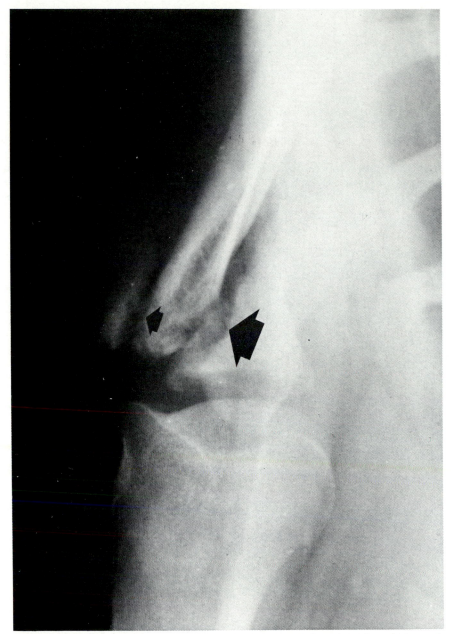

Figure 120–7 Caudocranial view of canine shoulder joint shows long oblique fracture of the scapular neck (*large arrow*) and longitudinal fracture of the scapular spine (*small arrow*). Diagnosis: fractures of the scapular neck and spine.

121

SHOULDER JOINT FRACTURES AND DISLOCATIONS

General Considerations

Fractures of the shoulder joint may involve either of its articular components—the glenoid or the proximal humerus—with the former being more frequent. Simple dislocations and fracture-dislocations are less common.

Major Radiographic Observations

Articular fractures of the glenoid depend primarily on their width for detection. They usually appear as longitudinal lucent lines or bands entering but not passing beyond the articular margin (Figs. 121–1 to 121–4). When an apparent fracture line goes beyond the joint, it is probably a superimposed and unrelated shadow. Shoulder dislocations typically appear as overlapping articular surfaces in lateral view, with more obvious displacement present in the caudocranial projection (Figs. 121–5 and 121–6).

Diagnostic Strategy

Make standard mediolateral and caudocranial views, centered on the shoulder joint. Sedate the animal if positioning results in pain. This is not only considerate of the animal's wellbeing, but it also results in much better images!

Pitfalls

The shoulder is a highly mobile joint and may demonstrate a wide range of normal angulations, especially in the caudocranial view. Consequently, great care must be taken in diagnosing dislocation based on this projection. Accessory ossification centers, represented as small, smooth ossicles located caudal to the glenoid, should not be mistaken as fractures or osteochondritis lesions. The width of the shoulder also varies considerably depending both on the amount of traction applied to the lower limb and on the degree of patient resistance. Generally the shoulder appears wider under anesthesia. The clavicles of the cat may be mistaken for fracture fragments or dystrophic calcification.

Alternative Diagnoses

Contusion, sprain, osteochondritis, or osteochondrosis.

Suggested Reading

Farrow CS. Osteochondrosis/osteochondritis of the shoulder. In: Farrow CS, ed. Decision making in small animal radiology. Toronto: BC Decker, 1987:24.

Kealy JK. Bones and joints. In: Kealy JK, ed. Diagnostic radiology of the dog and cat. 2nd ed. Philadelphia: WB Saunders, 1987:320.

Leighton RL, Robinson GW. Orthopedic surgery. In: Holzworth J, ed. Diseases of the cat. Philadelphia: WB Saunders, 1987:136

Newton CD. Dislocation of the shoulder. In: Newton CD, Nunamaker DM, eds. Textbook of small animal orthopedics. Philadelphia: JB Lippincott, 1985:343.

Owens JM. The shoulder. In: Owens JM, ed. Radiographic interpretation for the small animal clinician. Saint Louis: Ralston Purina Co, 1982:31.

Vasseur PB. Luxation of the scapulohumeral joint. In: Slatter DH, ed. Textbook of small animal surgery. Philadelphia: WB Saunders, 1985:2056.

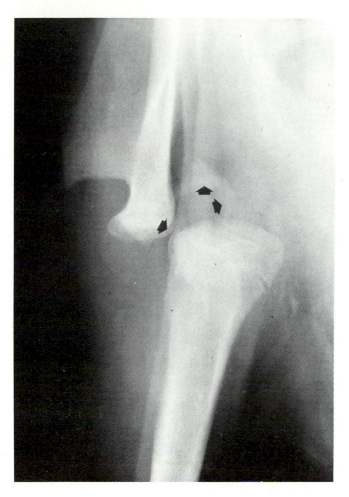

Figure 121–1 Caudocranial view of immature canine shoulder joint shows medial luxation with a severely fragmented, comminuted fracture of the medial aspect of the glenoid cavity (*arrows*). Diagnosis: articular fracture and dislocation of shoulder.

Figure 121–2 Lateral view of immature canine shoulder joint shows a vertically oriented fracture line entering the central part of the glenoid cavity (*arrows*). Diagnosis: articular fracture of the shoulder joint.

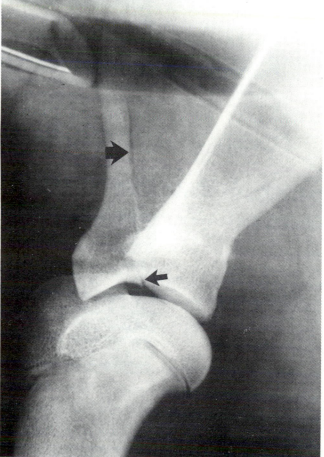

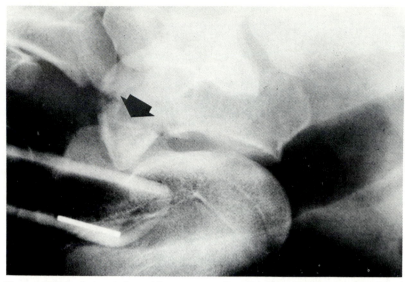

Figure 121–3 Lateral view of immature canine shoulder joint shows a displaced fracture of the supraglenoid tuberosity (*arrow*). Diagnosis: articular fracture of the shoulder joint.

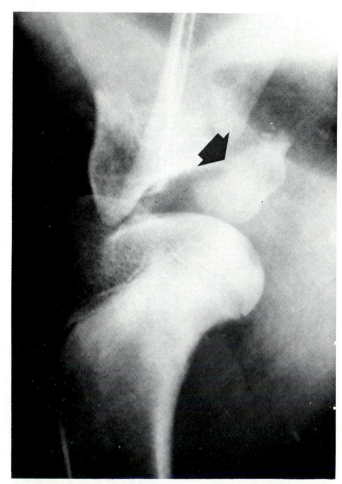

Figure 121–4 Lateral view of immature canine shoulder shows a displaced fracture of the infraglenoid tuberosity (*arrow*). Diagnosis: articular fracture of the shoulder joint.

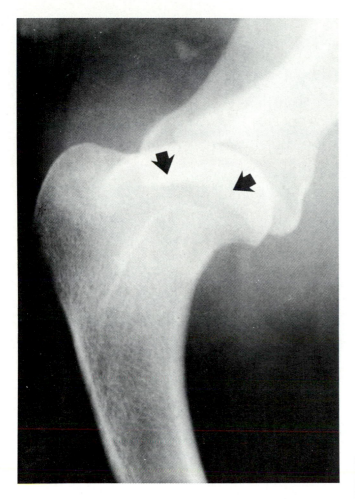

Figure 121–5   Lateral view of canine shoulder joint shows superimposition of the glenoid and humeral head (*arrows*).

Figure 121–6   Caudocranial view of patient seen in Figure 121–5 shows lateral luxation of the shoulder joint. Diagnosis: dislocated shoulder.

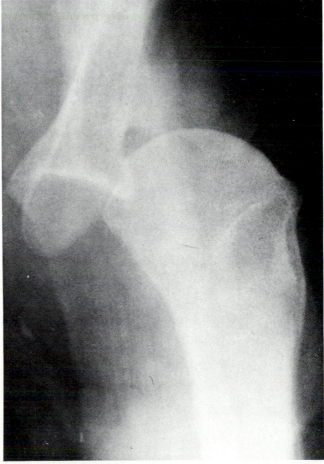

122

HUMERAL FRACTURE

General Considerations

Most humeral fractures involve the shaft, distal metaphysis, or epiphysis. Proximal injuries involving the metaphysis, tubercles, or humeral head are comparatively rare. Supracondylar, condylar, and epicondylar injuries are often associated with diagnostic uncertainty about whether the fracture enters the elbow joint—critical concern with regard to effective surgical treatment and rehabilitation.

Major Radiographic Observations

Moderately to severely displaced shaft fractures are usually obvious (Figs. 122–1 to 122–4). The same is true of metaphyseal and most proximal epiphyseal injuries (Figs. 122–5, 122–6, and 122–8). Nondisplaced or minimally displaced fractures are not as easily detected and may require additional views.

Diagnostic Strategy

Make lateral and caudocranial views of the entire humerus to include the shoulder and elbow joints. If the caudocranial view is too painful, make it when the animal is under anesthesia or later at the time of reduction. If the distal humerus is fractured, right and left caudocranial obliques centered on the distal humerus increase the likelihood of identifying articular injuries. These views may easily be included on a single film. If the elbow joint is obscured by one or more bone fragments, a traction-stress radiograph (caudocranial projection) performed under anesthesia usually improves joint clarity by drawing the offending bone fragments proximally.

Pitfalls

The relative difference in thickness between the proximal and distal aspects of the dog's forelimb frequently results in a marked exposure difference in the corresponding regions of the humerus.

Alternative Diagnoses

Shoulder and elbow fractures and dislocations, panosteitis (Fig. 122–7).

Suggested Reading

Berzon JL. Humeral fractures. In: Slatter DH, ed. Textbook of small animal surgery. Philadelphia: WB Saunders, 1985:2061.

Farrow CS. Stress radiography: applications in small animal practice. JAVMA 1982; 181:777–784

Farrow CS, Newton CD. Ligamentous injury(sprain). In: Newton CD, Nunamaker DM, eds. Textbook of small animal orthopedics. Philadelphia: JB Lippincott, 1985:843.

Kealy JK. Bones and joints. In: Kealy JK, ed. Diagnostic radiology of the dog and cat. 2nd ed. Philadelphia: WB Saunders, 1987:319, 384, 393.

Leighton RL, Robinson GW. Orthopedic surgery. In: Holzworth, ed. Diseases of the cat. Philadelphia: WB Saunders, 1987:102.

Nunamaker DM. Fractures of the humerus. In: Newton CD, Nunamaker DM, eds. Textbook of small animal orthopedics. Philadelphia: JB Lippincott, 1985:357.

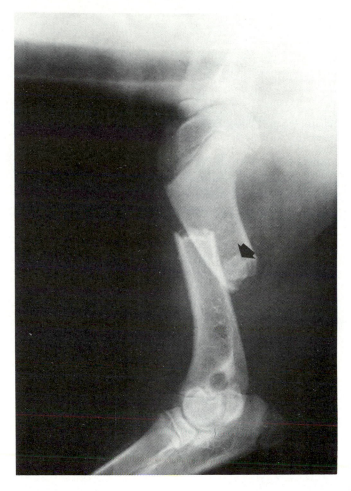

Figure 122–1 Lateral view of immature canine humerus shows overriding, transverse central diaphyseal fracture with a small rectangular fragment (*arrow*). Diagnosis: humeral diaphyseal fracture.

Figure 122–2 Lateral view of immature canine humerus shows overriding long, spiral, oblique, middle diaphyseal fracture (*arrows*). Diagnosis: humeral diaphyseal fracture.

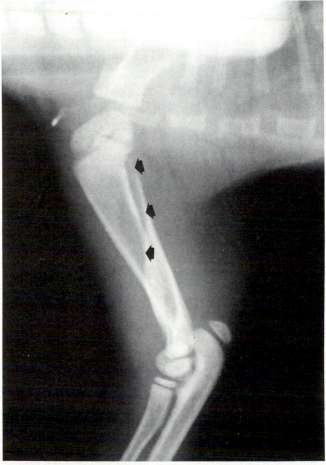

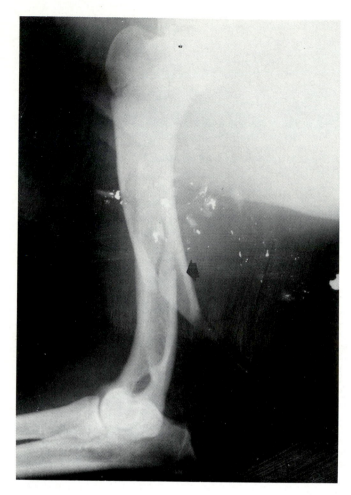

Figure 122–3 Lateral view of immature canine humerus shows comminuted central diaphyseal fracture with large butterfly fragment (*arrow*) and multiple bullet fragments. Diagnosis: gunshot fracture of humeral diaphysis.

Figure 122–4 Craniocaudal view of immature canine elbow shows displaced, transverse diaphyseal fracture of the distal humerus. Diagnosis: humeral diaphyseal fracture.

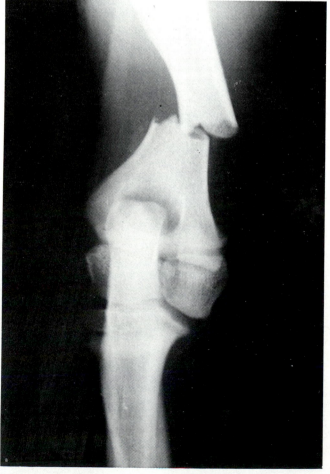

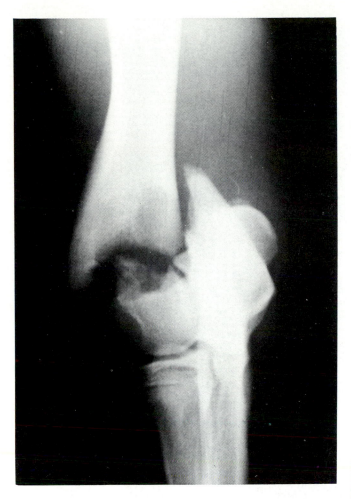

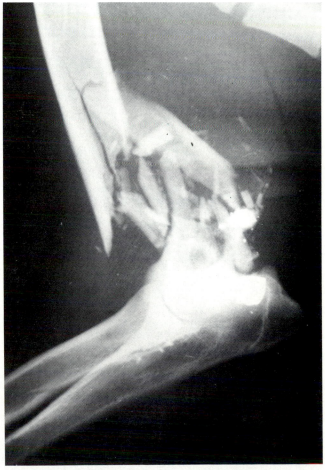

Figure 122–5   Craniocaudal oblique view of immature canine elbow shows displaced, transverse metaphyseal fracture of the distal humerus. Diagnosis: distal humeral metaphyseal fracture.

Figure 122–6   Lateral view of canine elbow shows severely comminuted and fragmented gunshot fracture of distal humeral diaphysis and metaphysis. The opposite projection indicated the epiphysis was intact. Diagnosis: distal humeral gunshot fracture.

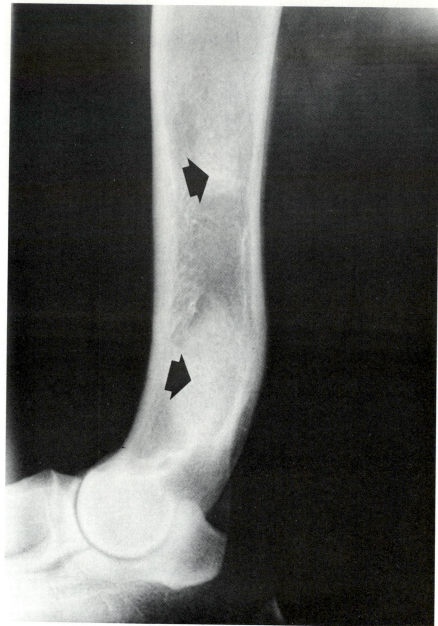

Figure 122–7 Lateral view of immature canine mid- and distal humerus shows patchy intramedullary densities (*arrows*). Diagnosis: panosteitis.

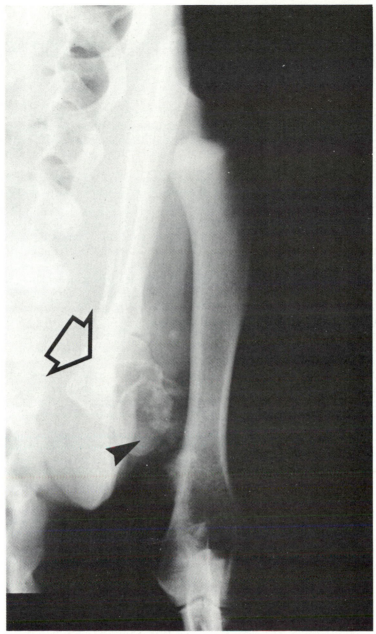

Figure 122–8 Caudocranial view of immature canine shoulder shows severely displaced, type I growth plate fractures of the humeral head (*large arrow*) and associated tubercles (*small arrow*). Diagnosis: severe proximal humeral fracture.

123

ELBOW JOINT FRACTURES AND DISLOCATIONS

General Considerations

Fractures of the elbow may be complex and confusing owing to such factors as the number of bones composing the joint (the humerus, radius, ulna, and occasionally one or more small sesamoidlike bones), the irregular and asymmetrical shape of the component parts, and the superimposition frequently resulting from elbow fractures, which can radically change the anticipated appearance of the elbow and hide one or more joint surfaces. Diagnosis is further complicated in immature animals because of their numerous growth plates, which may resemble fractures. Articular fractures of the distal humerus may assume a variety of shapes, which often are described according to the letter of the alphabet they most closely resemble when viewed in the frontal plane, i.e., T, V, or Y fractures. Growth plate injuries are specified according to the Salter-Harris system. Dislocations of the elbow may be associated with major or minor fractures, the latter often being avulsive and indicative of related second- or third-degree sprain injury.

Major Radiographic Observations

Articular fractures of the distal humerus often separate or spread the condyles, making the distal humerus appear abnormally wide in the caudocranial view. The articular margin of the humerus may appear disrupted, stepped, or angled, depending on the relative position and attitude of the humeral condyles. Nondistracted or minimally distracted articular fractures of the olecranon may be invisible if the proximal ulna is underpenetrated, or if the fracture line is not parallel to the x-ray beam. Major breaks in the distal humerus may be hidden by the superimposed olecranon or by overriding bone fragments. Sprain injuries may be associated with avulsion fractures, typically from the condylar regions of the distal humerus (Figs. 123–1 to 123–14).

Diagnostic Strategy

Because of the complexity of the elbow joint and its relatively wide range of pathology, four views are recommended: lateral, craniocaudal, and right and left craniocaudal obliques. All projections should be centered over the elbow rather than the central humerus. A traction-stress craniocaudal view often greatly improves visibility of the elbow joint.

Pitfalls

Oblique views of the elbow often make the radial head appear luxated. Some dogs have a small, smooth ossicle located lateral to the laterodistal margin of the humerus (usually present bilaterally), which may be mistaken for a fracture or a detached osteochondral fragment. The lateral aspect of the ulnohumeral articulation of the cat appears mildly luxated when compared to a comparable view in the dog.

Alternative Diagnoses

Osteochondrosis or osteochondritis, decompensated degenerative joint disease, distal humeral fracture, proximal radial or ulnar fracture, elbow sprain.

Suggested Reading

Farrow CS. Osteochondrosis of the elbow. In: Farrow CS, ed. Decision making in small animal radiology. Toronto: BC Decker, 1987:22.

Johnson RG, Hampel NL. Elbow luxation. In: Slatter DH, ed. Textbook of small animal surgery. Philadelphia: WB Saunders, 1985:2092.

Leighton RL, Robinson GW. Orthopedic Surgery. In: Holzworth J, ed. Diseases of the cat. Philadelphia: WB Saunders, 1987: 136.

Nunamaker DM. Fractures and dislocations of the elbow. In: Newton CD, Nunamaker DM, eds. Textbook of small animal orthopedics. Philadelphia: JB Lippincott, 1985:357.

Owens JM. The elbow. In: Owens JM, ed. Radiographic interpretation for the small animal clinician. Saint Louis: Ralston Purina Co, 1982:33.

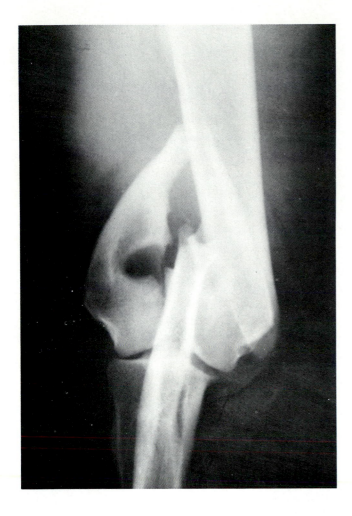

Figure 123–1 Craniocaudal view of canine elbow shows a Y-type articular fracture of the distal humeral metaphysis and epiphysis with an overriding distal humeral diaphysis. Associated fragment displacement has resulted in incongruency of the elbow joints (humeroulnar and humeroradial).

Figure 123–2 Lateral view of canine elbow shown in Figure 123–1 shows caudal displacement of the distal humeral fragments, radius, and ulna. Diagnosis: displaced, distal humeral articular fracture (also called supracondylar-intracondylar fracture).

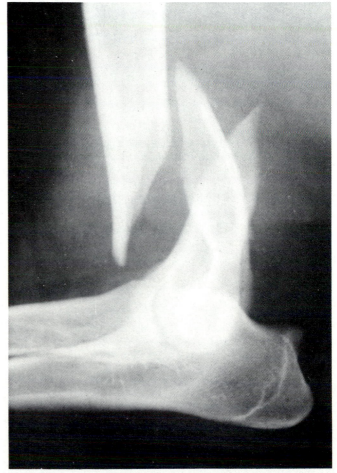

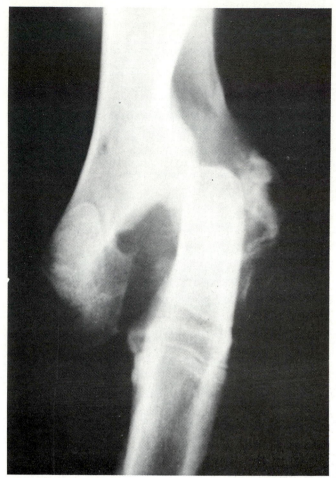

Figure 123–3 Craniocaudal oblique view of immature canine elbow shows displaced fractures of the lateral aspects of the distal humeral metaphysis and epiphysis (Salter-Harris IV) with resulting dislocation. Diagnosis: elbow luxation secondary to distal humeral fractures.

Figure 123–4 Craniocaudal oblique view of immature canine elbow shows a minimally displaced, T-type epiphyseal fracture of the distal humerus. Diagnosis: distal humeral articular fracture.

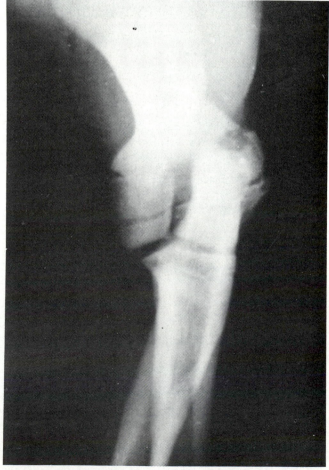

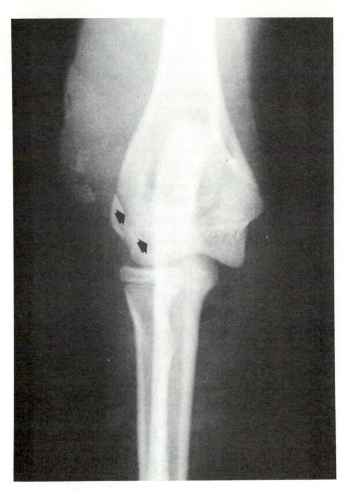

Figure 123–5 Craniocaudal oblique view of immature canine elbow shows a nondisplaced oblique fracture (Salter-Harris IV) of the lateral aspects of the distal humeral metaphysis and epiphysis (*arrows*). The elbow joints are mildly subluxated. Diagnosis: distal humeral articular fracture and subluxation.

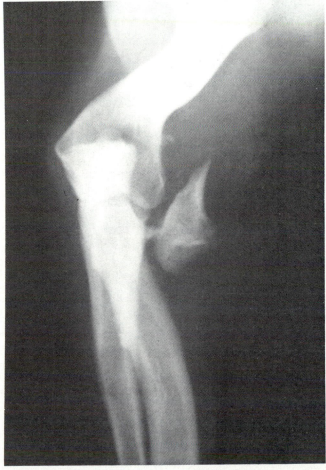

Figure 123–6 Craniocaudal oblique view of canine elbow shows a large bone fragment adjacent to the medial aspect of the elbow joint. There is some uncertainty about its origin.

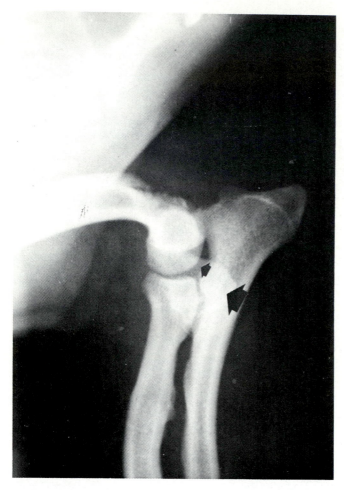

Figure 123–7 Lateral view of canine elbow shown in Figure 123–6 shows a severely displaced avulsion fracture of the medial humeral epicondyle and adjacent bone (*large arrow*). Mild to moderate luxation of the humeroulnar joint has resulted (*small arrow*). Diagnosis: elbow subluxation secondary to avulsion fracture of the distal humerus.

Figure 123–8 Lateral view of canine elbow shows a displaced proximal midshaft fracture of the ulna, luxated humeroradial joint (*small arrow*), and probable condylar fragment (*large arrow*).

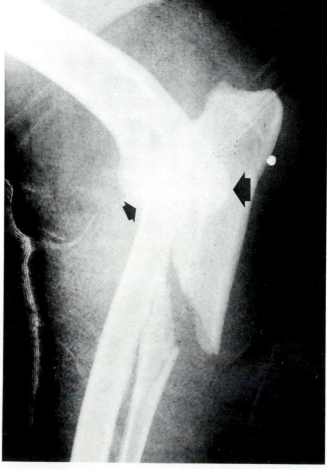

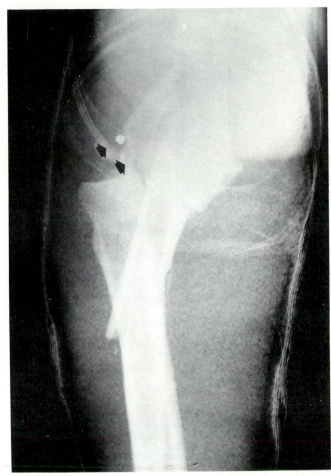

Figure 123–9 Craniocaudal view of canine elbow shown in Figure 123–8 confirms humeroradial luxation and fracture of the lateral humeral condyle, the latter being comminuted (*arrows*). Diagnosis: sprain-fracture-luxation of the elbow.

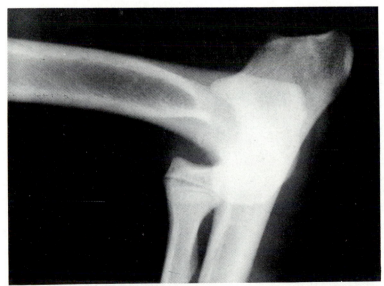

Figure 123–10 Lateral view of immature canine elbow shows cranial luxation of the radius and superimposition of the humerus on the ulna, which suggests humeroulnar luxation as well.

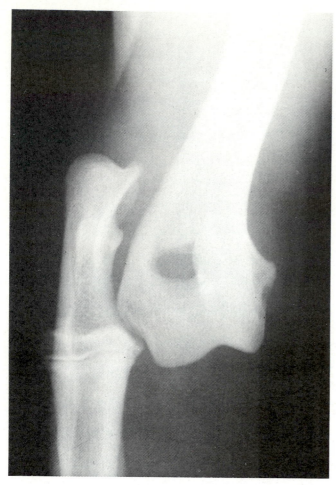

Figure 123–11 Craniocaudal oblique view of the elbow shown in Figure 123–10 confirms complete luxation without associated fracture. Diagnosis: sprain-luxation of the elbow.

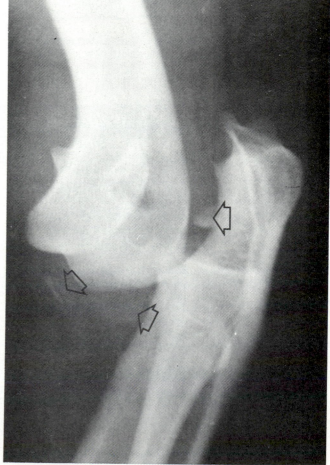

Figure 123–12 Craniocaudal oblique view of canine elbow shows complete dislocation of the elbow with associated avulsion fractures (*arrows*). Diagnosis: sprain-fracture-luxation of the elbow.

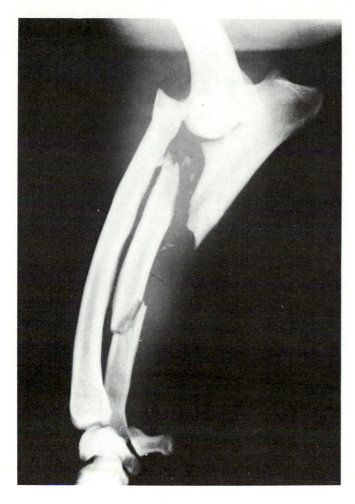

Figure 123–13   Lateral view of canine elbow shows multiple ulnar diaphyseal fractures and cranial radial luxation. Diagnosis: sprain-fracture-luxation of the elbow (Monteggia's fracture).

Figure 123–14   Lateral view of feline elbow shows comminuted fracture of proximal ulna, part of which is articular, and fracture-luxation of the proximal radius. Diagnosis: sprain-fracture-luxation of the elbow (modified Monteggia's fracture).

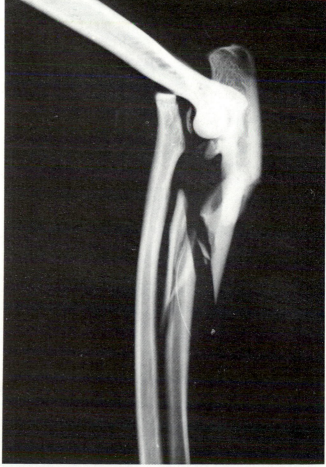

124

RADIAL FRACTURE

General Considerations

Radial fractures most often occur in conjunction with ulnar injuries, frequently at the same level in the respective diaphyses. Puppies often sustain greenstick fractures of the central radius, with or without a related ulnar injury. Growth plate fractures may involve either the proximal or distal radius, giving rise to premature closure, alteration or cessation of axial growth, and angular limb deformity.

Major Radiographic Observations

Radial fractures in young animals are often incomplete or minimally displaced depending on the view, appearing as a fine black or gray line in the central third of the diaphysis (Figs. 124–1 to 124–4). The associated cortical contour is often smooth or only mildly disrupted. Proximal radial dislocations are often associated with small flakes of bone, avulsion fractures resulting from sprain injury. Growth plate fractures may or may not be obvious, depending on their degree of displacement and the available views (Figs. 124–5 and 124–6). Following growth plate injury, it is usual for the associated metaphysis to lose density, falsely resembling epiphyseal displacement or infection.

Diagnostic Strategy

Make craniocaudal and lateral views of the radius and ulna including the elbow and carpal joints. Comparable views of the opposite limb are strongly advised in the case of immature animals. Make oblique views when there is an area of clinical or radiographic suspicion detected in the initial films, or when further lesion clarity is required. Additional views (standard or oblique projections) centered over the elbow or carpus are very helpful in evaluating subtle articular and growth plate injuries.

Pitfalls

Both proximal and distal radial fractures may be obscured by overlapping of the adjacent parts of the ulna. This problem may be partially overcome by making oblique views centered over the region of interest. Superimposition of the distal aspects of the radius and ulna, especially in young animals with open growth plates, may simulate a fracture. Bony superimposition may also result in edge enhancement or Mach lines, which resemble fractures.

Alternative Diagnoses

Bite wounds (especially cats), elbow or carpal sprains, fractures, or osteochondrosis (especially young animals), panosteitis.

Suggested Reading

Egger EL. Radius and ulna. In: Slatter DH, ed. Textbook of small animal surgery. Philadelphia: WB Saunders, 1985:2099.

Farrow CS. Angular limb deformity. In: Farrow CS, ed. Decision making in small animal radiology. Toronto: BC Decker, 1987:14.

Kealy JK. Bones and joints. In: Kealy JK, ed. Diagnostic radiology of the dog and cat. 2nd ed. Philadelphia: WB Saunders, 1987:394.

Leighton RL, Robinson GW. Orthopedic surgery. In: Newton CD, Nunamaker DM, eds. Textbook of small animal orthopedics. Philadelphia: JB Lippincott, 1985:373.

Toal RL. Fracture healing and complications. In: Thrall DE, ed. Textbook of veterinary diagnostic radiology. Philadelphia: WB Saunders, 1986:97.

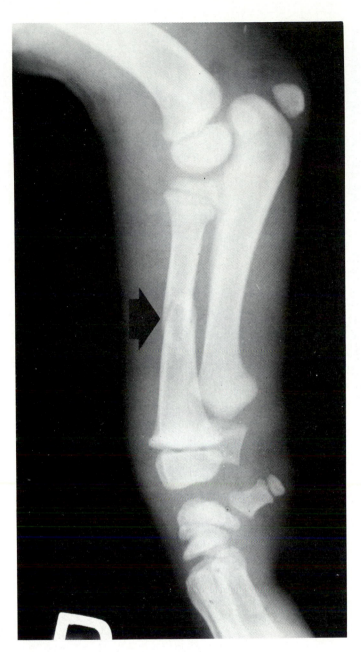

Figure 124–1 Lateral view of immature canine radius and ulna shows minimally displaced fracture of midshaft radius (*arrow*), without evidence of associated ulnar injury.

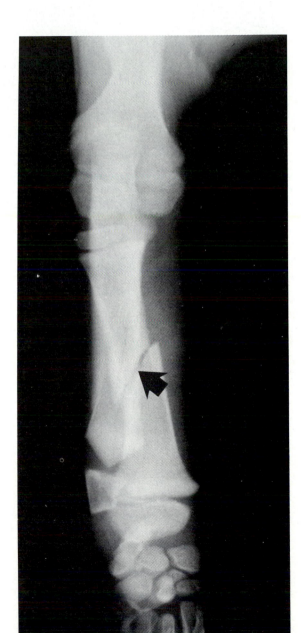

Figure 124–2 Craniocaudal view of radius and ulna shown in Figure 124–1 confirms mildly displaced oblique fracture of central radial diaphysis (*arrow*). Diagnosis: radial midshaft fracture.

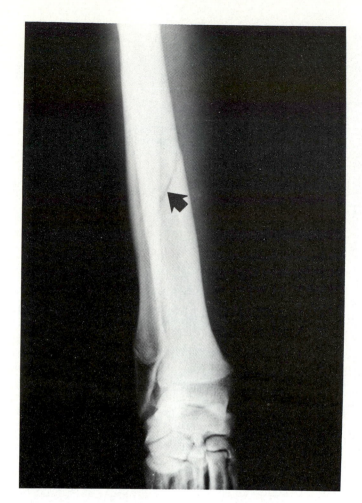

Figure 124–3 Craniocaudal view of immature canine radius and ulna shows nondisplaced oblique fracture of midshaft radius (*arrow*). Diagnosis: radial midshaft fracture.

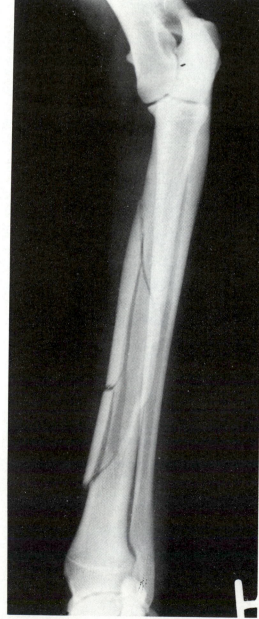

Figure 124–4 Craniocaudal view of immature canine radius and ulna shows extensive comminuted radial fracture. Diagnosis: severely comminuted radial fracture.

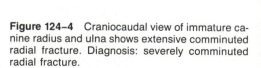

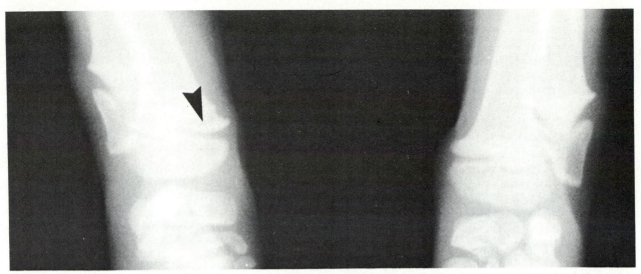

Figure 124–5 Craniocaudal view of immature canine right distal radius and ulna (with opposite side for comparison) shows nondisplaced medial metaphyseal fracture (*arrow*). Injury to the associated growth plate is inferred. Diagnosis: distal radial fracture.

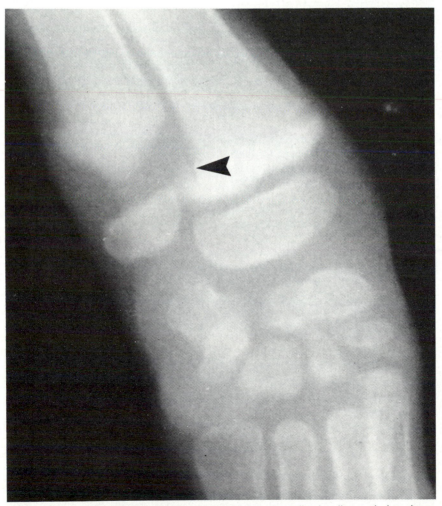

Figure 124–6 Craniocaudal oblique view of immature left distal radius and ulna shows minimally displaced fracture of lateral radial metaphysis (*arrow*). Related growth plate damage is probable. Diagnosis: distal radial fracture.

125
ULNAR FRACTURE

General Considerations

Ulnar fractures are often combined with radial injuries. Isolated dislocations are uncommon. Proximal fractures are most serious if articular and are frequently complicated by triceps-induced fragment distraction. Shaft fractures often occur in the distal third of the diaphysis because it is thinner and therefore structurally weaker. The styloid process is often broken in conjunction with carpal injuries. The distal ulnar growth plate is vulnerable to both compressive injury and fracture, both of which may halt growth and secondarily deform the limb.

Major Radiographic Observations

Avulsion fractures of the olecranon epiphysis are not always obviously displaced and may sometimes be proven only with stress radiography (Fig. 125–1). Like growth plate injuries elsewhere in the skeleton, physeal fractures may be very subtle and be discovered only by a slight widening or shift. Many ulnar shaft fractures are not identified until a callus has formed, a few weeks after the original injury. Distal ulnar growth plate injuries may also go undetected until premature closure begins some weeks later (Figs. 125–1A to 125–4).

Diagnostic Strategy

Make craniocaudal and lateral views to include the elbow and carpus. Make comparable views of the opposite limb if the animal has not reached skeletal maturity. If growth plate injury or articular fracture is suspected or suggested in the initial films, make standard or oblique views centered over the affected part, again with comparable projections of the opposite leg for comparison. If olecranon displacement is suspected and cannot be proven in standard films, make a flexed lateral view of the affected elbow and of the opposite side for comparison. Stress radiography is usually painful in the case of acute injuries and therefore should be done under sedation or anesthesia.

Pitfalls

The proximal edge of the distal ulnar epiphysis may resemble a transverse fracture in young animals. The distal ulna of the cat appears subluxated in the craniocaudal view when compared to the same area in a dog.

Alternative Diagnoses

Bite wounds (especially cats), elbow or carpal injury, metaphyseal osteopathy (Figs. 125–5 and 125–6).

Suggested Reading

Egger EL. Radius and ulna. In: Slatter DH, ed. Textbook of small animal surgery. Philadelphia: WB Saunders, 1985:2099.

Farrow CS. Stress radiography: applications in small animal practice. JAVMA 1982; 181:777–784.

Kealy JK. Bones and joints. In: Kealy JK, ed. Diagnostic radiology of the dog and cat. 2nd ed. Philadelphia: WB Saunders, 1987:325.

Leighton RL, Robinson GW. Orthopedic surgery. In: Holzworth J, ed. Diseases of the cat. Philadelphia: WB Saunders, 1987:105.

Nunamaker DM. Fractures of the radius and ulna. In: Newton CD, Nunamaker DM, eds. Textbook of small animal orthopedics. Philadelphia: JB Lippincott, 1985:373.

Owens JM. The teeth. In: Owens JM, ed. Radiographic interpretation for the small animal clinician. Saint Louis: Ralston Purina Co, 1982:65.

Toal RL. Fracture healing and complications. In: Thrall DE, ed. Textbook of veterinary diagnostic radiology. Philadelphia: WB Saunders, 1986:97.

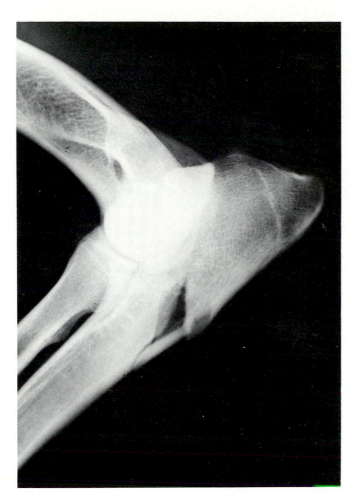

Figure 125–1   Lateral view of canine elbow shows comminuted fracture of the proximal ulna. Based on the location and direction of the major fracture line and the caudoproximal dislocation of the olecranon, an articular fracture may be inferred even though joint entry cannot be identified. Diagnosis: articular fracture of the proximal ulna.

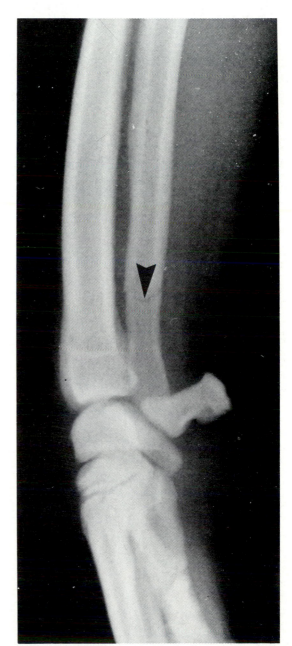

Figure 125–1A   Lateral view of canine left distal radius and ulna shows minimally displaced fracture of ulnar diaphysis (*arrow*). Diagnosis: distal ulnar fracture.

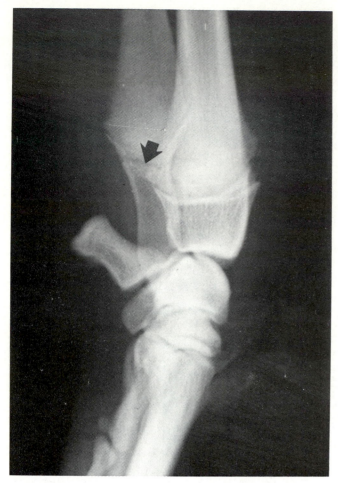

Figure 125–2 Lateral view of immature canine carpus shows nondisplaced fracture through part of distal ulna growth plate (*arrow*).

Figure 125–3 Dorsopalmar view of canine carpus shown in Figure 125–2 confirms distal ulnar fracture (*arrow*). Diagnosis: distal ulnar growth plate fracture.

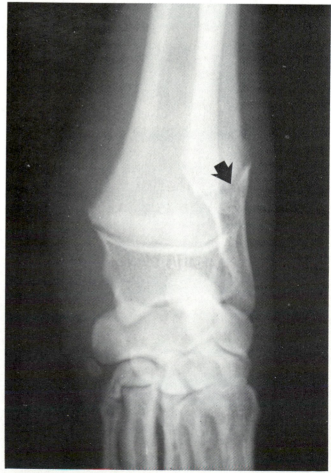

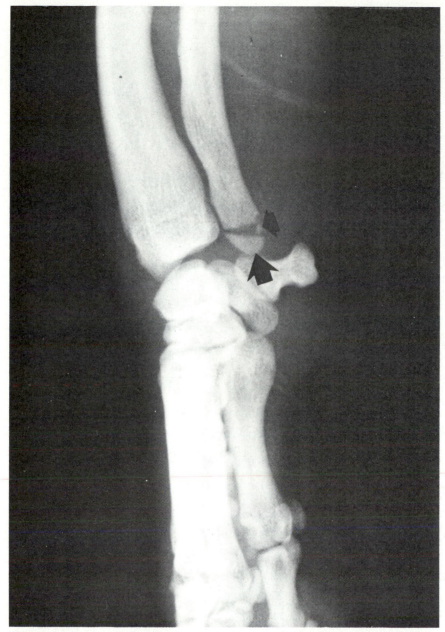

Figure 125–4   Lateral view of canine carpus shows displaced fracture of the ulnar styloid process (*large arrow*) and small secondary fragment (*small arrow*). Diagnosis: distal ulnar fracture.

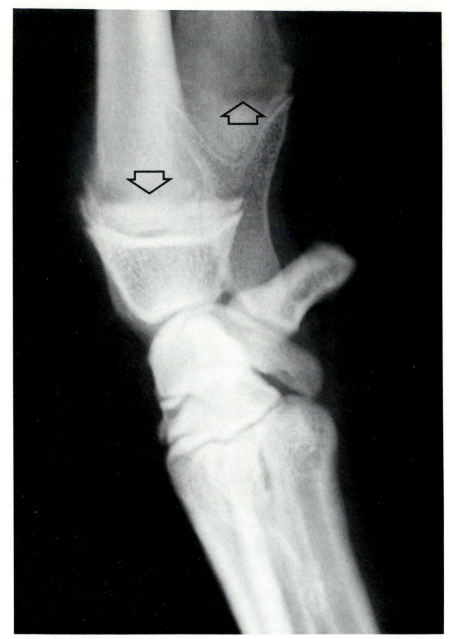

Figure 125–5   Lateral view of immature canine distal radius and ulna shows lucent bands in the metaphyses paralleling the growth plates (*arrows*) and resembling nondisplaced fractures. Diagnosis: metaphyseal osteopathy.

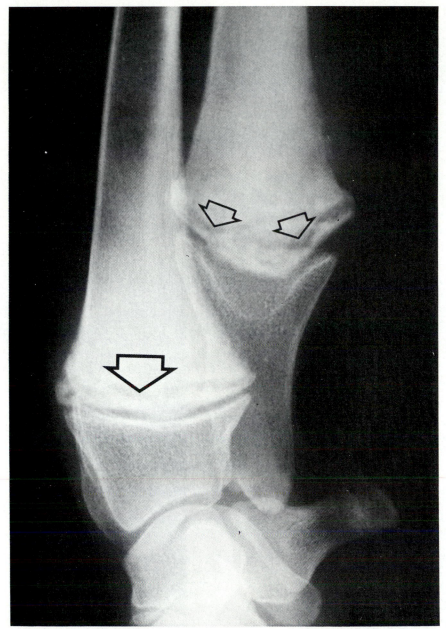

Figure 125–6 Lateral view of immature canine distal radius and ulna shows lucent bands in the metaphyses paralleling the growth plates (*arrows*) and resembling nondisplaced fractures. Compare with Figure 125–5. Diagnosis: metaphyseal osteopathy.

Combined Radial and Ulnar Fractures

The close proximity of the radius and ulna often results in both bones being fractured, although not always at the same anatomical level. Similar injury patterns occur in other paired or grouped bones such as the tibia and fibula and the paws. Consequently, the entire radius and ulna and their associated joints should be carefully checked for injuries other than the obvious. Figures 1 to 8 illustrate various types of combined radioulnar fractures.

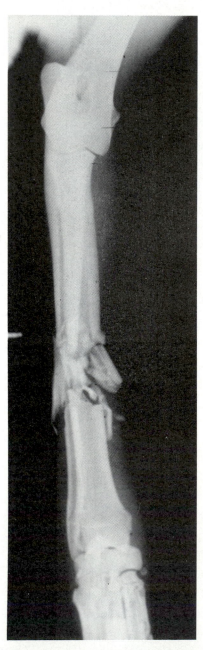

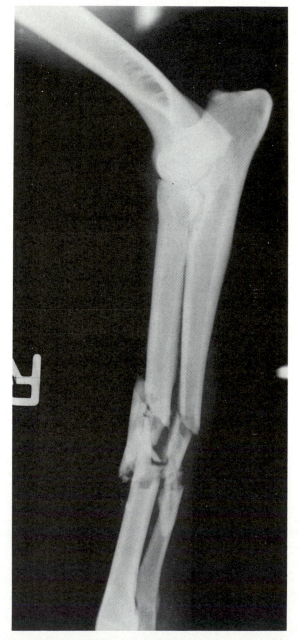

Figure 1 Lateral view of canine radius and ulna shows displaced, comminuted fractures of midshaft radius and ulna.

Figure 2 Craniocaudal view of radius and ulna shown in Figure 1 shows the full extent of lateral fragment displacement. Diagnosis: midshaft radial and ulnar fractures.

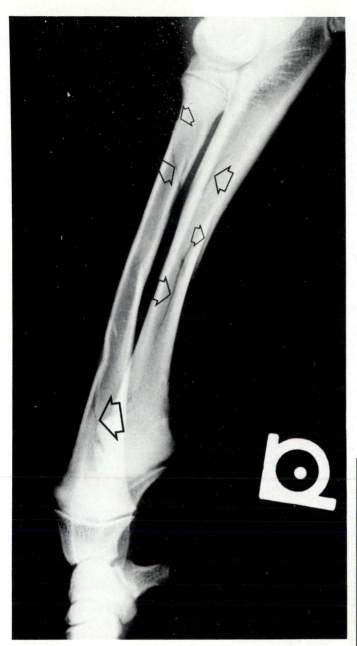

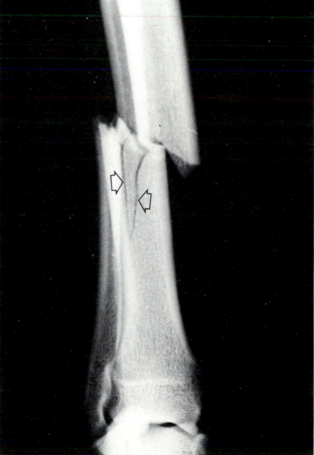

Figure 3 Lateral view of immature canine radius and ulna shows very long, minimally displaced spiral fractures (*arrows*).

Figure 4 Craniocaudal view of canine midshaft radius and ulna shows short oblique fractures with malalignment and disaposition. Medium-sized fissure lines (*arrows*) extend into the proximal part of the distal radial fragment. Diagnosis: displaced midshaft radial and ulnar fractures.

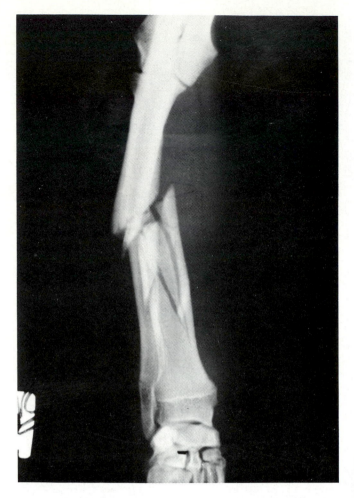

Figure 5 Craniocaudal view of canine midshaft radius and ulna shows comminuted fractures of the radius and ulna. The distal radial fragment is fragmented and deeply fissured. Diagnosis: displaced midshaft radial and ulnar fractures.

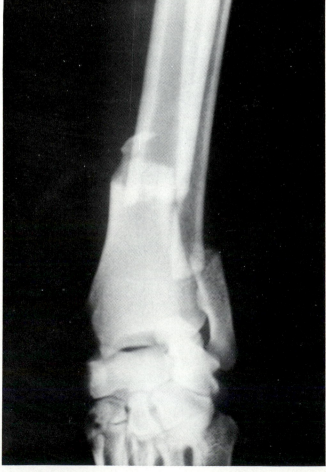

Figure 6 Craniocaudal view of canine distal radius and ulna shows a displaced transverse fracture of distal radial diaphysis associated with a small secondary fragment, and a sharp transverse fracture of the distal ulna proximal to the styloid process. Diagnosis: displaced distal diaphyseal radial and ulnar fractures.

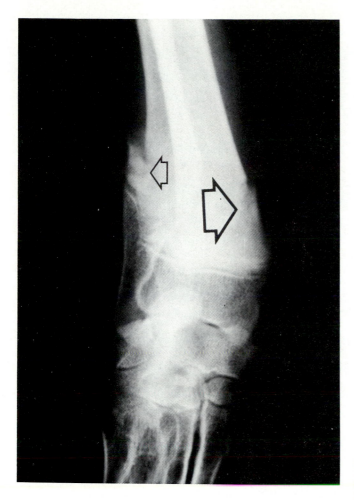

Figure 7 Craniocaudal view of immature canine distal radius and ulna shows nondisplaced fractures of the radial (*large arrow*) and ulnar (*small arrow*) metaphyses. Subsequent early closure of the associated distal ulnar growth plate is a strong possibilty. Diagnosis: nondisplaced distal radial and ulnar metaphyseal fractures.

Figure 8 Craniocaudal view of immature canine distal radius and ulna shows minimally displaced distal radial (*small arrow*) and moderately displaced ulnar (*large arrow*) metaphyseal fractures. Diagnosis: displaced radial and ulnar metaphyseal fractures.

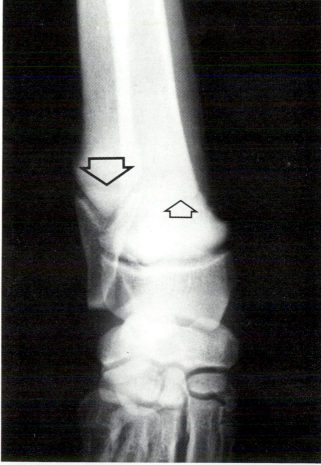

126

CARPAL JOINT FRACTURES, SPRAINS AND DISLOCATIONS

General Considerations

Sprain is the most common carpal injury in the dog. Third-degree sprains (complete separation of one or more ligaments) are usually associated with dislocations and frequently with small avulsion fractures. Second-degree sprains (internal tearing and lengthening without external separation) usually show subluxation on a stress film made after the swelling has subsided, but rarely involve avulsion fracture. First-degree sprains (internal hemorrhage and minor structural damage) are associated with neither dislocation nor fracture but nevertheless may result in severe lameness or even non-weightbearing. If reinjured before completely healed (aggravated), carpal ligments may be permanently lengthened, resulting in destabilization, cartilage damage, and arthritis. Carpal fractures are variable and may affect any single carpal bone or a combination of carpal bones. There is often accompanying subluxation and occasionally complete dislocation. Related joint effusions are typical and may persist, especially if the carpus is reinjured.

Major Radiographic Observations

Carpal sprains show subluxation or complete dislocation if severe, depending on which ligament or ligaments are injured and whether there are associated avulsion fractures. Mild carpal injury is typified by localized swelling, usually a combination of an increased production of joint fluid and hemorrhage, as well as extracapsular edema and bleeding. Carpal fractures are highly varied, ranging from small chips to large corner fragments, and less commonly, "slab" fractures (Figs. 126–1 to 126–9).

Diagnostic Strategy

Because of the anatomic complexity of the carpus, four views are advisable: dorsopalmar, lateral, and right and left dorsopalmar obliques. These films should be made with the x-ray beam centered directly over the carpus, not at the middle of the radius and ulna. Opposite-leg comparison views are very useful, often serving to rapidly distinguish between normal and abnormal anatomy, far better than a textbook comparison. Stress views made under anesthesia or sedation may demonstrate second- or third-degree sprain injuries, as well as small nondisplaced fractures.

Pitfalls

The radial and intermediate carpal bones are fused in the cat, appearing as a single large bone in the proximal carpal row. The sesamoid bone in the pollicis longus tendon, located proximal to the first digit, may be mistaken for a carpal chip fracture.

Alternative Diagnoses

Bite wound (especially cats), carpal strain, distal radial or ulnar fracture, metacarpal fracture.

Suggested Reading

Farrow CS. Stress radiography: applications in small animal practice. JAVMA 1982; 181:777–784.

Farrow CS, Newton CD. Ligamentous injury (sprain). In: Newton CD, Nunamaker DM, eds. Textbook of small animal orthopedics. Philadelphia: JB Lippincott, 1985:843.

Kealy JK. The skull and vertebral column. In: Kealy JK, ed. Diagnostic radiology of the dog and cat. 2nd ed. Philadelphia: WB Saunders, 1987:329, 396.

Leighton RL, Robinson GW. Orthopedic surgery. In: Holzworth J, ed. Diseases of the cat. Philadelphia: WB Saunders, 1987: 140.

Moore RW. Carpus and digits. In: Slatter DH, ed. Textbook of small animal surgery. Philadelphia: WB Saunders, 1985:2126.

Newton CD. Fracture and dislocation of the carpus. In: Newton CD, Nunamaker DM, eds. Textbook of small animal orthopedics. Philadelphia: JB Lippincott, 1985:381.

Owens JM. The carpus. In: Owens JM, ed. Radiographic interpretation for the small animal clinician. Saint Louis: Ralston Purina Co, 1982:37.

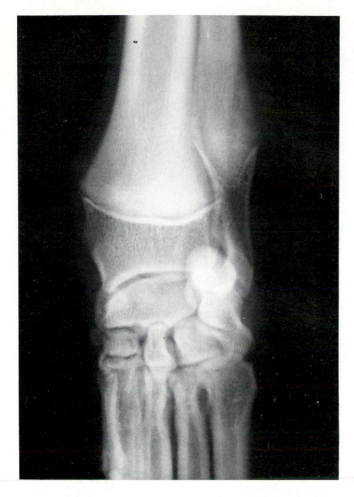

Figure 126–1 Dorsopalmar view of immature canine carpus. Diagnosis: normal.

Figure 126–2 Lateral view of immature canine carpus shown in Figure 126–1. Diagnosis: normal.

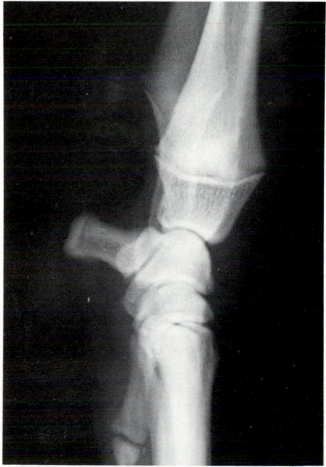

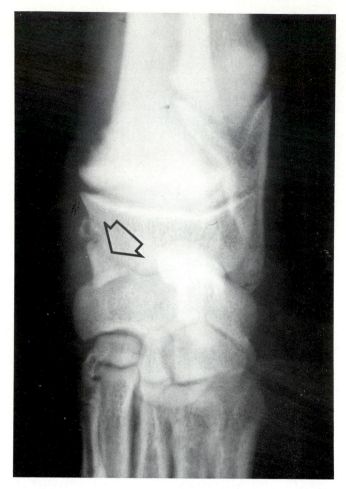

Figure 126–3 Dorsopalmar view of immature canine carpus shows displaced fracture of the radial styloid process (*arrow*). Diagnosis: distal radial articular fracture.

Figure 126–4 Dorsopalmar view of canine carpus shows tooth fragment (*arrow*) embedded within soft tissue and resembling a fracture fragment. Diagnosis: carpal foreign body.

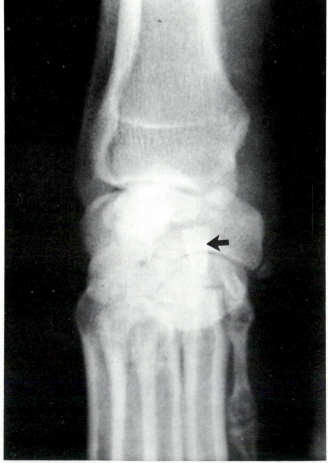

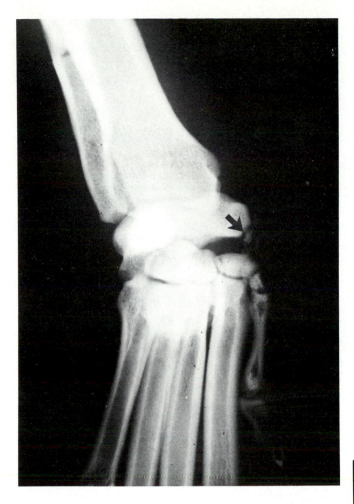

Figure 126-5 Dorsopalmar stress view (lateral wedge) of canine carpus shows small chip fracture of the mediodistal margin of the radiointermediate carpal bone (*arrow*), with widening of the medial aspect of the intercarpal joint. Diagnosis: carpal sprain-avulsion fracture.

Figure 126-6 Lateral view of canine carpus shows comminuted fracture of the radiointermediate carpal bone (*arrow*). Diagnosis: carpal fracture.

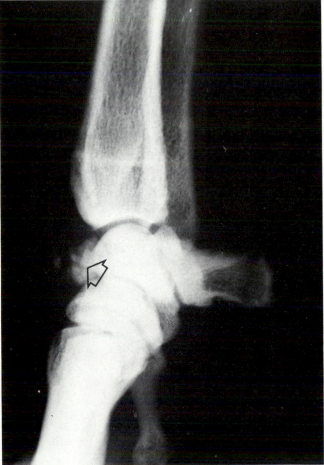

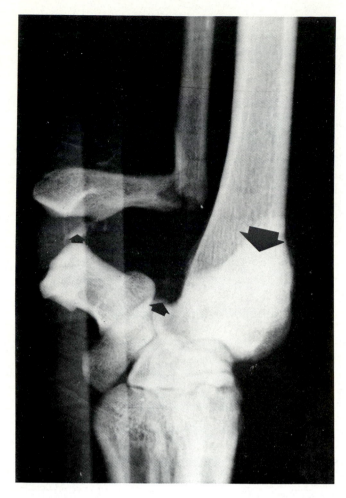

Figure 126–7 Craniomedial oblique view of canine carpus shows fracture-dislocation of the radiointermediate carpal bone (*large arrow*), fracture of the proximal part of the ulnar carpal bone (*medium arrow*), a displaced fracture of the distal ulnar diaphysis, and an avulsion fracture of the ulnar styloid (*small arrow*).

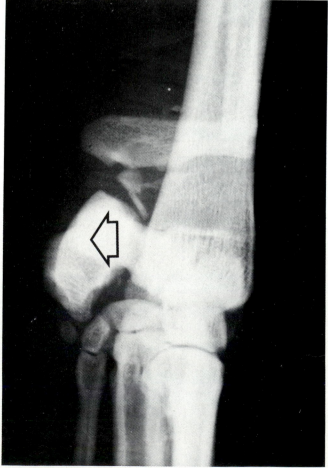

Figure 126–8 Craniolateral oblique view of canine carpus shown in Figure 126–7 provides an unobscured projection of the displaced radiointermediate carpal bone (*arrow*). Diagnosis: sprain-fracture-dislocation of the carpus.

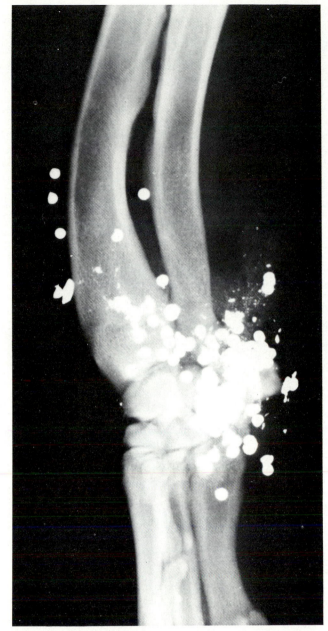

Figure 126–9 Craniomedial oblique view of canine carpus shows shotgun pellets, some of which are shattered, superimposed on the carpus and distal radius. Neither this projection nor any of the other views of the carpus revealed a fracture or intra-articular lead fragments. Diagnosis: carpal shotgun wound.

127

METACARPAL FRACTURE

General Considerations

Metacarpal fractures are typically multiple, usually deriving from a blow to the paw. Solitary metacarpal fractures are much less common. Growth plate fractures occur occasionally, and articular injuries are relatively rare. Hyperextension injuries are often associated with avulsion fractures of the caudoproximal parts of the fourth and fifth metacarpals.

Major Radiographic Observations

Typically best seen in dorsopalmar projection, metacarpal fractures are often of a short oblique nature, located in the central third of the diaphysis. Often multiple and displaced, such fractures may produce pronounced lateral angulation of the distal aspect of the paw when viewed frontally (Fig. 127–1). Younger animals often sustain greenstick diaphyseal fractures, which appear as fine diaphyseal lines that frequently pass through only a single cortex (see Fig. 127–1). Growth plate fractures may or may not be displaced and are accordingly more or less detectable (Fig. 127–2). Overlying paired sesamoid bones may obscure or mimic distal epiphyseal injuries. Comminuted fractures are rare (Fig. 127–3).

Diagnostic Strategy

Make dorsopalmar and lateral views. Proximal fractures of the second and fourth metacarpal bones are often best seen with 20-degree right and left dorsopalmar oblique projections. Visualization of questionable sesamoid and distal epiphyseal fractures may be improved with lateral oblique views or with postural radiography (standing lateral patient position, using a horizontal beam centered over the distal metatarsus). The latter view may also act as a stress maneuver and produce additional fragment distraction, making the injury more visible.

Pitfalls

Metacarpal sesamoids may produce edge enhancement, mimicking distal epiphyseal fractures. The normal variation of metacarpal sesamoids, with which many veterinarians are unfamiliar, may also falsely suggest fracture or at least constitute a questionable radiographic finding.

Alternative Diagnoses

Carpal fracture, sprain or strain, bite wounds in cats, digital injuries.

Suggested Reading

Kealy JK. Bones and joints. In: Kealy JK, ed. Diagnostic radiology of the dog and cat. 2nd ed. Philadelphia: WB Saunders, 1987:332.

Leighton RL, Robinson GW. Orthopedic surgery. In: Holzworth J, ed. Diseases of the cat. Philadelphia: WB Saunders, 1987:107.

Newton CD. Fracture and dislocation of metacarpal bones, metacarpophalangeal joints, phalanges, and interphalangeal joints. In: Newton CD, Nunamaker DM, eds. Textbook of small animal orthopedics. Philadelphia: JB Lippincott, 1985:387.

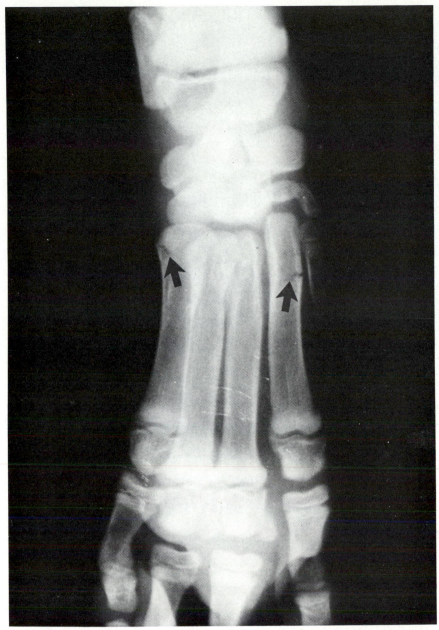

Figure 127–1 Dorsopalmar view of immature canine metacarpus shows incomplete (greenstick) fractures of the second and fifth metacarpal bones (*arrows*). Diagnosis: multiple metacarpal fractures.

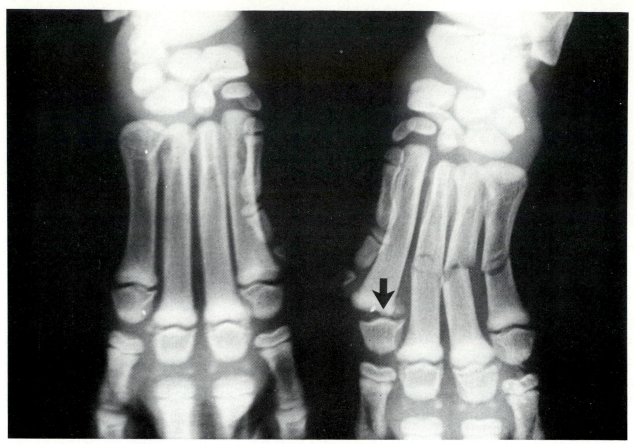

Figure 127–2 Dorsopalmar view of immature canine metacarpi shows displaced fractures of metacarpals 3 to 5 and a displaced growth plate fracture of the fourth metacarpal bone, Salter-Harris II (*arrow*). Diagnosis: multiple metacarpal fractures.

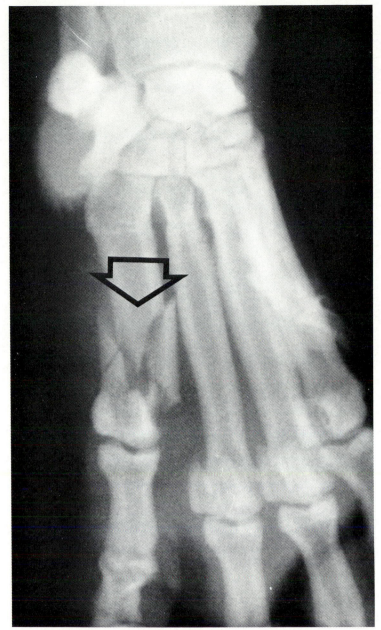

Figure 127–3 Dorsopalmar oblique view of canine right metacarpus shows impacted-type, comminuted fracture of fifth metacarpal bone (*arrow*). Diagnosis: metacarpal fracture.

128

METACARPOPHALANGEAL JOINT FRACTURES AND DISLOCATIONS

General Considerations

Metacarpophalangeal joint fractures are uncommon. Many are of the avulsive variety and are associated with sprain dislocation. Corner fractures of the proximal aspect of the first phalanx and avulsion fractures of the caudal protuberance are most typical, with longitudinally oriented, articular fractures of the distal metacarpal bones being less frequent. The first metacarpal bone is rarely fractured because of its reduced size and relatively protected position, although it may be dislocated if the first digit is caught and the associated ligament is torn. The palmar (caudal) sesamoid bones are occasionally fractured, usually centrally, with surprisingly little separation; the dorsal sesamoids are rarely injured.

Major Radiographic Observations

Typically, the dislocated metacarpophalangeal joint is widened, asymmetrical, or offset. Articular fractures usually produce a visible disruption in the affected joint margin. (Fig. 128–1). Sesamoidian fractures usually show distraction.

Diagnostic Strategy

Make dorsopalmar and lateral views centered on the metacarpophalangeal joints. A dorsopalmar comparison view of the opposite leg is valuable in immature dogs. Oblique views are useful, particularly in the case of the most lateral joints. The lateral projection is often severely compromised by superimposition, to the extent that individual joints are very difficult to isolate; for this reason, right and left lateral obliques are often substituted. Stress or postural projections are useful in sesamoidian injuries.

Pitfalls

Because of the considerable anatomic variability among sesamoids, as well as developmental anomalies such as bipartite and tripartite sesamoids, it is highly advisable to radiograph the opposite side first before establishing a diagnosis of fracture.

Alternative Diagnoses

Bite wounds (especially cats), carpal, metacarpal, and digital injuries.

Suggested Reading

Farrow CS, Newton CD. Ligamentous injury(sprain). In: Newton CD, Nunamaker DM, eds. Textbook of small animal orthopedics. Philadelphia: JB Lippincott, 1985:843.

Newton CD. Fracture and dislocation of metacarpal bones, metacarpophalangeal joints, phalanges, and interphalangeal joints. In: Newton CD, Nunamaker DM, eds. Textbook of small animal orthopedics. Philadelphia: JB Lippincott, 1985:387.

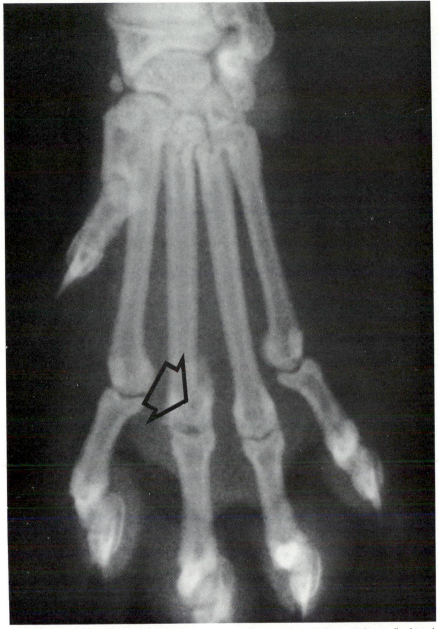

Figure 128–1 Dorsopalmar view of feline right metacarpus and phalanges shows displaced, vertically oriented, articular fracture of distal aspect of third metacarpal bone (*arrow*). Diagnosis: metacarpophalangeal joint fracture.

129

DIGITAL FRACTURE

General Considerations

The digit, perhaps more than any other functional bone group in the body, often *falsely* appears abnormal. This is primarily due to its normal angulation, which results in varying degrees of anatomic magnification and distortion when radiographed. The problem is further aggravated when selective digital radiography is attempted, because this often results in nonstandard positioning and raises the question of what is positional variation and what is injury.

Major Radiographic Observations

Young animals often sustain incomplete (or incomplete-appearing) diaphyseal fractures, as well as displaced and nondisplaced epiphyseal fractures (Fig. 129–1). A normal comparison radiograph is often necessary to differentiate such injuries from normal developmental variation. Digital fractures in mature dogs are less difficult to diagnose, resembling for the most part, other long-bone injuries (Fig. 129–2). As with younger animals, comparison films are useful in questionable cases.

Diagnostic Strategy

Begin with a standard examination with a lateral and dorsoplantar view. If the injuries are unusual or complex, include right and left dorsoplantar obliques. When superimposition is a problem in the lateral view, isolate the affected digit from the remaining digits with a gauze loop using gentle traction. Cotton balls are useful in separating the digits in the dor-

soplantar projection. Stress radiography may be required to establish sprain injury involving the interphalangeal joints.

Pitfalls

Dorsoplantar views of the digits are difficult to assess accurately owing to the considerable natural angulation in both the proximal and distal intertarsal joints, which produces both distortion and magnification of many of the component parts. The lateral view is flawed by extensive digital superimposition, which may conceal surprisingly large injuries.

Alternative Diagnoses

Bite wounds (especially cats), broken or avulsed claw, tarsal injuries.

Suggested Reading

Farrow CS, Newton, CD. Ligamentous injury(sprain). In: Newton CD, Nunamaker DM, eds. Textbook of small animal orthopedics. Philadelphia: JB Lippincott, 1985:843.

Newton CD. Fracture and dislocation of metacarpal bones, metacarpophalangeal joints, phalanges, and interphalangeal joints. In: Newton CD, Nunamaker DM, eds. Textbook of small animal orthopedics. Philadelphia: JB Lippincott, 1985:387.

Owens JM. The digits. In: Owens JM, ed. Radiographic interpretation for the small animal clinician. Saint Louis: Ralston Purina Co, 1982:39.

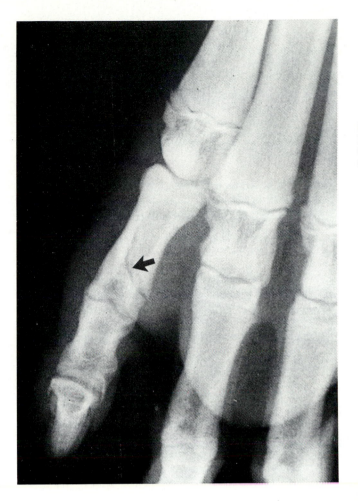

Figure 129–1 Dorsopalmar view of immature canine third to fifth digits shows long nondisplaced diaphyseal fracture of the proximal phalanx (*arrow*) of the fifth digit. Diagnosis: digital fracture.

Figure 129–2 Dorsopalmar view of canine third to fifth digits shows a displaced epiphyseal fracture (*arrow*) of the fifth digit with associated subluxation of the proximal interphalangeal joint. Diagnosis: digital sprain-fracture-luxation.

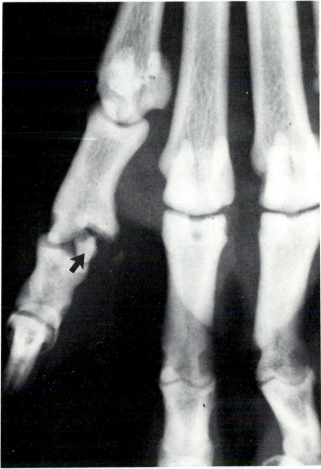

ACCESSORY SKELETON

130
HYOID FRACTURE

General Considerations

Hyoid fractures are rare; most occur as a result of bite wounds to the throat. Occasionally the hyoid is avulsed secondary to a tearing neck wound or massive blunt trauma. Hyoid fractures may also result from a sharp blow to the ventral aspect of the neck.

Major Radiographic Observations

In severe injuries the hyoid apparatus may appear disrupted or distorted, often being elongated and relatively flattened in lateral projection. Normal symmetry, typically able to be seen in lateral projection, is often absent, and one side of the hyoid complex is positioned differently from the other. Occasionally, individual hyoid bones may be identified as fractured, although it is more common to see an abnormal hyoid configuration or location secondary to ligamentous injury. In massive avulsive trauma the hyoid is often displaced in a caudoventral direction (Fig. 130–1).

Diagnostic Strategy

Hyoid trauma is usually associated with difficulty in breathing or swallowing. Hence animals with suspected hyoid fractures should not be stressed! A lateral radiograph centered over the larynx and using *reduced* radiographic technique is adequate. A ventrodorsal view is typically of little diagnostic help and is uncomfortable for most animals.

Pitfalls

Rotation of the head typically results in asymmetry of the hyoid bones, resembling fracture. Likewise, extension and flexion of the head and proximal neck may produce unusual hyoid configurations, potentially resembling injury.

Alternative Diagnoses

Blunt, puncture, or lacerative throat injuries, certain snake and insect bites, pharyngeal or laryngeal foreign bodies, and abscesses (Fig. 130–2).

Suggested Reading

Newton CD. Fractures of small bones. In: Newton CD, Nunamaker DM, eds. Textbook of small animal orthopedics. Philadelphia: JB Lippincott, 1985:457.

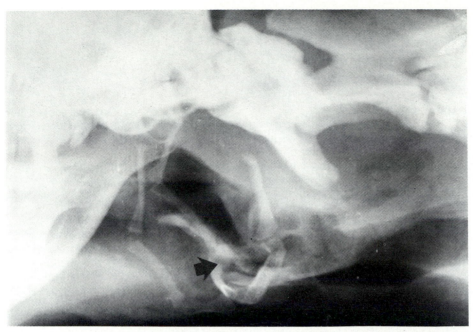

Figure 130–1 Lateral oblique view of canine throat region shows dislocation of the caudal hyoid elements secondary to fracture-luxation of the basihyoid bone (*arrow*). Diagnosis: fracture of the hyoid apparatus.

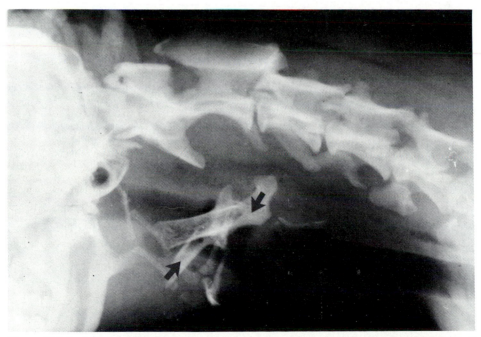

Figure 130–2 Lateral oblique view of canine throat region shows multiple bone fragments (*arrows*) superimposed on the hyoid apparatus, mimicking a hyoid fracture. Diagnosis: pharyngeal foreign bodies.

131

RIB FRACTURES AND DISLOCATIONS

General Considerations

Rib fractures generally occur in groups, typically within the central third of the rib cage, at or near their point of greatest lateral extension. Most rib injuries are unilateral, resulting from automobile accidents, and they cause considerable pain. Associated lung injuries are common, most often including contusions and pneumothorax. Lung lacerations secondary to rib fracture or displacement are comparatively rare. Flail chest, or chest wall instability resulting from multiple segmental rib fractures, is also a comparative rarity. Dislocations from the spine are unusual; avulsions of the cartilaginous rib elements occur more frequently, often in conjunction with sternal injury. (For additional information on rib fractures, see page 2).

Major Radiographic Observations

There is often some fragment displacement of the central elements in a group of rib fractures, whereas segmental rib fractures are usually associated with large gaps in the rib cage and defects in the chest wall (Fig. 131–1). Nondisplaced rib fractures are often difficult to identify. Both types of fractures are seen better in the dorsoventral or ventrodorsal view, because each side of the rib cage is seen separately. Avulsion fractures of the chondral ribs, usually from their sternal attachments, are best seen in lateral or lateral oblique projections. Intercostal tearing (as evidenced by widened intercostal space) and chest wall bruising (typified by narrowed rib spaces) are optimally visualized in the dorsoventral or ventrodorsal projections.

Diagnostic Strategy

Make lateral and dorsoventral or ventrodorsal views of the entire rib cage, being careful not to overpenetrate the ribs. Attempt to obtain true lateral and dorsoventral or ventrodor-

sal positions to facilitate comparison between a suspected lesion and an anatomic variation. Check the right and left halves of the rib cage separately, and each rib individually, comparing questionable findings with both adjacent and contralateral ribs.

Pitfalls

The shape, size, attitude, and degree of curvature of the ribs differ considerably from the thoracic inlet to the diaphragm. Many of these differences are accentuated by nonstandard positioning and x-ray beam decentering. A struggling animal can mimic a "position of protection," which is indicative of chest wall or rib injury.

Alternative Diagnoses

Chest wall bruising, intercostal tearing.

Suggested Reading

Burk RL, Ackerman N. The thorax. In: Burk RL, Ackerman N, eds. Small animal radiology. New York: Churchill Livingstone, 1986:30.

Kealy JK. The thorax. In: Kealy JK, ed. Diagnostic radiology of the dog and cat. 2nd ed. Philadelphia: WB Saunders, 1987:250.

Newton CD. Fractures of small bones. In: Newton CD, Nunamaker DM, eds. Textbook of small animal orthopedics. Philadelphia: JB Lippincott, 1985:457.

Owens JM. Thoracic wall and rib cage. In: Owens JM, ed. Radiographic interpretation for the small animal clinician. Saint Louis: Ralston Purina Co, 1982:114.

Root CR, Bahr RJ. The thoracic wall. In: Thrall DE, ed. Textbook of veterinary diagnostic radiology. Philadelphia: WB Saunders, 1986:238.

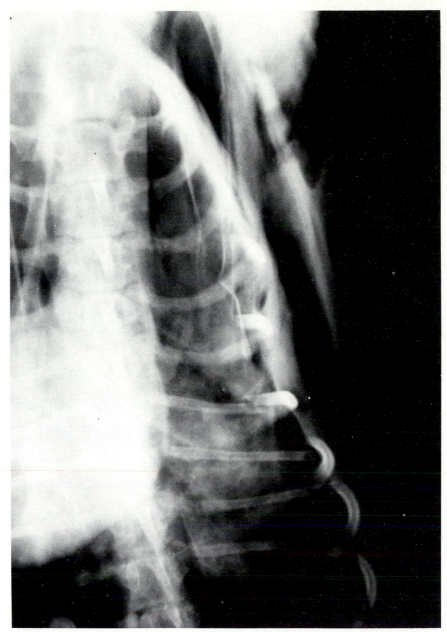

Figure 131–1 Right ventrodorsal oblique view of thoracic wall shows displaced fractures of ribs 5 to 9 with associated widening of the intercostal spaces centrally, deep and superficial gas accumulation, and soft-tissue swelling. There is also pleural air and abnormal lung density. Diagnosis: multiple rib fractures, intercostal muscle tearing, chest wall contusions and emphysema, pneumothorax, and pulmonary contusion.

132

STERNAL FRACTURE

General Considerations

Sternal fractures and dislocations are relatively rare. The cranial aspect of the manubrium (first sternabra), and the distal aspect of the xiphoid (last sternabra) are relatively vulnerable to fracture because of their unprotected positions. Fractures of the central sternabrae often occur as a result of a direct blow to the sternum, or in cats and small dogs secondary to bites.

Major Radiographic Observations

Fractures of the manubrium or xiphoid are often moderately to severely displaced (Fig. 132–1). Nondisplaced fractures may be very hard to recognize, especially if there is associated soft-tissue swelling and gas.

Diagnostic Strategy

Begin by making lateral and dorsoventral views of the entire thorax to include the sternum. Then, if the lesion is unclear or incompletely visualized, make a lateral spot film directly over the injury site using bone (as opposed to thoracic) technique. If additional information is needed, make paired right and left dorsoventral oblique films approximately 45 degrees off center.

Pitfalls

Enormous, undocumented, normal individual variations exist in the canine sternum; fewer anatomic differences are present among cats.

Alternative Diagnoses

Peristernal abscess, regional cellulitis, chest wall bruising, intercostal muscle tear, fracture or dislocation of one or more chondral ribs.

Suggested Reading

Newton CD. Fractures of small bones. In: Newton CD, Nunamaker DM, eds. Textbook of small animal orthopedics. Philadelphia: JB Lippincott, 1985:458.

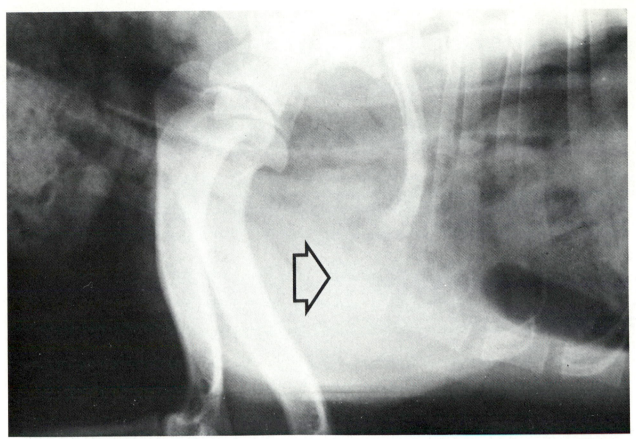

Figure 132-1 Lateral view of canine cranioventral thorax shows absence of cranial aspect of first sternabra and manubrium (*arrow*). Diagnosis: displaced fracture of the manubrium.

133
PENIS BONE FRACTURE

General Considerations

Fractures of the penis bone are, fortunately, rare, owing both to its protected position and to the flexibility of the tissues within which it lies. Most such injuries result from bite wounds or entrapment or tearing of the penis. Occasionally, fracture occurs during breeding. Because of the great anatomic variation in the appearance of the os penis, false-positive diagnosis is common, especially in the context of penile injury. Partial or complete urethral obstruction accompanies most displaced penile fractures. Nondisplaced fractures may also result in urethral obstruction, but usually do not; hematuria is a more common sequela. Occasionally, penile fractures go unrecognized until after the original trauma, being detected finally because of urethral stenosis secondary to callus entrapment or malunion displacement.

Major Radiographic Observations

Fractures of the os penis may occur anywhere in the bone but are most apt to be located in the structurally weaker, cranial third. A large fracture gap is usual, although it is not present in every case.

Diagnostic Strategy

Make a lateral radiograph centered directly over the central part of the penis, using *reduced* radiographic technique.

If the animal is large or there is swelling, employ a grid. Gentle compression with a wooden spoon or paddle further improves radiographic detail and better isolates the penis from the adjacent abdomen.

Pitfalls

Some normal individual variations of the os penis may resemble a recent fracture.

Alternative Diagnoses

Normal anatomic variation, osteomyelitis (usually secondary to bite wound).

Suggested Reading

Newton CD. Fractures of small bones. In: Newton CD, Nunamaker DM, eds. Textbook of small animal orthopedics. Philadelphia: JB Lippincott, 1985:457.
Owens JM. The genitourinary system. In: Owens JM, ed. Radiographic interpretation for the small animal clinician. Saint Louis: Ralston Purina Co, 1982:193.

RELATED SOFT-TISSUE INJURIES

134

SOFT - TISSUE INJURIES

The Meaning of Soft-Tissue Swelling

Soft-tissue swelling, when used as a radiology descriptor, indicates increased soft-tissue area, often associated with increased density. The term is otherwise nonspecific, indicating nothing of the nature of the swelling, its composition, activity, or duration. In proximity to a joint, it may be *inferred* to be the result of an increased synovial volume (intracapsular), although extracapsular swelling may appear identical.

Contusions

Contusions (or bruises) are caused by blows to the soft tissues, which result in capillary disruption and produce varying degrees of heat, pain, and swelling followed by a period of stiffness and soreness. Tissue discoloration may be evident in light-skinned animals and may persist as long as a month. Radiographically, the injury is nonspecific, appearing as soft-tissue swelling and often temporarily displacing or eliminating surrounding fascial planes. The phrase "bone bruise" is a misnomer that actually refers to a subperiosteal hematoma.

Hematoma

Like any soft-tissue swelling, a hematoma lacks radiographic specificity; however, hematomas do possess certain characteristics which, although shared by other lesions, may be employed inferentially to arrive at a diagnosis. These highly suggestive indicators include a localized or regional occurrence, an oval or circular shape, and an outward displacement of surrounding fascial planes. Abscesses and soft-tissue tumors may have a similar appearance.

Compartmental Syndrome

Compartmental syndrome is a rare (or at least rarely reported) condition that develops following a large, acute hemorrhage into a relatively small soft-tissue space or compartment, usually one located close to a major long bone. The resulting distention places pressure on the surrounding vasculature, causing ischemia and, if applied long enough, necrosis. Affected bone typically responds with a periosteal new-bone deposition 7 to 14 days later. Such reactions cannot be differentiated from infection.

Lacerations

Lacerations may be detected radiographically, depending on the size of the tissue defect, its air content, and whether the injury is viewed in profile or frontally. Blood, mud, gravel, and other kinds of road debris adhering to the hair coat add greatly to the lesion's density. Embedded wooden stakes and other radiographically transparent foreign bodies usually cannot be detected.

Strains

Strains may affect a muscle, its tendon, or both. They are graded according to increasing severity as first, second, or third degree. This classification is useful not only in defining the extent of injury but also in providing a prognosis.

Sprains

Sprains are injuries to ligaments and, like strains, are classified according to increasing severity as first-, second- or third-degree injuries. This categorization provides valuable prognostic information. Many second- and third- degree injuries require as much as or more healing time than a complete long-bone fracture.

Torn Muscles

Muscle tears are often associated with sudden bursts of speed or exceptional effort. Although they may be associated with insufficient warm-up, this is not a prerequisite. A large localized hemorrhage often results, which can be painful and, if great enough, can produce a mild degree of shock.

Gas

Gas within the soft tissues is of either intrinsic or extrinsic origin. In the context of recent injury, atmospheric contamination is most common, with air reaching the subcutaneous tissues and deeper fascial planes through skin punctures and lacertions. By a similar mechanism, air may be inoculated directly into muscle and occasionally into a joint. Gas accumulations from inoculation do not remain in the tissues long before being absorbed, usually less than 24 hours. Intrinsic gas is much less common and is usually the result of infection. Such findings should not be anticipated in fresh injuries; if they are, the accuracy of the history should be questioned.

Foreign Bodies

Foreign bodies may be divided into those that are visible and those that are not, with visibility being primarily a function of the object's density. For example, a bullet is highly visible because of its metallic composition, whereas a plant awn is invisible because of its low-density, fibrous make-up. Some things that are visually transparent, such as glass, may be radiographically opaque because of their lead content. Other foreign bodies that are normally radiographically transparent, such as wood, may be detectable if surrounded by air fortuitously carried into the wound at the time of injury.

Note: The letter f following a page number indicates a figure.

A

Abdomen, gunshot wound to, 132, 133f
Abdominal hernia, 124, 125f
Abscess
  dental, 224
  intrapelvic, 179f
  periapical, 224
  pleural, 10, 11f
  prostatic, 198, 199f
  pulmonary, 5f, 56, 57f
  renal, 184, 184f–185f
Acetabulum, fractures of, 272, 273f–274f
Adenocarcinoma
  of lung, 17f
  of prostate gland, 203f
  pyloric, 161f
Adenopathy, pseudoperihilar, 14
Air-space hemorrhage, 60, 62f–63f
Aspiration, of drowning fluid, 80, 81f
Aspiration pneumonia, 54
Asthma, feline, 68, 69f
Atelectasis, postural, 90, 91f–93f
Atrium, hemangiosarcoma of, 116, 117f
Axial hiatal hernia, 158

B

Bacterial pneumonia, acute, 52, 53f
Ballooning, tracheal, 28
Bile duct, ruptured, causing peritonitis, 130, 131f
Bite wound, peritonitis and, 128, 129f
Bladder, urinary. See Urinary bladder
Bone bruise, 369
Bone loss, in dental infection, 224
Bronchus(i), collapse of, 30, 31f
Bruise(s), 369
  of chest wall, 2, 3f
Bulla(e)
  infections of, 246, 247f
  traumatic, 64, 65f
Burn, oral-cavity, 74

C

Calcaneus, fractures of, 296, 300f–301f
Calculus(i), bladder, 190, 191f
Canine cardiomyopathy, 100, 101f–103f
Canine dirofilariasis, 108, 109f–111f
Canine heartworm disease, 108, 109f–111f
Canine parvoviral enteritis, 174, 175f
Carcinoma, annular, 173f
Cardiomyopathy
  in cat, 104, 105f–107f
  dilated, 100, 104
  in dog, 100, 101f–103f
  hypertrophic, 104
  restrictive, 104
Carinal collapse, 30, 31f
Carnassial tooth, 220
Carpal joint, fractures, sprains, and dislocations of, 348, 349f–353f
Caudal mediastinal mass, 16, 17f

Cervical spine, fractures of, 248–249, 250f–251f
Cervical spondylopathy, 262, 264f
Chemodectoma, 118, 119f
Chest, gunshot wound to, 72, 73f
Chest wall trauma, 2, 3f
"Choking," 36
Cicatrix, 26
Closed pneumothorax, 4, 5f
Coccidioidomycosis, 15f
Collapse
  carinal, 30, 31f
  tracheal, 28, 29f
Colon, ruptured, 176, 177f–179f
Compartmental syndrome, 369
Compartmentalization, of stomach, 152
Congenital megaesophagus, 42–43, 42f–45f
Congestive heart failure
  acquired mitral insufficiency and, 98, 99f
  ventricular septal defect and, 94, 95f–97f
Contusion(s), 369
  of chest wall, 2, 3f
  pulmonary, 60, 61f–63f
Cor pulmonale, 108
Cranial fracture, 242, 243f–245f
Cranial mediastinal mass, 12, 13f
Craniomandibular osteopathy, 231f
Cystitis, emphysematous, 192, 193f

D

Death, fetal, early-term, 206
  late-term, 206, 207f
Dental fracture(s), 220, 221f–223f
Dental infection, 224, 225f
Diaphragmatic hernia, 46, 47f–49f
Digital fracture
  forelimb, 360, 361f
  hindlimb, 308, 309f
Dilatation, gastric, 150, 151f
Dirofilariasis
  canine, 108, 109f–111f
  feline, 112, 113f
Disk herniation, 256, 257f–261f
Dislocation(s)
  of carpal joint, 348, 349f–353f
  of elbow joint, 326, 327f–333f
  of hip joint, 272, 275f–277f
  of metacarpophalangeal joint, 358
  of metatarsophalangeal joint, 306, 307f
  of shoulder joint, 316, 317f–319f
  of stifle joint, 286, 287f–289f
  of tarsus, 296, 297f–301f
  of temporomandibular joint, 228, 229f–231f
Dyspnea, acute, 66, 67f
Dystocia, 204, 205f

E

Edema, pulmonary, electrocution producing, 74, 75f
  secondary to strangulation, 76, 77f

Effusion, pericardial, benign, 114, 115f
  hemangiosarcoma producing, 116, 117f
Elbow joint, fracture and dislocation of,
  326, 327f–333f
Electrocution, producing pulmonary
  edema, 74, 75f
Embolus(i), fibrocartilaginous, spinal
  disorders and, 262
Emphysema
  associated with tracheal perforation,
    22, 23f
  of chest wall, 2, 3f
  secondary to bite wound, 19f
Emphysematous cystitis, 192, 193f
Enema, colonic ruptured following, 176
Enteritis, parvoviral, canine, 174, 175f
Eosinophilia, peripheral, pulmonary
  infiltrates with, 70, 71f
Epiphysis, fractures of, 278, 279f–280f
Escherichia coli, 192
Esophagus
  foreign bodies of, 36, 37f–39f
  perforation of, 40, 41f

F

Facial fracture, dental fracture-dislocation
  following, 223f
Feline asthma, 68, 69f
Feline cardiomyopathy, 104, 105f–107f
Feline dirofilariasis, 112, 113f
Feline heartworm disease, 112, 113f
Feline infectious peritonitis,
  intussusception and, 140, 141f
Femoral head, avulsion fractures of, 272,
  276f–277f
Femur, fractures of, 278, 279f–283f
Fetal death
  early-term, 206
  late-term, 206, 207f
Fibrocartilaginous embolus(i), spinal
  disorders and, 262
Fibrosarcoma, peritoneal, disseminated,
  142, 143f
Fibula, fractures of, 290, 291f–295f
Flail chest, 2
Fluid overload, 86, 87f–89f
Foreign body(ies), 370
  esophageal, 36, 37f–39f
  gastric, 144, 145f–147f
  gastrointestinal, 148, 149f
  granuloma induced by, 138, 139f
  intestinal
    linear, 162, 163f
    nonlinear, penetrating, 164, 165f
    pancreatitis secondary to, 216, 217f
  peritoneal, gastroesophageal
    perforation and, 136, 137f
  tracheal, 24, 25f
Foreign body pneumonia, 56, 57f
Forelimb digital fracture, 360, 361f
Fracture(s)
  of carpal joint, 348, 349f–353f
  combined radial and ulnar, 338, 344,
    344f–347f
  compression, nondisplaced, 248
  of cranium, 242, 243f–245f
  dental, 220, 221f–223f
  digital
    of forelimb, 360, 361f
    of hindlimb, 308, 309f
  of elbow joint, 326, 327f–333f
  of femur, 278, 279f–283f
  of frontal sinus, 236, 236f–237f
  greenstick, 278
  of hip, 267f–268f, 272, 273f–277f
  of humerus, 320, 321f–325f
  of hyoid apparatus, 362, 363f
  mandibular, 226, 227f
  maxillary, 232, 233
  of metacarpophalangeal joint, 358,
    359f
  of metacarpus, 354, 355f–357f
  of metatarsophalangeal joints, 306,
    307f
  of metatarsus, 302, 303f–305f
  of nasal cavity, 234, 235f
  of orbit, 240, 241f
  of patella, 284, 285f
  of pelvis, 266, 267f–271f
  of penis bone, 368
  of radius, 334, 335f–337f
  of ribs, 2, 3f, 364, 365f
  of scapula, 310, 311f–315f
  of shoulder joint, 316, 317f–319f
  of spine, 248–250, 250f–255f
  of sternum, 366, 367f
  of stifle joint, 286, 287f–289f
  of tarsus, 296, 297f–301f
  of temporomandibular joint, 226, 228,
    229f–231f
  of tibia and fibula, 290, 291f–295f
  of ulna, 338, 339f–341f
  of zygomatic arch, 238, 238f–239f
Frontal sinus(es), fractures of, 236,
  236f–237f

G

Gallbladder, ruptured, causing peritonitis,
  130, 131f
Gas, in soft tissues, 369
Gastric dilatation, 150, 151f
Gastric dilatation volvulus syndrome
  (GDVS), 152
Gastric torsion, 152, 153f
Gastric ulcer, penetrating, 156, 157f
Gastritis, hemorrhagic, 154, 155f
Gastroenteritis, hemorrhagic, 154, 155f
Gastroesophageal perforation, peritoneal
  foreign body and, 136, 137f
Gastrointestinal foreign bodies, 148, 149f
Glenoid fracture, 310
Granuloma, foreign body, induced by
  surgical sponge, 138, 139f
Greenstick fractures, 278
Growth plates, fracture of, 278
Gunshot wound
  to abdomen, 132, 133f
  to chest, 72, 73f
  dental loss following, 222f

H

Heart base tumor, 118, 119f
Heart failure, congestive, acquired mitral
  insufficiency and, 98, 99f
    ventricular septal defect and, 94,
      95f–97f
  heart base tumor producing, 118, 119f
  left-sided, 94
  right-sided, 94
Heartworm disease
  in cat, 112, 113f
  in dog, 108, 109f–111f
Hemangiosarcoma, pericardial, 116, 117f
Hematoma, 369
Hemomediastinum, ruptured subclavian
  artery and, 20, 21f
Hemorrhage
  intrapulmonary capillary, 60, 62f–63f
  of liver tumors, 212, 213f

mediastinal, 20, 21f
retroperitoneal, ruptured kidney
   producing, 182, 183f
of splenic tumor, 214, 215f
Hepatomegaly, 212, 213f
Hernia
   abdominal, intestinal herniation and,
      124, 125f
   diaphragmatic, 46, 47f–49f
   hiatal, incarcerated, 158, 159f
   inguinal, 126, 127f
   pericardioperitoneal, 50, 51f
Herniation, disk, 256, 257f–261f
Hiatal hernia, incarcerated, 158, 159f
Hindlimb digital fracture, 308, 309f
Hip, fractures of, 267f–268f, 272,
      273f–277f
Humerus, fracture of, 320, 321f–325f
Hyoid apparatus, fracture of, 362, 363f
Hypoplasia, tracheal, 32, 33f

I

Ilium, fractures of, 266, 269f
Incarceration, intestinal, 168, 169f
Infection
   dental, 224, 225f
   tympanic bulla, 246, 247f
Inguinal hernia, 126, 127f
Inhalation, smoke, 78, 79f
Inhalation pneumonia, acute, 54, 55f
Intestinal foreign body(ies)
   linear, 162, 163f
   nonlinear, 164, 165f
Intestinal herniation
   abdominal hernia producing, 124, 125f
   inguinal hernia producing, 126, 127f
Intestinal incarceration, 168, 169f
Intussusception, 166, 167f
   feline infectious peritonitis and, 140,
      141f

J

Joint(s). *See named joints*

K

Kidney
   abscess of, 184, 184f–185f
   ruptured, retroperitoneal hemorrhage
      following, 182, 183f

L

Laceration(s), 369
Leiomyoma, 161f
Liver tumor, hemorrhaging, 212, 213f
Lung. *See also* Pulmonary *entries*
   traumatic bullae of, 64, 65f
Lung lobe torsion, 58, 59f
Lymphadenopathy, perihilar, 14, 15f
Lymphoma, thymic, 12, 13f

M

Malleolus, fractures of, 296, 298f–299f
Mandibular fracture, 226, 227f
   dental dislocation following, 221f
Manubrium, fracture of, 366, 367f
Mass(es), mediastinal. *See* Mediastinal
      mass
Maxilla, fractures of, 232, 233
Mediastinal mass, 14, 15f
   caudal, 16, 17f
   cranial, 12, 13f
Mediastinitis, esophageal perforation
      and, 36, 40

Megacolon, post-traumatic, 180, 181f
Megaesophagus, congenital, 42–43,
      42f–45f
Metacarpophalangeal joint, fractures and
      dislocations of, 358, 359f
Metacarpus, fractures of, 354, 355f–357f
Metaphyseal osteopathy, 342f–343f
Metastasis, pulmonary, 66, 67f
Metatarsophalangeal joint, fractures and
      dislocations of, 306, 307f
Metatarsus, fractures of, 302, 303f–305f
Mitral valve(s), insufficiency of, acquired,
      98, 99f
Monteggia's fracture, 333f
Muscle(s), torn, 369

N

Nasal cavity, fractures of, 234, 235f
Near drowning, 80, 81f
Necrotic pyometritis, 210, 211f
Nephritis, 197f

O

Obstruction
   bladder stones leading to, 190, 191f
   bladder tumors causing, 194, 195f
Occult hernia, 46
Odontoid process, aplasia of, 263f
Open pneumothorax, 6, 7f
Oral-cavity burn, 74
Orbit, fractures of, 240, 241f
Os penis, fracture of, 368
Otitis externa, 246
Otitis media, 246
Overhydration, 86, 87f–89f

P

Pancreatitis, following penetrating foreign
      body, 216, 217f
Paraesophageal hiatal hernia, 158
Paraquat poisoning, 84, 85f
Parvoviral enteritis, canine, 174, 175f
Patellar, fractures of, 284, 285f
Patent ductus arteriosus, 94, 97f, 100
Pelvis, fractures of, 266, 267f–271f
Penis bone, fracture of, 368
Perforation
   esophageal, 40, 41f
   gastroesophageal, peritoneal foreign
      body and, 136, 137f
   tracheal, 22, 23f
Pericardial effusion
   benign, 114, 115f
   hemangiosarcoma producing, 116, 117f
Pericardioperitoneal hernia, 50, 51f
Perihilar lymphadenopathy, 14, 15f
Peritoneal fibrosarcoma, disseminated,
      142, 143f
Peritonitis
   bite wounds and, 128, 129f
   feline infectious, intussusception and,
      140, 141f
   ruptured bladder and, 186, 187f
   ruptured gallbladder and, 130, 131f
   ruptured prostate and, 200, 201f
Peritracheal tumor, 34, 35f
Pleural abscess, 10, 11f
Pleuropneumonia, 8, 9f
Pneumomediastinum, 18, 19f
   esophageal perforation and, 36, 40
Pneumonia
   aspiration, 54
   bacterial, acute, 52, 53f
   following near drowning, 80

following smoke inhalation, 78
foreign body, 56, 57f
inhalation, acute, 54, 55f
secondary to megaesophagus, 42,
44f–45f
Pneumonitis, 52. *See also* Pneumonia
Pneumopericardium, traumatic, 120, 121f
Pneumoperitoneum, spontaneous, 134,
135f
Pneumothorax
spontaneous, 4, 5f
tension, 6, 7f
Poisoning
paraquat, 84, 85f
warfarin, 82, 83f
Prostate gland
abscess of, 198, 199f
ruptured, peritonitis following, 200,
201f
tumors of, 202, 203f
Prostatitis, 198
Pseudoperihilar adenopathy, 14
Pubis, fractures of, 266
Pulmonary. *See also* Lung *entries*
Pulmonary abscess, 5f, 56, 57f
Pulmonary contusion, 60, 61f–63f
Pulmonary edema
electrocution producing, 74, 75f
overhydration and, 86
secondary to strangulation, 76, 77f
Pulmonary heart disease, 108
Pulmonary infiltrates, with peripheral
eosinophilia, 70, 71f
Pulmonary metastasis, 66, 67f
Pyloric tumor, 160, 161f
Pyometra, 208, 209f
draining, 210
Pyometritis, necrotic, 210, 211f

R

Radius
fractures of, 334, 335f–337f
and ulnar, combined fractures of, 338,
344, 344f–347f
Renal insufficiency, uremia and, 196,
197f
Respiratory distress syndrome, adult
(ARDS), 78, 80, 84, 85f
Retroflexion, of urinary bladder, 188,
189f
Retroperitoneal hemorrhage, ruptured
kidney producing, 182, 183f
Rhabdomyosarcoma, 195f
Rib(s), fractures and dislocations, of, 2,
3f, 364, 365f

S

Sacrococcygeal spine, fractures of, 248,
249, 255f
Sacroiliac joint, fractures of, 266,
267f–268f
Salter-Harris fracture, 278, 295f, 328f,
329f
Sarcoma, intestinal, 173f
Scapula, fractures of, 310, 311f–315f
Sesamoidian fracture, 358
Shoulder joint, fracture and dislocation
of, 316, 317f–319f
Silhouette sign, 11f, 50, 51f, 55f, 63f
Skull, fractures of, 242, 243f–245f
Small intestine
tumors of, 172, 173f
volvulus, 170, 171f
Smoke inhalation, 78, 79f
Soft-tissue injury, 369

Spine
disorders of, subacute and chronic,
262, 263f–265f
fractures of, 248–250, 250f–255f
tumors of, 262, 264f–265f
Splenic tumor, hemorrhaging, 214, 215f
Sprain(s), 369
of carpal joint, 348, 349f–353f
Sprain-avulsion injury, 284
Stenosis, tracheal, 26, 27f
Sternum, fractures of, 366, 367f
Stifle joint, fractures and dislocations of,
286, 287f–289f
Stomach, foreign bodies in, 144,
145f–147f
Stones, bladder, 190, 191f
Strain(s), 369
Strangulation, 76, 77f
Subclavian artery, ruptured,
hemomediastinum and, 20, 21f
Supracondylar-intracondylar fracture, 327f
Surgical sponge, foreign body granuloma
induced by, 138, 139f
Swelling, soft-tissue, 369
Symphysis, fractures of 226, 227f

T

Talus, fractures of, 296
Tamponade, 114, 115f
Tarsometatarsal joint, subluxation of,
302, 303f–304f
Tarsus, fractures and dislocations of, 296,
297f–301f
Teeth, fractures of, 220, 221f–223f
Temporomandibular joint, fractures of,
226, 228, 229f–231f
Tension pneumothorax, 6, 7f
Thoracolumbar spine, fractures, of, 248
249, 251f–254f
Thymic lymphoma, 12, 13f
Tibia, fractures of, 290, 291f–295f
Tibiotarsal joint, fractures of, 296,
297f–301f
Torsion, gastric, 152, 153f
Trachea
ballooning of, 28
collapse of, 28, 29f
foreign bodies in, 24, 25f
hypoplasia of, 32, 33f
perforation of, 22, 23f
stenosis of, 26, 27f
tumors of, 34, 35f
Trauma
chest wall, 2, 3f
soft tissue, 369
Trochanter, fracture of, 278, 280f–281f
Tumor(s)
bladder, 194, 195f
heart base, 118, 119f
hepatic, hemorrhaging, 212, 213f
intestinal, 172, 173f
lymphoreticular, 12
peritracheal, 34, 35f
prostatic, 202, 203f
pyloric, 160, 161f
spinal, 262, 264f–265f
splenic, hemorrhaging, 214, 215f
Tympanic bulla infection, 246, 247f
Tympanitis, 246

U

Ulcer(s), gastric, penetrating, 156, 157f
Ulna
fractures of, 338, 339f–341f

and radius, combined fractures of, 338,
    344, 344f–347f
Uremia, renal insufficiency and, 196,
    197f
Urinary bladder
    retroflexion of, 188, 189f
    ruptured, peritonitis following, 186,
187f
    stones in, 190, 191f
    tumors of, 194, 195f

V

Valsalva's maneuver, 188
Vena caval syndrome, 108, 111f
Ventricle(s), septal defect of, 94, 95f–97f
Volvulus, 152, 153f
    intestinal, 170, 171f

W

Warfarin poisoning, 82, 83f
Wobbler disease, 262
Wound(s)
    bite, peritonitis and, 128, 129f
    gunshot
        to abdomen, 132, 133f
        to chest, 72, 73f
        dental loss following, 222f

X

Xiphoid, fracture of, 366

Z

Zygomatic arch, fractures of, 238,
    238f–239f